49.50

D1545354

SECOND EDITION

Radiographic Technique
in VETERINARY
PRACTICE

JAMES W. TICER, D.V.M., Ph.D.

Diplomate, American College of Veterinary Radiology
Veterinary Radiologist,
Santa Cruz, California
Formerly Professor and Chairman,
Department of Veterinary Radiology
and Assistant Dean for Instruction,
College of Veterinary Medicine
University of Florida
Gainesville, Florida

1984
W. B. SAUNDERS COMPANY
PHILADELPHIA/LONDON/TORONTO/MEXICO CITY/RIO DE JANEIRO/SYDNEY/TOKYO

W. B. Saunders Company: West Washington Square
                          Philadelphia, PA   19105

                          1 St. Anne's Road
                          Eastbourne, East Sussex BN21 3UN, England

                          1 Goldthorne Avenue
                          Toronto, Ontario M8Z 5T9, Canada

                          Apartado 26370—Cedro 512
                          Mexico 4, D.F., Mexico

                          Rua Coronel Cabrita, 8
                          Sao Cristovao Caixa Postal 21176
                          Rio de Janeiro, Brazil

                          9 Waltham Street
                          Artarmon, N.S.W. 2064, Australia

                          Ichibancho, Central Bldg., 22-1 Ichibancho
                          Chiyoda-Ku, Tokyo 102, Japan

Library of Congress Cataloging in Publication Data

Ticer, James W.

Radiographic technique in veterinary practice.

Rev. ed. of: Radiographic technique in small animal practice. 1975.

Includes index.

1. Veterinary radiography.   I. Title.

SF757.8.T52   1984   636.089'607572   82-42600
ISBN 0–7216–8861–6

Listed here is the latest translated edition of this
book together with the language of the translation
and the publisher.

Japanese (*1st Edition*) — Japanese Veterinary Radiology Society

Radiographic Technique in Veterinary Practice   ISBN   0-7216-8861-6

Last digit is the print number: 9   8   7   6   5   4   3   2   1

To my wife, Vivian

Contributors

LOUIS A. CORWIN, JR., D.V.M., PhD.
Diplomate, American College of Veterinary Radiology, Professor of Veterinary Medicine and Surgery, College of Veterinary Medicine; Professor of Radiology, School of Medicine, University of Missouri, Columbia, Missouri.
Radiation Protection

NEIL KOOYMAN, M.B.A.
Sales Manager, California X-Ray Company, Concord, California.
Equipping Your Radiology Department
Planning Your Radiology Department

ROBERT E. LEWIS, D.V.M., M.S.
Diplomate, American College of Veterinary Radiology, Professor and Chairman, Department of Anatomy and Radiology; Director of the Veterinary Medical Teaching Hospital, College of Veterinary Medicine, The University of Georgia, Athens, Georgia.
Economics of Your Radiology Department

CHARLES R. ROOT, D.V.M., M.S.
Diplomate, American College of Veterinary Radiology, Professor of Veterinary Radiology, Chief of Radiology Section, Boren Veterinary Medical Teaching Hospital, Department of Medicine and Surgery, College of Veterinary Medicine, Oklahoma State University, Stillwater, Oklahoma.
Contrast Radiography of the Alimentary Tract
Contrast Radiography of the Urinary System

SAM SILVERMAN, D.V.M., Ph.D.
Diplomate, American College of Veterinary Radiology, Veterinary Radiologists, San Francisco, California.
Avian Radiographic Technique

STEPHEN J. ETTINGER, D.V.M.
Fellow, American College of Cardiology; Diplomate, American College of Veterinary Internal Medicine, Cardiology and Internal Medicine; Practitioner, California Animal Hospital Corporation, Los Angeles, California.
Angiocardiography
Pneumopericardiography

GARY L. WOOD, D.V.M.
Diplomate, American College of Veterinary Internal Medicine, Cardiology. Veterinary Cardiologist, Oregon Veterinary Specialty Clinic, Portland, Oregon. *Angiocardiography*

EDWARD A. RHODE, D.V.M.
Diplomate, American College of Veterinary Internal Medicine. Professor of Medicine and Dean, School of Veterinary Medicine, University of California, Davis, California. *Angiocardiography*

Preface to the Second Edition

The second edition of this book has been retitled to reflect the addition of radiographic technique in large animal practice. It is my hope that the book will now become a more useful resource for veterinary students and for general practitioners.

Several chapters and sections on seldom used special procedures from the first edition have been eliminated to make room for the expanded material.

The addition of a small chapter on radiograph duplication and slide making should provide a reference for the practitioner who wishes to use radiographs to illustrate talks or to satisfy client requests. The chapter on economics should prove useful to those who wish to understand how income is derived and expenses incurred in the radiology department.

I wish to thank Mrs. Sharon Martin for her assistance in typing the manuscript for this edition, Mr. Mark Hoffenberg for his skilled photographic assistance, and Ms. Jeanne Clark and Mrs. Sybil Smith-Adams for their assistance and technical advice during the production of the position illustrations. Without these able people, this new edition would not have been possible.

The people of W. B. Saunders Company were, as usual, extremely helpful. Mr. R. W. "Sandy" Reinhardt, Veterinary Editor; Mr. Raymond R. Kersey, Associate Veterinary Editor; Mr. Dan Ruth, Copy Editor; and Mrs. Laura Tarves, production manager, provided much encouragement and assistance.

My wife Vivian continues not only to tolerate but also to encourage my writing of books. Without her assistance and understanding, this book would not have become a reality.

Preface to the First Edition

Six years ago I left the rewards and frustrations of teaching and the shelter of academia to establish a consultative and referral practice in veterinary radiology. During these years I have had the privilege and probably the unique opportunity of working closely with many practicing veterinarians as a consultant in radiographic technique and radiologic diagnosis. Generally, I have found that the ability to render an accurate radiologic diagnosis is compromised by referral radiographic examinations that are technically deficient. Some of these are a result of improper exposure or darkroom techniques or of inadequate equipment, but by far the most common error encountered is improper patient preparation or positioning. From these observations, this book was conceived.

The purpose of this book is to provide a source of information on radiographic technique in small animal practice for use by veterinary students, by practitioners and by their technical assistants. The format presents the more theoretical aspects of radiographic technique in the first part of the book and an atlas on technique and positioning in the second part. I have tried to keep the theoretical concepts that are necessary for an understanding of radiographic technique in practical perspective in an effort to make their consumption more tolerable. The atlas on technique and positioning is arranged according to regional anatomy and, in most cases, pertinent radiographic anatomy is illustrated by line drawing overlays and labels. No attempt has been made to illustrate pathologic anatomy except where illustration of a particular technique is enhanced by its use.

I am very fortunate in having obtained contributions in specific areas from several experts in their fields. Without their efforts, this book would not have been possible and I am deeply indebted to them.

The errors and omissions that may be present in this book should be brought to my attention, since improvement can only be made with knowledge.

The effort necessary to produce this volume required the assistance of several individuals. In addition to my colleagues who gave so generously of their time and knowledge to provide contributions for the text, many other persons gave me encouragement and technical help. My partners at the Berkeley Veterinary Medical Group, Drs. S. Gary Brown and Steve Ettinger, have continually provided me with the necessary stimulation to remain abreast of the current trends in our profession. Without the editorial assistance of Ms. Barbara Warren, the original manuscript would have remained a clutter of extraneous verbiage.

The advice and direction provided by Mr. Carroll Cann has been outstanding. As veterinary editor for the W. B. Saunders Company, his encouragement and friendship were a vital stimulus in undertaking the task of producing this book. Miss Catherine Fix of the editorial department, Mr. Ray Kersey of the illustration department, and Ms. Lorraine Battista of the design department of the W. B. Saunders Company have been extremely helpful during the production of the book. Mrs. Laura Tarves, as production manager for veterinary titles, has made the flow from manuscript to printed page go smoothly.

There is nothing that I can write that would adequately express my gratitude for the efforts of my wife, Vivian, during the production of this book. She possesses the unique ability of translating my handwritten hieroglyphics into a typewritten page, which she did with great skill. Her encouragement and assistance have made my career and this book possible.

JAMES W. TICER

Contents

SECTION I

Physical Principles

1

X-Ray Generation

INTRODUCTION

Medical x-rays are generated within a vacuum tube that consists of a source of electrons and a target with which the electrons can interact after being accelerated across a space. The resultant electron-target interaction generates x-rays and heat. The electron source is usually a cathode that has been heated to a temperature required to impart escape velocities to the electrons. Electrons are thereby made available in a semifree state, as a cloud adjacent to the cathode surface.

By applying a positive electrical potential to the target (anode) side of the tube through a voltage source that has its negative side attached to the cathode, the electron cloud can be accelerated across the vacuum and caused to collide and interact with the target material. By controlling the number of electrons moving from the anode to the cathode per unit time and the time that the positive potential is applied to the anode, the total number of generated x-rays may be regulated. The three basic components of a functional x-ray generator are an electron source, a voltage difference between the cathode and anode and a timing mechanism.

TYPES OF ELECTRON-TARGET INTERACTIONS

Usually, an accelerated electron must undergo several interactions with target atoms before losing all its energy. Two types of energy losses occur—collisional losses and radiation losses. Stated simply, collisional losses involve the outer electrons of the target atom and generate heat, whereas radiation losses involve the nucleus of the target atom and are responsible for the x-radiation generated (Johns, 1961; Christensen et al., 1978). The number of these individual interactions may be as high as many thousands for an accelerated electron used in diagnostic radiography.

Collisional Interactions

Two types of collisional interactions take place. In the first type, an incoming electron may excite an outer orbital electron of the target atom by passing in near proximity to its orbit, thus transferring energy. This allows the orbital electron to increase its distance from the nucleus, or raise its orbit. When the excited orbital electron returns to its original orbit, energy is irradiated as heat (Johns, 1961; Christensen et al., 1978).

A second type of collisional interaction may occur if the incoming electron possesses sufficient energy to remove an outer orbital electron from a target atom. The target atom is then ionized. The ejected electron (if it possesses energies in excess of the order of 100 electron volts) and the incoming electron then undergo additional interactions with target atoms. The total energy loss is eventually dissipated as heat (Johns, 1961; Christensen et al., 1978).

Heat Losses

When an accelerated electron beam interacts with a tungsten x-ray tube target, more than 99 per cent of the energy dissipated is in the form of heat from collisional interactions. The remaining energy is irradiated in the form of x-rays.

Tungsten targets are usually used in diagnostic x-ray tubes because they possess a high melting point and have the ability to generate x-ray energies that are useful in diagnostic radiography. In stationary anode x-ray tubes, the tungsten target is usually embedded in copper, since this metal has the ability to conduct heat away from the target efficiently. Heat loss also occurs by direct radiation to surrounding material.

In order to appreciate the magnitude of the energy that must be dissipated as heat, one should review the principle of power distribution in an electrical circuit. Energy developed in the anode of an x-ray tube is given by:

$$P = VI$$

where P is the power expressed in joules[1] per second or watts, V is the potential difference in volts across the circuit, and I is the current in amperes flowing through the circuit. As an example, a diagnostic x-ray tube operating at 100 kilovolts (kv) (100,000 volts) and 300 milliamperes (ma) (0.3 amperes) has a rate of energy dissipation of $VI = 100,000 \times 0.3 = 30,000$ watts. This is approximately five times the rate of energy dissipation that is created by a large cooking element of an electric stove.

It is obvious that prolonged current flow (amperage) created by exposures that exceed the capabilites of an x-ray tube should not be

---

[1]The joule is 10 million ergs. Power is the rate of doing work and is measured in joules per second (1 joule per second = 1 watt).

permitted. Excessive heating of the target results in melting and vaporization of the tungsten element, with its secondary effect of decreased x-ray output for a given number of electrons interacting with the tungsten element. Figure 1–1 illustrates damage caused by target overheating. Diagnostic x-ray tubes should, therefore, never be used for x-ray therapeutic purposes.

Generally, the larger the target, the more efficient will be the heat dissipation. For purposes of constructing a diagnostic x-ray tube, however, a small target size is desirable (Cahoon, 1965; Fuchs, 1966; Christensen et al., 1978; Gillette et al., 1977; Selman, 1977).

Tube Rating Charts

Tube rating charts are provided for all x-ray tubes to assist the operator in determining the maximum exposure characteristics that permit safe operation. By maintaining exposure factors below these factors, heat developed at the anode will not result in target damage. Figure 1–2 illustrates a typical chart for an anode size of 2.0 mm². An upper limit of exposure time may be determined by following the milliamperage value on the ordinate to the appropriate kilovoltage value curve. The maximum exposure time for safe operation is then determined by drawing a vertical line to the abscissa, where the scale of time in seconds is recorded. For example, a tube operated at 300 ma and 80 kv would have an exposure time limit of approximately 1.5 seconds to remain within safe operating limits. Prolonged tube life may be assured by operating the x-ray equipment within safe limits.

Multiple exposures made during a short period of time, as in angiographic proce-

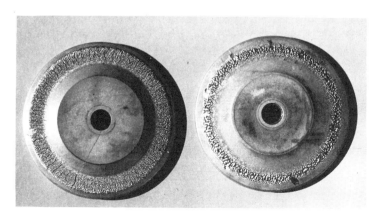

Figure 1–1. Damaged anodes. Heat damage (melting) to x-ray tube targets (rotating anodes) due to improper use.

RATING CHART FOR SINGLE-PHASE FULL-WAVE RECTIFICATION

Figure 1–2. Tube rating chart for a tube operated with a single-phase, full-wave rectified generator. Maximum ma and exposure times for a given KV operation for safe x-ray tube operation may be calculated from this chart. Rating charts are characteristic for each tube type and are not interchangeable.

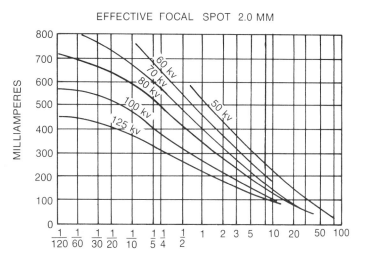

EFFECTIVE FOCAL SPOT 2.0 MM

MAXIMUM EXPOSURE TIME IN SECONDS

dures, result in the production of large amounts of heat in the anode. The target surface may be overheated by repeated exposures and may not have sufficient time to dissipate the heat to the body of the anode. Likewise, anode and tube housing heat can build up and not have sufficient time to radiate into the surrounding structures. To control rapid exposure technique, the concept of the heat unit must be understood. The heat unit is a measure of total heat produced by an exposure or series of exposures and is a product of the kv, ma and exposure time (Christensen et al., 1978). For example, an exposure made with 80 kv, 300 ma for one second would result in:

$$80 \times 300 \times 1 = 24,000 \text{ heat units.}$$

Heat units are usually used to express heat build-up in a single-phase x-ray generator, that is, one that uses single-phase alternating current as its power source.

Some tubes with a high-speed rotating anode and a three-phase generator have exposure limits expressed in terms of their power rating or kilowatt (kw) rating (Christensen et al., 1978). For conventional use, the kilowatt rating of an x-ray tube is 1/1000 of the maximum kv × ma at 0.1 second exposure for a particular tube. For example, a tube rated to withstand exposures of 125 kv at 500 ma for 0.1 second would be rated at:

$$\frac{125 \times 500}{1000} = 62.5 \text{ KW.}$$

Angiographic rating charts are usually available for equipment that is capable of producing multiple exposures in a short period of time. These charts or tables should be consulted before establishing a technique chart for rapid multiple exposure examinations.

Most x-ray tubes are also rated for heat storage capacity. Charts are also available that indicate the maximum heat units that may be safely stored in the anode and the time between examinations that is required for cooling to occur. If rapid exposure technique is used, careful study of this chart is required.

Radiative Interactions

One type of radiative interaction occurs when the incoming electron has sufficient energy to remove an inner (K or L shell) orbital electron from the target atom (Johns, 1961; Christensen et al., 1978). The ejected electron is replaced by an outer orbital electron, and the difference in the binding energies of the ejected electron and the replacement electron is irradiated as characteristic x-ray radiation. The term "characteristic" is derived from the fact that these radiations are characteristic for a given target atom, since the differences in orbital electron-binding energies are unique.

A second type of radiative interaction occurs when incoming electrons approach the nucleus of a target atom and are attracted toward the positive nucleus. The attraction of these two opposite charges causes the incoming electron to orbit partially around the nucleus. The change in electron direction results in reduced velocity (Johns, 1961; Christensen et al., 1978).

The energy lost by decreasing the velocity is irradiated in the form of x-radiation. The sudden deceleration, or "braking," of the incoming electron gives rise to the German term "bremsstrahlung," or braking radiation. This type of x-radiation is more probable with increased energies of incoming electrons.

The energy of the resulting bremsstrahlung radiations varies with the energy of the incoming electron and the angle of the interaction with the target atom. In contrast to characteristic radiations, bremsstrahlung radiations have a spectrum of energies.

Spectrum of X-ray Energies Generated

With the energies used in diagnostic radiography (40 to 120 kv), the majority of the x-radiation generated is in the form of bremsstrahlung radiation. Bremsstrahlung radiation energies vary with the energies of the accelerated electrons and are a function of the magnitude of the voltage applied between the anode and cathode of the x-ray tube (kv) as well as of the proximity to the nucleus where the reaction occurs. Thus, a wide range of x-ray energies is generated.

Figure 1–3 illustrates the spectrum of characteristic and bremsstrahlung radiations generated by a tungsten target for accelerating voltages of 65, 100, 150 and 200 kv (Johns, 1961). Note that the energy of the peaks created by the characteristic radiations of tungsten does not vary with the voltage applied across the x-ray tube. Only the relative number increases with increased accelerating voltage (kv).

The bremsstrahlung radiation spectrum, on the other hand, shows an increase in the maximum energy as the accelerating voltage

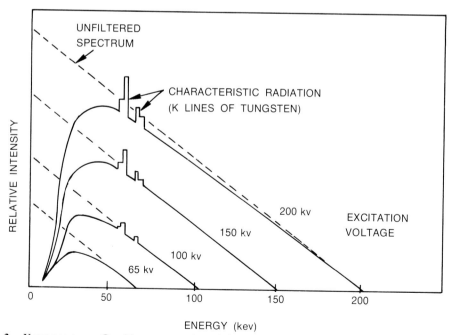

Figure 1–3. X-ray spectrum. Graphic representation of the variation of x-ray energies generated as a function of the energy of bombarding electrons interacting with a tungsten target. (From Johns, H. E., *The Physics of Radiology*, 2nd ed., 1961. Courtesy of Charles C Thomas, Publisher, Springfield, Illinois.)

(kv) is increased. This phenomenon accounts for the relative increase in x-ray beam energy as the kv of the x-ray machine is increased.

The dashed lines in Figure 1–3 represent the theoretical distribution of bremsstrahlung radiation. In the low energy region, the curve decreases rapidly to zero at approximately 10 kv. This phenomenon occurs because the lower energy levels of bremsstrahlung radiations below 10 kv are not able to penetrate the target metal, vacuum tube wall and other filtering material placed in the x-ray beam.

The usefulness of the x-ray beam spectrum for diagnostic radiography decreases rapidly below 40 kv, since penetration of the patient's body parts is not easily accomplished below this energy level. To prevent absorption of relatively nonpenetrating, low energy x-rays by the superficial layers of a patient's body, they are removed from the primary x-ray beam by the addition of a thin layer (2 to 3 mm) of aluminum (added filtration).

It is important to recall that the distribution of the low energy x-rays is not affected by increased operating voltages. Increasing the voltage applied across the tube only increases the maximum energy of the x-ray spectrum and does not increase the minimal energy. Filtration of the x-ray beam with aluminum to remove the less penetrating x-rays, therefore, remains as important for high voltages as it is for low voltages.

Heel Effect

There is an unequal distribution of the x-ray beam intensity as it leaves the x-ray tube (Fig. 1–4). This variation has a definite relationship to the angle of the x-ray tube target. When the angle of the target is 20 degrees from the central ray, distribution of beam intensity decreases rapidly toward the anode (positive) side of the tube. This phenomenon is due to absorption of the x-ray beam by target and anode material. The x-ray beam on the cathode (negative) side of the tube is slightly more intense than the central ray. This is the so-called "heel effect."

This phenomenon may be used to good advantage when radiographing parts of unequal thickness. By placing the thickest part of the patient toward the cathode of the x-ray tube, a more uniform density of the radiograph may be obtained. The heel effect can be used most effectively when radio-

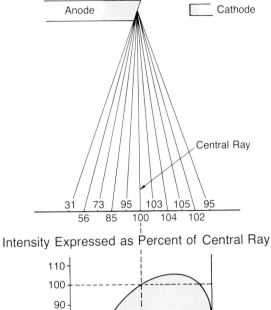

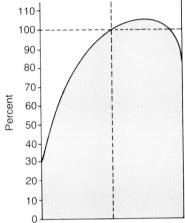

Figure 1–4. Heel effect. The unequal distribution of x-ray beam intensity is shown to decrease rapidly toward the anode of the x-ray tube, producing the so-called heel effect. This phenomenon is due to absorption of the x-ray beam by the target and the anode material.

graphing relatively long patients with marked differences in part thickness, such as the abdomen of a dog with a deep thorax. This method should always be considered when using a 14 × 17 inch cassette. The heel effect is not noticeable when radiographing parts that are less than 12 inches in length.

X-RAY TUBE CONSTRUCTION

An x-ray tube is essentially a large diode-type electronic tube. The heated cathode acts as a source of electrons and the anode acts as the positive plate that contains an embedded tungsten target (Fig. 1–5). These elements are placed within a glass envelope

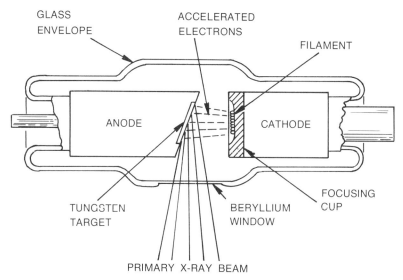

Figure 1–5. Diagram of simple x-ray tube.

which is then evacuated to form a vacuum. This vacuum will prevent rapid oxidation of the elements. A thin window area is formed in the glass envelope to act as an exit for the x-ray beam by decreasing the x-ray-absorbing qualities of the glass. The entire tube is then enclosed in a metal container to control the escape of stray radiation and to protect the glass envelope from physical damage.

The cathode is usually placed in a shallow depression called a focusing cup. A negative electrical potential is applied to the focusing cup to control the beam diameter, thereby confining the electron beam to the target area. A decreased target area (focal spot) increases the detail of the resultant radiographic image, and, therefore, the focal spot should remain as small as possible. The lower

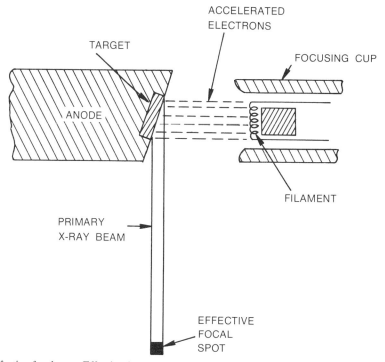

Figure 1–6. Effective focal spot. Effective focal spot is decreased by placing the target at an angle to the cathode.

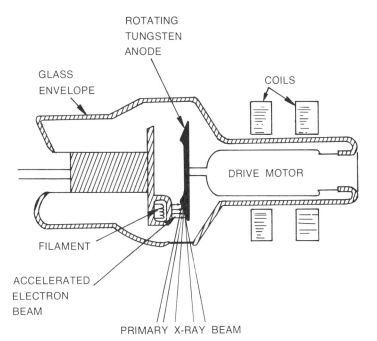

Figure 1–7. Rotating anode. Dissipation of heat is enhanced by placing the target material in the form of a strip around the circumference of a high-speed rotating disc.

ROTATING
TUNGSTEN
ANODE

GLASS
ENVELOPE

COILS

DRIVE MOTOR

FILAMENT

ACCELERATED
ELECTRON
BEAM

PRIMARY X-RAY BEAM

limit of focal spot size is governed by the ability of the anode to dissipate the heat of collisional electron interactions within the target material.

The effective focal spot size may be decreased by placing the face of the target at approximately 20 degrees to the cathode (Fig. 1–6). The effective focal spot size is made smaller than the actual focal spot size owing to an artifact of geometric projection. Manufacturers of x-ray tubes designate the size of the effective focal spot. The so-called 1.0 mm focal spot tube, therefore, has a *projected* focal spot measuring 1 mm × 1 mm.

Dissipation of heat may also be enhanced by placing the tungsten target material in the form of a strip around the circumference of a high-speed rotating disk (Fig. 1–7). This device prevents continuous bombardment of the same target surface and thus allows cooling of the target element. Rotating anode tubes may contain a focal spot of approximately one sixth the size required for stationary anode tubes. X-ray machines with high milliamperage capabilities require the use of rotating anode x-ray tubes to prevent excessive heat damage to the target surface. Rotating anode x-ray tubes, therefore, are a good investment despite their increased cost.

Some x-ray tubes have two cathodes and focusing cups, each producing a different electron beam diameter for use in differing target sizes. Thus, when decreased milliamperage is used, the smaller effective focal spot may be used to increase radiographic detail.

ELECTRICAL CIRCUITS FOR X-RAY TUBE CONTROL

High Voltage Circuit

Relatively simple electrical circuitry is necessary to provide the x-ray tube with a source of high voltage potential for accelerating electrons from the cathode to the anode. High voltage is generated by a step-up transformer. By adding an appropriate number of windings to the transformer's secondary, the input of 60 cycles alternating voltage may be increased from 110 or 220 volts to the required 40 to 120 kv.

Variation of the voltage applied to the primary winding of the high voltage transformer permits one to control the output voltage in the secondary winding, and thereby to control the voltage applied across the x-ray tube. This is accomplished by an autotransformer. An autotransformer differs from other step-up transformers by having both the primary and secondary windings contained on one core. A switching device allows voltages to be obtained from various levels on the winding. The kilovoltage selection switch on the x-ray machine control panel is connected to this switching mechanism on the autotransformer.

Most x-ray machines used in veterinary practices have single-phase generators; that is, they use alternating voltage that varies from a maximum positive to a maximum negative potential 60 times per second. More efficient generators are available, however, that utilize a three-phase alternating voltage. Three-phase alternating voltage produces an almost constant potential difference across the x-ray tube, since the pulsating or ripple effect of the rectified single-phase voltage is decreased markedly. Three-phase alternating voltages are generated by superimposing three separate 60-cycle alternating wave forms that are out of phase with each other by 120 degrees; that is, the second wave is started after the first wave has cycled 120 degrees, and the third wave is started after the first wave has cycled 240 degrees. By superimposing these three wave forms, a nearly constant maximum positive and negative potential difference is applied across the x-ray tube.

The major advantage of three-phase generators is a much higher tube rating for very short exposures, thereby allowing tube currents of up to 2000 ma. It is then possible to perform high quality rapid sequence filming, such as in angiography, when very short exposure times must be made at a high repetition rate.

Filament Circuit

A simple stepdown transformer is applied between the input voltage of the x-ray machine and the cathode filament. The filament voltage supply must be relatively low, while the current flow or amperage must be high. The number of electrons available for transport to the target of the x-ray tube is a function of cathode heat.

Increased cathode heat results in increased electron availability and thus in an increased electron flow and an increased number of x-rays generated.

Decreasing the amperage in the cathode filament results in decreased heat and, thereby, decreased availability of electrons. Control of the amperage in the cathode filament therefore accomplishes direct control over the number of x-rays produced in a given time period.

Amperage control is accomplished by inserting a choke coil in the input side of the primary filament transformer winding. The impedancy (resistance in an alternating current circuit) may be varied by inserting or retracting the core of the coil. This mechanism is connected to the milliampere control of the x-ray control console.

Timer

Completion of a functional x-ray machine requires only the addition of an accurate timer switch in the primary windings of the high voltage transformer. This device will control the amount of time that high voltage is applied across the x-ray tube and thereby control the duration of x-ray generation.

Various mechanical and electronic devices have been manufactured for this purpose. Electronic timing devices are necessary for the short exposure times required in diagnostic veterinary radiography (Ticer, 1969). Though these are more expensive, the increased expense must be accepted as a necessary investment.

Rectification Circuits

Rectification of the alternating voltage applied to the x-ray tube increases the efficiency of the unit. Basically, "self-rectification" is a term used to describe the limitation of current flow across the x-ray tube in one direction, that is, from the cathode to the anode. The inefficiency of a self-rectified x-ray machine can only be tolerated in portable equipment.

When an alternating 60-cycle voltage is applied to the x-ray tube, electrons flow from the cathode to the anode only when a positive voltage is applied to the anode. During one half of every cycle, a negative potential is applied to the anode, resulting in no electron flow and no x-ray generation. The result is 60 pulses of x-rays generated every second.

If a valve tube (diode) is placed in the high voltage supply, the anode of the x-ray tube can be protected from the extremely high negative voltages , and the cathode from high positive potentials, by removing the negative half of the voltage cycle. This protection becomes important when high milliamperage generators are used, because increased current (electron) flow results in anode heating sufficient to make some electrons available in the form of an electron cloud, similar to the phenomenon occurring at the heated cathode. If a high positive voltage is applied to the cathode, an electron beam will be accelerated toward the filament of the cathode, causing severe damage from electron bombardment.

Prolongation of x-ray tube life is accomplished by the addition of valve tube rectification. The efficiency of a valve-rectified x-ray generator is, however, not appreciably increased over the self-rectified system, since one half of the voltage input cycle is wasted. The resultant x-ray generation is pulsed at a rate of 60 pulses per second.

By adding four valve tubes to the high voltage supply in such a manner that positive voltage is always applied to the anode of the x-ray tube, the efficiency of operation is increased by 100 per cent. A pulsing positive voltage is then applied to the x-ray tube anode at the rate of 120 times per second. This results in twice the x-ray output than is achieved with the half-wave rectified units. The advantage of the full-wave rectified generator becomes obvious when one considers that exposures can be made in half the time— a consideration that is extremely important in veterinary radiography, where patient movement is always a problem (Ticer, 1969).

Condenser Discharge Units

An alternate method of generating the extremely high voltages necessary to produce diagnostic radiographs is by the use of a condenser discharge generator. High voltage is generated by charging a relatively large condenser with a low-power circuit taken from the input voltage available. This voltage input may be from a standard 110-volt supply. A charge is allowed to build up to the desired kilovoltage.

The voltage is then switched to the x-ray tube, where it discharges in a fraction of a second. The resulting electron flow generates x-rays as the electrons bombard the target. Condenser discharge generators give high voltage performance from low voltage supplies. This is an obvious advantage in mobile equipment and should find a use in veterinary radiography, in which mobility and high voltage performance often are needed.

REFERENCES

Cahoon, J. B.: Formulating X-ray Techniques. 7th ed. Durham, North Carolina, Duke University Press, 1970.
Christensen, E. E., Curry, T. S., III, and Dowdey, J. E.: An Introduction to the Physics of Diagnostic Radiology. 2nd ed. Philadelphia, Lea and Febiger, 1978.
Gillette, E. L., Thrall, D. E., and Lebel, J. L.: Carlson's Veterinary Radiology. 3rd ed. Philadelphia, Lea and Febiger, 1977.
Johns, H. E., and Cunningham, J. R. : The Physics of Radiology. 3rd ed. Springfield, Ill., Charles C Thomas, Publisher, 1974.
Selman, J.: The Fundamentals of X-ray and Radium. 6th ed. Springfield, Ill., Charles C Thomas, Publisher, 1977.
Ticer, J. W.: Production of diagnostic radiographs in veterinary medicine. I. Machine factors. Calif. Vet., 23:18–21, 1969.

2

Image Formation and Recording

INTRODUCTION

The usefulness of a radiographic examination is limited by the quality of the image recording process. Distortion caused by faulty geometric projection of the part examined is frequently a cause of poor quality radiographs. The vast majority of unsatisfactory radiographic examinations are, however, caused by poor radiographic density, contrast or detail. Multiple factors relating to the patient type, radiographic equipment and technique and darkroom methods affect the production of high quality radiographic examinations.

GEOMETRY OF IMAGE FORMATION

An accurate recording of patient shape is necessary in order to obtain quality radiographs. Distortion of the projected image may result in inaccurate interpretation. It is therefore important to understand the effect of geometric projection of the subject onto the recording surface.

To preserve accurate geometric projection, the subject to be examined and the recording surface must be parallel. Figure 2–1 A illustrates this effect. Note that when relatively large areas are radiographed, it is not necessary for the x-ray source to be directly above the part examined if the part and the recording surface are parallel (Eastman Kodak Co., 1980). If the part being examined is not parallel to the recording surface, geometric

distortion results (Fig. 2–1 B). This becomes important in veterinary radiography when the long bones of the appendicular skeleton are examined. An example of the artifactual shortening of the femur that may occur if the bone is not parallel to the recording surface is illustrated in Figure 2–2 A and B.

Although geometric shape is preserved by a parallel positioning of subject and recording surface, a significant enlargement in the recorded image occurs when the distance between the subject and the recording surface is increased (Fig. 2–3 A and B) (Gillette et al., 1977; Eastman Kodak Co., 1980). Figure 2–4 illustrates this magnifying effect when a lateral recumbent radiographic view of both scapulohumeral articulations is produced simultaneously. Note that the humerus lying farther from the recording surface is artifactually enlarged.

The geometric relationships between areas of radiolucency and radiodensity are important to consider, especially when the vertebral column is radiographed. Figure 2–5 A and B illustrates these relationships in the radiographic examination of the caudal cervical vertebrae in a ventrodorsal projection. Note that either elevating the caudal cervical vertebrae or shifting the angle of the x-ray tube caudally results in an improved projection of the intervertebral spaces, as shown in Figure 2–6 A and B.

Accurate projection of interfaces between a series of radiolucent and radiodense objects, such as vertebrae, requires that these parts be parallel to the recording surface. Figure 2–7 A shows the inaccurate projection

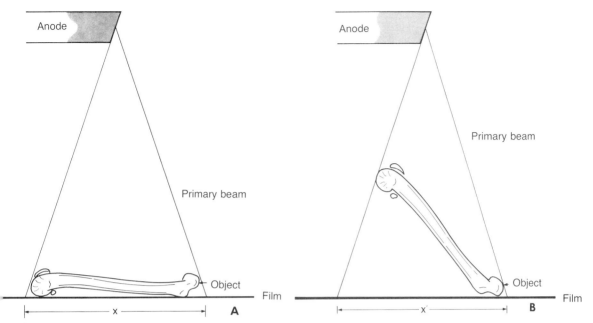

Figure 2–1. *A*, Diagram of the radiographic projection when a long bone such as a femur is placed parallel to a recording surface such as a film. Note that there is only a minor artifactual recorded length increase, especially when the part is placed close to the film. *B*, Diagram of the radiographic projection when a femur is placed at an angle to the film. Note that there is an artifactual shortening when projected onto the recording surface.

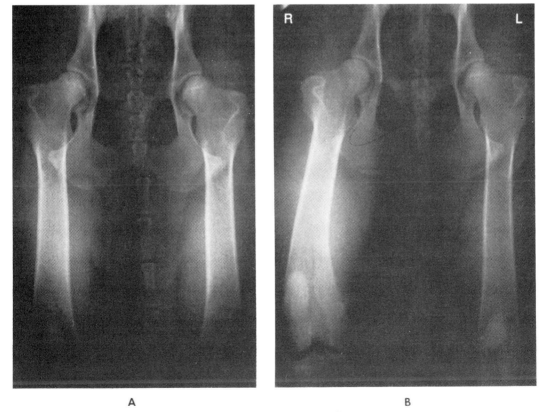

Figure 2–2. *A*, A radiograph produced with both femurs placed parallel to the film. *B*, A radiograph produced with the left femur placed parallel to the film and the right femur placed at an increased angle by allowing the hip to flex. This is the same dog as in *A*.

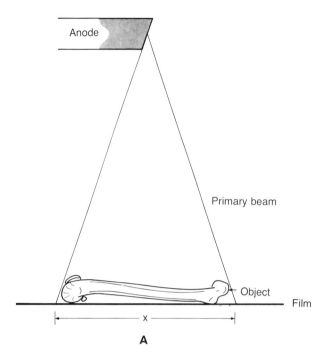

A

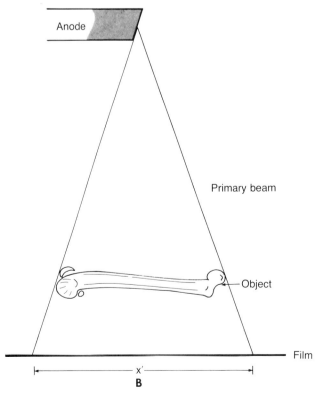

B

Figure 2–3. *A*, Diagram of the effect of placing the patient in close proximity to the film. Note that very little magnification occurs. *B*, Diagram of the magnification effect produced by increasing the distance between the patient and film.

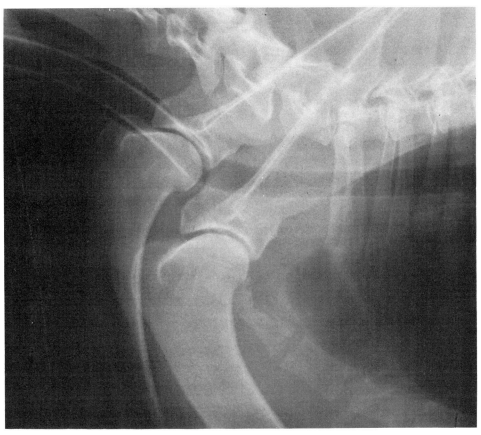

Figure 2–4. A lateral radiographic projection illustrates the principle shown in Figure 2–3. Note that the humerus and ribs that are farthest from the film are magnified. Radiographic detail is also decreased by increasing the distance between the patient part and the film, which is also illustrated in this study.

of cervical vertebrae in a lateral recumbent view when these parts are allowed to sag toward the recording surface, thus producing artifactually narrowed intervertebral spaces (Bartels and Hoerlein, 1971; Gillette et al., 1977). If the midcervical region is elevated, a more accurate projection is obtained (Fig. 2–7 *B*). Note that the intervertebral spaces are now nearly the same width.

A further example of the geometric projection of radiolucent-radiodense planes is found in the artifactual narrowing of intervertebral disk spaces that occurs as the distance from the central ray of the x-ray beam is increased (Bartels and Hoerlein, 1971). Figure 2–8 illustrates this principle in a lateral recumbent radiograph of a lumbar vertebral column. Note that the intervertebral spaces appear to decrease caudal to the L1, L2 interspace, where the central ray of the x-ray beam was placed. This becomes particularly important when evaluating radiographs for possible intervertebral disk herniations. Mul-

tiple lateral recumbent views of the vertebral column, with the central ray of the x-ray beam placed at several different levels, are necessary for accurate evaluation of a series of intervertebral spaces.

RADIOGRAPHIC CONTRAST

The differences in the densities of the various subjects on a finished radiograph are termed radiographic contrast (Gillette et al., 1977; Eastman Kodak Co., 1980). These differences are a function of both film contrast and subject or patient contrast.

Modern medical x-ray film usually exaggerates the differences in x-ray image contrast by a factor of two (Eastman Kodak Co., 1980). This means that for a given density difference between two tissues, such as bone and muscle, approximately twice this difference will be recorded on a finished radiograph, compared with the original image dis-

Text continued on page 19.

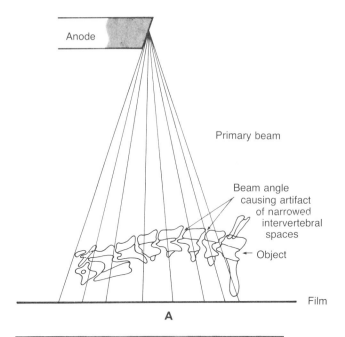

A

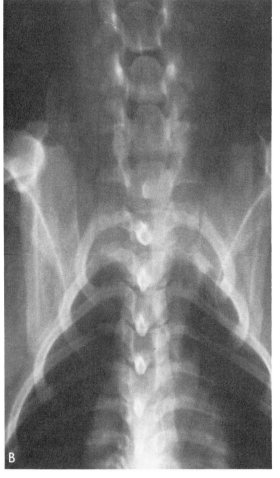

Figure 2–5. *A*, Diagram of the radiographic projection produced when the patient is placed in a ventrodorsal position and the x-ray beam is placed perpendicular to the film. *B*, A radiograph produced under these conditions. Note the artifactually narrowed intervertebral spaces in the caudal cervical and cranial thoracic region.

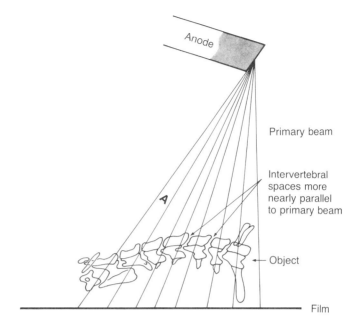

Primary beam

Intervertebral spaces more nearly parallel to primary beam

Object

Film

Figure 2–6. *A*, Diagram of the radiographic projection produced when the patient is placed in a ventrodorsal position and the x-ray beam is directed approximately 15 degrees caudal from the perpendicular. *B*, A radiograph produced under these conditions. Note the nearly accurate projection of the intervertebral spaces.

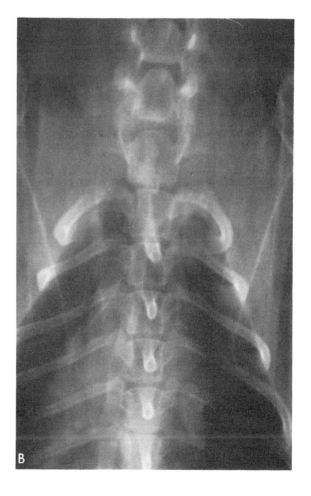

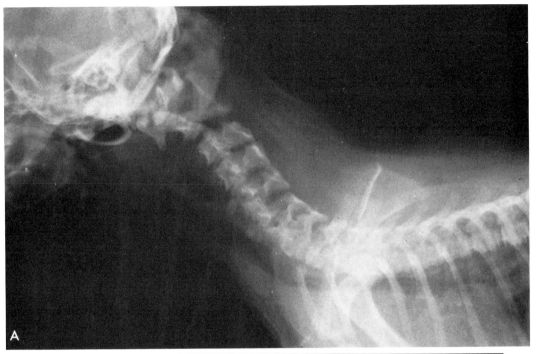

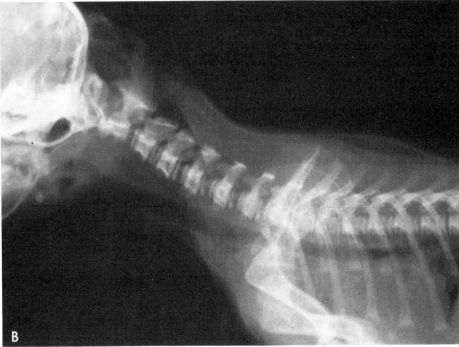

Figure 2–7. *A*, A lateral radiograph of the cervical region of a 7-week-old Dachshund produced by allowing the central cervical vertebrae to sag toward the film. Note that this position artifactually produces a bizarre appearance of the central and caudal vertebral bodies and intervertebral spaces which does not allow for adequate radiographic interpretation. *B*, A lateral radiograph of the cervical vertebrae in the same position as in *A* produced by maintaining a parallel relationship between the film and the vertebral bodies of the entire cervical and thoracic region. Note the normal appearance of the epiphyseal lines and the narrowed intervertebral space between C-3 and C-4.

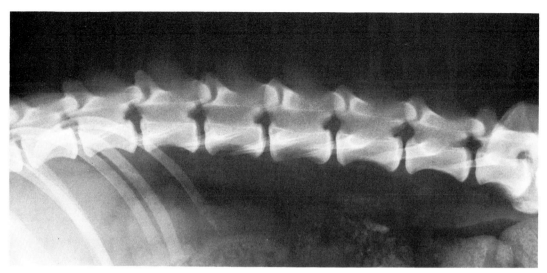

Figure 2–8. A lateral radiograph of the lumbar vertebrae produced with the central x-ray beam centered at L-2. Note the artifactually narrowed intervertebral spaces both cranial and caudal to this body, produced by the increased angle of x-ray beam incidence.

played on a fluoroscopic screen. Proper developing technique must also be maintained to preserve this contrast created by the x-ray film.

Differences in density found on a finished radiograph are, in part, a function of the differences in x-ray absorption by the tissues of the patient. These differences depend upon the thickness of the part being examined and upon the average atomic number of the components of the various tissues (Johns, 1950). This is true only for x-ray absorption in the energy range used in medical radiography, when the principal mode of x-ray absorption is by the photoelectric effect (Johns and Cunningham, 1974). This mechanism of electromagnetic energy absorption varies with the number of electrons per gram of absorbing material, which in turn varies with atomic number (Johns and Cunningham, 1974). An increased average atomic number of the absorbing material will, therefore, result in increased x-ray absorption. (Recall that a higher atomic number represents an increase in the proton number and, therefore, an increase in the number of orbital electrons, since the proton number and the atomic number are equal to the orbital electron number in electrically neutral atoms.) It is easy to see that calcium- and phosphorus-containing bone will absorb a greater number of x-rays than muscle, which contains relatively more atoms of low atomic numbers, such as nitrogen, oxygen, and hydrogen.

These differences in absorption of x-rays with energies used in medical radiography make possible the recording of contrast on a finished radiograph.

Increased x-ray energies (produced by increased accelerating voltage applied across the x-ray tube) result in both increased penetrability of the x-ray beam and decreased difference in contrast at subject interfaces, such as bone and muscle (Glasser et al., 1961). Figure 2–9 shows graphically that the number of electrons per gram of absorbing material becomes less important to the differential absorption of x-rays as the energy of the x-ray beam increases. This phenomenon is caused by a relative decrease in the photoelectric mode of electromagnetic energy absorption (which is a function of the number of electrons per gram of absorbing material) as x-ray energy is increased. In the upper range of x-ray energies used in medical radiography, the Compton absorption mechanism becomes increasingly important (Johns, 1950). This absorption mechanism is independent of the number of electrons per gram of absorbing material and therefore produces decreasing density differences at subject interfaces recorded on a finished radiograph (Johns and Cunningham, 1974).

Increased x-ray energies result in a finished radiograph with a increased scale of contrast (Cahoon, 1970); this means that there are relatively more shades of grey and fewer contrasting black and white surfaces. This

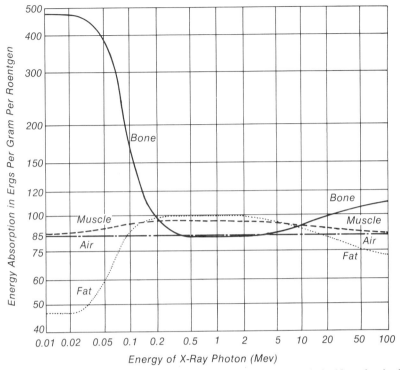

Figure 2–9. A graph of the absorption of x-ray photons by bone, muscle, fat and air. Note that in the range below 0.2 Mev (200 Kev) the difference in absorption ability between these media increases rapidly with decreasing electromagnetic energy. This is due to the photoelectric absorption effect and accounts for the selection of this energy range for use in medical radiography, since the resultant radiographic image depends on the different absorption rates of various tissues. (After Johns, H. E.: Radiation therapy: depth dose. *In* Glasser, O. (Ed.), *Medical Physics*, Vol. II. Chicago, Year Book Publishers, Inc., 1950.)

effect is best illustrated by radiographing a series of aluminum blocks of increasing thickness with x-ray beams of increasing energies (Fig. 2–10). Note that as the voltage used to generate the x-ray beam is increased from 40 to 100 kv, the ability to determine differences in the aluminum block thickness is improved. The relatively low energy x-ray beam generated with 40 kv produces fewer tones of grey on the finshed radiograph, whereas increased x-ray energies produce more tones of grey and possess an increased scale of contrast (Cahoon, 1970; Eastman Kodak Co., 1980). The decreasing differential absorption effect of increasing kilovoltage becomes particularly important when an increased scale of contrast is desired for the radiographic examination of subjects that have subtle differences in density, such as fascial planes of muscle and the serosal surface–peritoneal fat interfaces of the abdomen. Generally, the examination of bone structures requires a relatively low kilovoltage (low scale of contrast) in order to differentiate the interfaces of bone and soft tissue. Soft tissue structures should be ex-

amined with a relatively higher kv x-ray beam, which produces the increased scale of contrast necessary to differentiate subtle density differences.

Other factors that affect subject contrast are voltage waveform and filtration. Recall that utilization of a three-phase generator increases the average energy of an x-ray beam and therefore has the effect of decreasing the scale of contrast when compared with that of a single-phase generator. Filtration of the x-ray beam also has the effect of increasing the average beam energy by removing the relatively low-energy, nonpenetrating x-rays (see p. 26), and therefore decreases the scale of contrast when compared with that of a nonfiltered beam.

EXPOSURE LATITUDE

Radiographs produced with high kilovoltage result in increased exposure latitude as well as an increased scale of contrast. Latitude is a term used to describe the range of

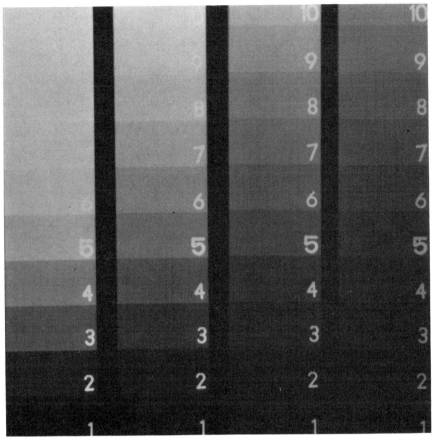

Figure 2–10. Radiograph of four aluminum step wedges produced with increasing kilovoltage from left to right. Kilovolt values of 40, 60, 80 and 100 were used. Milliampere second (mas) values were lowered simultaneously to ensure constant density. Note the increasing penetrability of the more energetic beams, illustrated by number 10 step visualization. There is also better differentiation between the steps as kv is increased, resulting in the production of more shades of grey (increased scale of contrast).

exposure that will produce film density within an acceptable quality for a diagnostic radiograph (Christensen et al., 1978). Thus, radiographs produced with high kilovoltage (and latitude) allow a greater variation in exposure factors that result in diagnostic quality. Conversely, low kilovoltage technique requires more precision in selecting exposure factors, since there will be less exposure latitude.

RADIOGRAPHIC DENSITY

Radiographic density is defined as the degree of blackness on a finished radiograph. Dark areas on a finished radiograph are produced by deposits of metallic silver in the film emulsion. These areas appear dark when light is transmitted through a radiograph.

In a finished radiograph, increased silver retention occurs in areas where increased x-ray beam penetration has occurred. It follows that such body parts as air-containing lungs will produce a radiographic image that is blacker than the bones of the thoracic cage.

Increased radiographic density may be produced by increasing the number of x-rays penetrating the patient or by increasing developing time or temperature. The number of x-rays available to produce an exposure may be increased by increasing the milliamperage (electron flow from the x-ray tube cathode to the anode), or by increasing the time of exposure. Both techniques result in increased total x-ray production per exposure. Figure 2–11 illustrates the effect of doubling the milliamperage during a given exposure time. Note that the overall blackness or density has increased, but the scale of contrast is not affected—i.e., the number

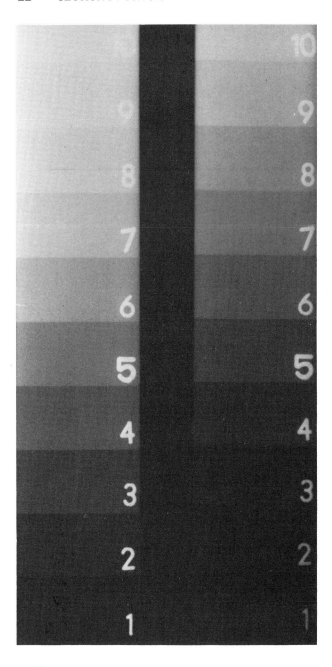

Figure 2–11. Radiograph of two aluminum step wedges produced by 6.7 and 13.3 mas at 60 kv. Note that with a constant kv setting, the number of shades of grey (steps penetrated) does not change with increasing mas values. Only the overall radiographic density has increased as a result of an increase in the total number of x-rays available to expose the film.

of shades of grey has not changed. The same effect could be produced by doubling the time of exposure, thereby also producing twice the number of x-rays. Increasing the milliamperage or the time of exposure therefore determines the quantity of x-rays available to penetrate the patient and expose x-ray film but does not affect the quality of the resultant image (Cahoon, 1970; Eastman Kodak Co., 1980).

Increased kilovoltage results in increased penetrability of the x-ray beam and increases the overall density of the finished radiograph, since more x-rays penetrate the patient and are made available to be recorded on the film. This effect, unlike the increases in milliamperage or time, is accompanied by an increase in the scale of contrast (Fig. 2–10).

RADIOGRAPHIC DETAIL

Radiographic detail is essentially a visual quality. Radiographs possess good detail when the tissue interfaces, such as the junc-

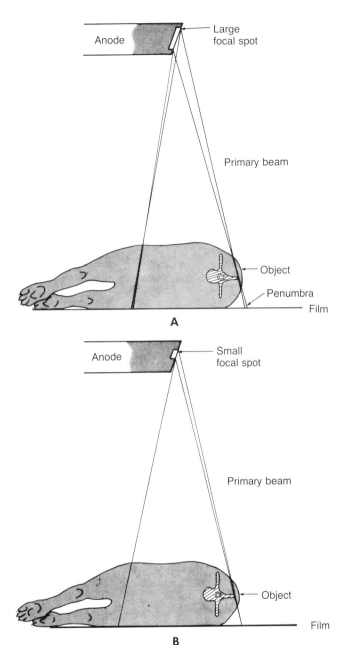

Figure 2–12. *A*, Diagram of the effect of increased x-ray tube focal spot (target) size on the production of a penumbra, which results in blurring of the edges of the various radiographic densities. *B*, Decreasing the x-ray tube focal spot size produces less penumbra effect, with the result that there is decreased blurring at the edges of various radiographic densities. This yields increased radiographic detail.

ture of bone and soft tissue, are sharp (clearly delineated) and possess good contrast (Cahoon, 1970; Ticer, 1969).

Good detail in radiographs depends upon many factors. Sharpness of definition may be increased by using an x-ray tube with an effective focal spot that is as small as is practical, consistent with heat tolerance of the x-ray tube target (Eastman Kodak Co., 1980; Christensen et al., 1978). This principle is illustrated diagrammatically in Figure 2–12 *A* and *B*. Note that the larger the effective

focal spot, the more pronounced will be the penumbra effect, which produces a blurred tissue interface.

The magnitude of the penumbra effect may also be decreased by increasing the focal-film distance (FFD) (Cahoon, 1970). The FFD is the distance from the x-ray tube target to the recording surface, or film. There is, however, an upper practical limit to the FFD, which is governed by the marked decrease in the x-ray beam intensity at the recording surface as the FFD is increased. This intensity decrease occurs at a rate inverse to the square of the distance, so that by doubling the distance, the x-ray beam intensity will be decreased by a factor of four and will have one fourth the original intensity (see Chap. 4). In practice, this means that the exposure must be increased four times if the FFD is doubled to maintain equal density. This factor becomes very important in veterinary radiography, where short exposure times are needed to decrease detail loss caused by recording imperceptible patient motion on the finished radiograph. A practical FFD is 36 to 40 inches (Ticer, 1969); this distance seems to be sufficient to avoid noticeable detail loss due to the penumbra effect.

The penumbra effect may also be diminished by decreasing the distance between the subject and the recording surface. This factor is of practical importance when producing lateral oblique views of the mandible or temporomandibular articulation or lateral views of limbs, where a minimal distance between the subject and the film may be maintained by placing the part being examined closest to the film.

High detail x-ray film and intensifying screens also increase the sharpness of the recorded image, thereby improving radiographic detail. Good film-intensifying screen contact is also necessary for preservation of sharpness (see p. 31). The use of nonscreen x-ray film will eliminate the two variables of intensifying screen detail loss and poor screen-film contact. However, the increased exposure time required to produce radiographs with nonscreen technique renders this method of increasing radiographic detail impractical for general veterinary radiographic technique, since longer exposure times increase the chances that patient motion will cause loss of detail. For this reason, nonscreen technique should be reserved for high detail radiography of the peripheral appendicular skeleton and skull.

The detail of veterinary radiographic examinations is often limited by imperceptible patient motion during exposure (Gillette et al., 1977; Ticer, 1969). This is particularly true when examining the thorax or cranial abdomen, because diaphragmatic movement often causes blurring of tissue interfaces. Since control of patient movement is often not possible in veterinary radiography, fast exposure times should be used.

Subject contrast also affects radiographic detail (Eastman Kodak Co., 1980). Skeletal structures may be examined using a relatively low kilovoltage technique that produces a shortened scale of contrast that improves radiographic detail. Some loss of detail must be accepted when high kilovoltage technique is used for examining soft tissue structures, since subtle differences in density require radiographs with a longer scale of contrast.

Mottle. Although not strictly a modifier of radiographic detail, radiographic mottle does affect image quality. Radiographic mottle is the density variation in a radiograph made with intensifying screens that have been given a uniform exposure. Radiographic mottle is the result of quantum mottle, structure mottle, and film graininess.

Quantum mottle is usually the principal contributor to the density fluctuation (Rossmann, 1962). X-rays can be described as bundles or packets of energy known as quanta or photons as well as waves. Quantum mottle is the variation in density of a uniformly exposed radiograph that results from the random spatial distribution of the x-ray quanta absorbed in the screen (Eastman Kodak Co., 1980). A better understanding of this phenomenon may be had by using a raindrop analogy. Think of a sidewalk, with its many squares, as corresponding to the film-screen combination, the raindrops as x-ray quanta and the sidewalk wetness as radiographic density. If a given wetness is produced by a shower that is composed of many fine droplets, it is difficult to see the individual droplets and the sidewalk looks uniformly wet. Now consider the situation in which the same amount of moisture is applied by large drops. The individual drop can readily be seen. There will be square-to-square differences in the distribution and number of the drops.

The same phenomenon occurs during the production of a radiograph. Radiographs produced with a large number of x-rays are more nearly uniformly dense than are those produced with similar density by fewer x-rays. As faster film speed and intensifying screen speed have become available (see pp. 30 and 32), fewer x-rays are required to produce a given radiographic density and therefore the effect of quantum mottle becomes more apparent.

Structure mottle is the density fluctuation caused by nonuniform structure of intensifying screens. Slight variations in screen thickness or in the distribution of crystals and other components may cause structure mottle.

Film graininess is due to random distribution of deposits of developed silver. Film graininess usually does not affect radiographic quality unless the image is magnified.

Subject contrast and, subsequently, radiographic detail may also be improved by decreasing the scatter radiation, which reduces the contrast of finished radiographs (Cahoon, 1970; Gillette et al., 1977). Beam restrictors and grids are used to control stray radiation.

X-ray Beam Restrictors. Controlling the volume of the patient's body irradiated during radiography not only increases the safety factor by preventing unnecessary patient exposure but also decreases scatter radiation to which the operator may be exposed unnecessarily. Limiting the area of the primary x-ray beam also has the effect of reducing fog-producing scatter radiation from reaching the recording surface (Christensen et al., 1978). An unrestricted, primary x-ray beam irradiates a large volume of patient tissue, which, in turn, causes an excessive amount of scatter radiation to reach the recording surface (Fig. 2–13 A).

Control of the patient volume being irradiated during an exposure is accomplished by placing a cone, a diaphragm or a collimator containing an adjustable diaphragm in the primary beam (Fig. 2–13 B and C). The major disadvantage of the use of cones or a nonadjustable diaphragm to restrict the primary beam is that they are available in fixed sizes and must be changed when a different area of the patient is radiographed. The chance of error or misuse is inherent in the mechanical maneuver required to change these devices.

The most satisfactory method of limiting the primary x-ray beam is the use of a collimator, which contains moveable lead leaves that may be adjusted to conform precisely to the area being examined. The collimator has the added advantage of usually having a localizing light incorporated within its structure. This light illuminates the area to be examined and has dimensions similar to the limited x-ray beam. This mechanism has the obvious advantage of aiding in accurate patient positioning within the area of the primary x-ray beam.

Filters. A thin sheet of aluminum called a filter may be placed over the window of the x-ray tube for the purpose of removing the less energetic, less penetrating x-rays from the primary beam. The resultant filtered x-ray beam is free of this useless portion of the x-ray spectrum. Filtered, primary x-ray beams decrease the amount of undesirable exposure to patient skin, thereby reducing the relative radiation hazard (see Chap. 6).

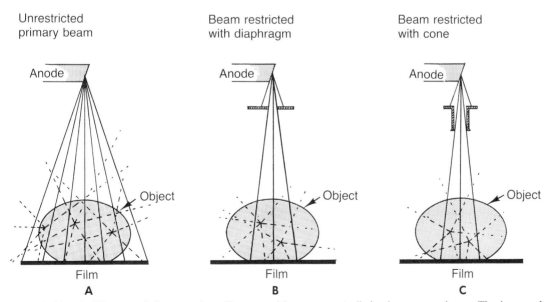

Unrestricted primary beam

Beam restricted with diaphragm

Beam restricted with cone

Anode

Anode

Anode

Object

Object

Object

Film

Film

Film

A

B

C

Figure 2–13. *A,* Diagram of the scattering effect caused by an uncontrolled primary x-ray beam. The increased volume of tissue irradiated results in increased scatter radiation. *B,* Decreased scatter radiation obtained when the area of exposure is controlled by means of a diaphragm. *C,* Decreased scatter radiation produced when the area of exposure is controlled by means of a cone.

Figure 2–14. A 17 × 17 inch grid encased in a rectangular wafer of aluminum.

Filtered x-ray beams also have the advantage of reducing fog-producing scatter radiation, thus increasing radiographic detail.

Grids. As thickness of the part of the patient's body being examined increases, there is an increase in the amount of secondary scatter radiation produced (Gillette et al., 1977). Generally, subjects greater than 9 cm thick produce sufficient secondary scatter radiation to cause detail loss on the finished radiograph, even when proper beam restriction and filtration have been accomplished. This requires devices that will limit exposure of the x-ray film to the primary beam by removing those scattered x-rays that cause loss of detail. This is accomplished by the addition of a grid between the patient and the film.

A grid is a series of thin, linear strips of alternating radiodense and radiolucent materials that are encased in a rectangular wafer (Fig. 2–14). Generally, the radiodense strips are made of lead, and the radiolucent strips are made of plastic. The placement of the strips, their height, and the number of strips per linear inch of grid width are variables that are adjusted to the specific requirements of the examination being performed.

Placing a grid between the patient and the x-ray film results in removal of a large portion of the x-rays available to produce a radiographic image of a given density. To compensate for this loss, an increased number of x-rays must be made available by increasing milliamperage, exposure time or kilovoltage (see Chap. 4).

PARALLEL GRIDS. Parallel grids are those grids composed of strips that are placed perpendicular to the grid surface (Fig. 2–15). These parallel lead strips absorb oblique, scattered radiation, while the radiolucent strips allow the x-rays traveling perpendicular to the grid surface to pass through and expose the film (Johns and Cunningham, 1974). Grid efficiency is governed by the grid ratio. Grid ratio is defined as the ratio of the height of the strips to the width between the opaque strips (Johns and Cunningham, 1974). For example, a grid with lead strips that are 2.5 mm high and 0.5 mm apart has a 5:1 ratio. Increased efficiency of scatter radiation cleanup occurs with grids of increased ratio. A

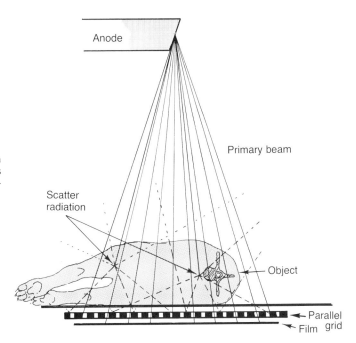

Figure 2–15. Diagram of a cross section of a parallel grid. Note that all lead strips are placed perpendicular to the grid surface.

grid with a 5:1 ratio is therefore less efficient than a 10:1 ratio grid.

Increased grid ratios necessitate increased exposure, since the percentage of radiographic density caused by scattered radiation decreases. Grids with increased ratio also remove a relatively greater number of primary beam x-rays. Therefore, to obtain the same radiographic density, a greater number of primary x-rays is needed for a 10:1 ratio grid compared with a grid with a 5:1 ratio (see Chap. 4).

Parallel grids have a distinct disadvantage in that an x-ray beam emanating from a tube target interacts with the periphery of the grid at an increasing angle, thus reducing the number of primary x-rays reaching the film near the grid edges. This disadvantage increases with increased grid ratio, thus limiting the use of parallel grids of small size and small ratios (5:1 or 6:1).

FOCUSED GRIDS. To compensate for the decreasing peripheral radiographic density produced with parallel grids, the so-called focused grid was designed (Fig. 2–16). This grid is constructed so that the lead strips are placed parallel to the primary x-ray beam and at decreasing angles to the grid surface near the periphery of the grid. This design allows the primary beam to expose the periphery of the film with nearly the same intensity as the central ray.

Placing a series of leads strips in the pri-

mary beam causes the recording of an image of the grid on the radiograph. This image appears as a series of thin white lines. Decreasing the width of these lines results in a less objectionable effect on the radiograph and may be accomplished by increasing the number of lines per linear inch of grid width. A grid of 80 to 100 lines per inch provides radiographic images of the lead strips that are so fine that they do not produce interference with the diagnostic quality of the radiograph. Increasing the number of lines per inch obviously increases the cost of these fine-lined grids. An increased number of lines per inch also increases the ratio of the grid, since the space between the lead strips is decreased. Hence, increased exposure is required. Since increased exposure requirements generally dictate increased exposure time, high ratio, fine-lined grids have a distinct disadvantage in veterinary radiography, because patient movement is sometimes difficult to control. However, with high milliamperage x-ray machines, short exposure times may be maintained, thus eliminating this disadvantage (see Chap. 4).

BUCKY DIAPHRAGM. By moving the grid at right angles to the grid strips during exposure, the white line images of the lead strips may be blurred and thereby made indistinguishable. This is accomplished by a Potter-Bucky diaphragm, sometimes called a Bucky. This mechanism is usually suspended

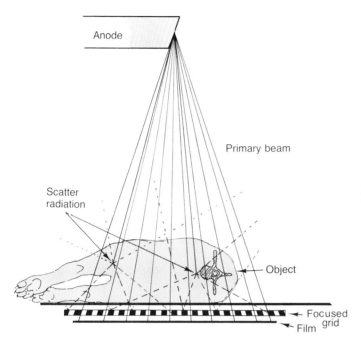

Figure 2–16. Diagram of a cross section of a focused grid. The lead strips are placed at decreasing angles to the grid surface as the distance from the center is increased. This serves to maintain the parallel relationship between the x-ray beam and the grid strips for the entire distance across the grid.

in a cabinet beneath the x-ray tabletop. A tray is placed in this cabinet for holding an x-ray film cassette.

Movement of the grid may be produced by several methods. Older equipment utilizes a spring-loaded slide. After the spring device is compressed, release must be coordinated with exposure so that the grid is in motion during the time of the exposure. Travel time for the grid must therefore be longer than the exposure time. On the other hand, the speed of travel must be sufficient to cause blurring of the lines. Mechanical or, preferably, electrical release that is coordinated with exposure is available with some older x-ray equipment. Reciprocating Bucky mechanisms are driven by a solenoid that works against a spring tension on the opposite end of the slide. This mechanism oscillates continuously without manual loading. Minimum exposure time with the use of this mechanism is 1/20 sec, since faster exposure times tend to produce visualization of grid lines owing to a relatively slow grid travel speed (Selman, 1977). Some modern electric motor driven mechanisms provide constant motion of the grid. This type of device is called a reciprofmatic Bucky. Exposure times as short as 1/60 sec are possible without grid visualization when this mechanism is used (Selman, 1977).

By rendering grid lines indistinguishable,

Bucky mechanisms allow the use of grids with fewer lines per inch, which results in decreased exposure requirements.

There are several causes for the appearance of grid lines on radiographs made with moving grids. If exposures are made before or after grid movement occurs, grid lines will appear. Similarly, grid lines will appear if exposures are made before the grid reaches full speed. In all but the very old equipment, this problem has been eliminated by an electric contactor that prevents exposure until the grid is moving at full speed. Uneven or irregular movement of the grid may produce grid lines. Grid lines may also be visualized if the x-ray tube is not centered above the grid (particularly with a high ratio grid). Grid lines may appear if there is inadvertent synchronization of the peak x-ray output pulses and grid travel speed—i.e., a lead grid strip is present over the same point on the x-ray film during each maximum x-ray output (maximum x-ray output occurs in pulses of 120 times per second in full-wave rectified generators).

A disadvantage to the use of Bucky diaphragms in veterinary radiography is the noise produced by certain mechanisms. Motor-driven mechanisms (particularly reciprocating or reciprofmatic devices) are quieter and tend not to frighten the nonsedated patient.

Figure 2–17. Diagram of a cross section of x-ray film.

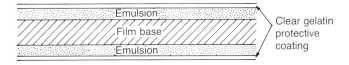

Emulsion

Film base

Emulsion

Clear gelatin protective coating

X-RAY FILM

X-ray film is formed by a layering a silver halide–containing emulsion on each side of a supporting polyester sheet (Fig. 2–17). When exposed to radiant energy, silver halide (mostly silver bromide) crystals become more susceptible to chemical change. These chemically susceptible crystals form the so-called latent image. Reduction of the sensitized silver halide crystals to metallic silver is accomplished by a developer solution in a darkroom. Removal of the unreduced silver halide crystals is accomplished by a separate fixer solution. The remaining metallic silver appears as black particles, which compose the negative image of a finished radiograph.

The sensitivity of x-ray film allows latent image formation when the film is exposed to all forms of radiant energy, including x-rays, gamma rays, particulate radiations (alpha and beta particles), heat and light. Latent image formation can also occur in the presence of excessive pressure. Handling and storage of film to avoid exposure of these elements obviously becomes important in the production of diagnostic radiographs.

X-ray film used in medical radiography is available in various sensitivity ranges, depending upon the requirements of the examination. X-ray film that can be used with intensifying screens is designed to be most sensitive to light emitted by the screen. Most film is designed to have maximum sensitivity to the light spectrum emitted by calcium tungstate crystals, which are used in most intensifying screens. These films are usually called blue-sensitive film, since the light emitted by calcium tungstate crystals is in the ultraviolet and blue-violet range of visual light. Blue-sensitive film may also be used with the new rare earth phosphor screens that emit ultraviolet or blue visible light such as terbium- and thulium-activated lanthanum oxybromide and with the new non–rare earth phosphor, europium-activated barium fluorochloride.

Special green-sensitive (orthochromatic) films have been developed for use with green-emitting rare earth (terbium-activated gadolinium and lanthanum) phosphors. When using these orthochromatic films, the usual amber darkroom safelight filter that is used for blue-sensitive film must be changed to a filter shifted toward the red portion of the visible spectrum. These filters can be used with both blue-sensitive and green-sensitive films.

X-ray film designed to be used without intensifying screens is more sensitive to x-ray energies than to light. This nonscreen film may be used when increased detail is needed, such as in examinations of the peripheral appendicular skeleton.

The sensitivity rating of an x-ray film is determined by the exposure required to produce a radiograph of a given density (degree of blackness). Film that is very sensitive is referred to as being fast or high-speed. High-speed films are therefore those films that require less total exposure to produce a given density than film of average (par) speed.

Increased film speed is generally accomplished by increasing the size of the silver halide crystals. Although larger black particles of reduced silver impart more density per unit of exposure, they also result in a radiograph with a more granular appearance because these particles are within the range of easy visibility. This increased granularity decreases radiographic detail considerably. The use of high-speed film should therefore be reserved for situations in which low milliamperage x-ray equipment is necessary. For most other examinations, par speed film should be used.

Film Latitude. X-ray film that has an inherent long scale of contrast—that is, records images with many shades of gray—has increased latitude. Film with increased latitude allows a greater exposure error while recording an image of diagnostic quality. Conversely, film with a short scale of contrast has decreased latitude and will tolerate less exposure error in the production of diagnostic radiographs. The use of film with increased latitude (usually designated simply as *latitude film*) is recommended for radiographing the distal extremities of horses and other large animals with portable equipment, since, for practical purposes, it is difficult to accurately reproduce the same FFD for each exposure. This is especially true if the patient moves around the room between exposures, thus requiring repositioning of the equipment. Changes in FFD affect the number of x-rays available to produce radiographic density and therefore result in exposure error (see Chapter 4). The use of latitude film makes these errors tolerable. Additionally, latitude film allows visualization of periosteal reactions, periarticular changes and other soft tissue abnormalities on the same radiograph as bony structures. High-contrast film produces a relatively dense soft tissue image when sufficient exposure is obtained to visualize the bony structures; additional radiographs are therefore needed to adequately examine soft tissue structures of a limb.

Automatic Processor Film. X-ray film designed specifically for use in automatic processors has several special characteristics, including heat tolerance and increased hardness, which allow the film to be transported by a roller system. These films are sometimes called rapid processor film. In the current x-ray film market, these films cost about 20 per cent less than conventional manual process film and are therefore recommended for use in manual systems. They may be processed with conventional developer and fixer solution; however, because automatic processor solutions have a chemical composition designed specifically for this rapid processor film, it is recommended for use in manual processing. By using automatic processor film and solutions, rapid, high-temperature manual processing can be performed (see Chapter 3).

INTENSIFYING SCREENS AND CASSETTES

X-ray intensifying screens are sheets of luminescent chemical applied to a supporting base. These screens fluoresce when irradiated and emit foci of light in areas in which x-rays have penetrated a patient. By placing film in direct contact with the surface of these screens, an accurate recording of the resulting image may be made. Approximately 95 per cent of the film's silver halide crystal exposure occurs from the light of fluorescing crystals in the screens. About 5 per cent of the total film exposure is accomplished by direct x-ray

interactions. The use of intensifying screens allows the total exposure to be decreased to a small fraction of that which would be required if screens were not used. Intensifying screens also increase the contrast of the resultant radiograph and thereby improve radiographic detail.

Intensifying screens are mounted in pairs in a cassette (Fig. 2–18). The cassette is a light-tight metal or plastic case designed to support a pair of intensifying screens and x-ray film, and to apply moderate pressure to insure good screen-film contact. The front of the cassette is made of plastic or a low atomic number metal such as magnesium, and the back of the cassette is a hinged metal or plastic lid. A pad of oil-free felt, glass fiber, or isocyanate foam is placed between the lid and the back screen. This pad forms a light seal around the edges and serves as a means of evenly distributing moderate pressure on the screens and film. A second screen is mounted on the inside of the cassette front in such a way that when film is placed in the cassette, a screen is in direct contact with the emulsion on each side of the x-ray film. The lid is equipped with springs or other types of latches that are designed to prevent light leaks and to exert uniform pressure to preserve good screen-film contact. Figure 2–19 diagrammatically illustrates a cross section of a loaded cassette.

Film exposure is accomplished by passing an x-ray beam through the patient, the front of the cassette, the front screen, the film and the back screen. Since x-rays are absorbed by the front screen, this screen is thinner than the back screen. The x-rays interact with screen crystals (usually calcium tungstate), which fluoresce ultraviolet and visible blue-violet light, which then exposes the silver halide crystals of the x-ray film, thus forming the latent image. The use of par (average) speed screens allows the production of radiographs with as much as 25 times less exposure than those made without intensifying screens.

Cardboard cassettes for holding nonscreen x-ray film are designed to provide a light-tight envelope and support. A sheet of lead on the back side increases radiographic detail by preventing back-scatter x-rays from exposing the film. Medical nonscreen film is available in ready-to-use, light-tight envelopes and does not require the use of cardboard cassettes. These ready-to-use packs are recommended for low volume radiology de-

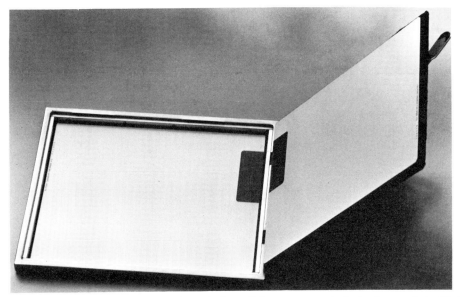

Figure 2–18. Film cassette with lid open to show the intensifying screens on both the front and the lid. The lead blockers are seen on the screens. These prevent film exposure in the regions covered both by physically blocking x-ray exposure and through the lack of fluorescing crystals in the underlying areas. This unexposed area may then be used to imprint identification material with a light flasher.

partments. Nonscreen film is extremely pressure sensitive and should be protected with a cardboard sheet if used without cardboard cassettes. This protection is essential when radiographing the peripheral limbs of dogs and cats, where toenail pressure may cause artifacts.

Intensifying screens are available in various speeds and are designed for specific purposes. The primary factor affecting speed and radiographic detail of conventional screens is the thickness of the chemical layer of luminescent calcium tungstate (Johns and Cunningham, 1974). X-radiation interacts with the luminescent crystals both on the surface and within the depth of the screen. Fluorescence from the underlying crystals is reflected and refracted toward the surface, thereby causing a diffusion of light from the point of x-ray interaction, which results in the recording of an unsharp image with consequent loss of radiographic detail. With increasing screen thickness, less exposure is required to produce a given radiographic density, since there will be a greater number of fluorescing crystals for each x-ray interaction. The speed of the intensifying screen is then increased at the expense of radiographic detail. It is evident, therefore, that a compromise is necessary between screen speed and radiographic detail.

Crystal size also is a factor in determining screen speed, just as it is with film speed. However, this factor is of less importance than screen thickness. Within certain limits, the larger the luminescent crystal, the greater will be the fluorescent emission, since x-radiation impinging upon any part of a crystal causes the entire crystal to fluoresce (Johns and Cunningham, 1974). Increased crystal size therefore results in both greater granularity of the finished radiograph and

Figure 2–19. Diagram of a cross section of a loaded cassette, showing the relationship of the film to the intensifying screens.

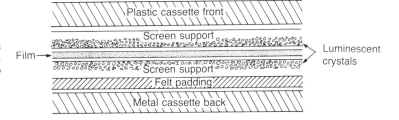

increased speed of the intensifying screen. High-speed screens usually have increased luminescent crystal size with consequent sacrifice of radiographic detail. Conversely, slow or detail screens use smaller crystals and produce greater radiographic detail.

A dye may be added to the luminescent layer in order to absorb refracted and reflected light from the deeper underlying screen crystals, thereby improving radiographic detail. These dyes tend to absorb the deeper, less direct light rays, while those rays emitted from the surface tend to expose the x-ray film. The use of a dye results in a decreased light emission for a given x-ray interaction, and this decreases the speed of the screen. Dyes are therefore generally used for slow-speed detail screens.

By combining in various ways the factors of layer thickness, dyes, and crystal size and type, a correct balance of speed and detail may be produced. Various screen speeds, generally designated as detail, fast detail, par (average) and high, are available commercially. Exposure requirements to produce a given radiographic density usually double between the various speed screens. For example, twice as much exposure is required for the use of par speed screens compared with that needed for high-speed screens.

Recently, the so-called rare earth phosphor screens have been made available for medical radiography. These phosphors are used instead of calcium tungstate to increase the speed of intensifying screens. This technology is a spinoff from the electronics industry, in which rare earth phosphors have been used extensively for color television tubes. Rare earth phosphors emit light when excited by x-rays in a way similar to that seen in calcium tungstate crystals. Terbium-activated gadolinium and lanthanum phosphor emit green light and require the use of orthochromic x-ray film (see p. 30). Terbium- and thulium-activated lanthanum oxybromide and the non–rare earth phosphor europium-activated barium fluorochloride emit ultraviolet and blue-violet visible light and may be used with conventional blue-sensitive film.

Rare earth phosphors offer advantages over calcium tungstate phosphors in that they have an increased x-ray absorption efficiency and have a greater conversion efficiency (x-ray energy to light energy conversion). Because more x-rays are absorbed by rare earth phosphors, the light emitted is in-

creased without significant loss of image quality. X-ray absorption of a phosphor depends upon the predominant heavy element present in the screen. Lanthanum, for example, has greater absorption capability than does calcium tungstate for x-ray energies in the middle of the diagnostic kv range; gadolinium is better at a higher kv range. Conversion of x-ray energy to light has an efficiency of approximately 5 per cent for calcium tungstate and almost 20 per cent for rare earth phosphors (Buchanan et al., 1972).

When compared with a combination of par speed, calcium tungstate screens and par speed film, various rare earth phosphor screens and film combinations can yield speeds as much as 12 times as fast. This can only be accomplished, however, with a sacrifice of sharpness and an increase in mottle (see p. 25).

For routine veterinary radiography of large patients, film-screen combinations that result in speeds 4 times ($4\times$ systems) those of par-speed screens and par-speed film are recommended. The increased information on the finished radiograph is a direct result of decreasing the motion unsharpness by allowing exposures to be made in one fourth the time. The resultant radiographic mottle does not cause objectionable distraction (Skucas and Gorski, 1980). An additional benefit of using rare earth screens is that with decreasing exposure requirements there is a marked increase in radiation safety. Scatter radiation levels recorded during abdominal radiography of a dog were shown to decrease by as much as 70 per cent when rare earth phosphor screens were used as compared with results from par-speed calcium tungstate screens (Koblik et al., 1980).

Radiographic examinations of the large animal thorax, skull, cervical region and the thicker portions of the extremities can be produced using the $4\times$ system and, at times, the $8\times$ system to good advantage, especially when low-milliamperage equipment is used. With the relatively high exposure required for adequate radiographic density, mottle does not appear to be as prominent as when examinations of small animals are made using these high-speed systems. These high-speed systems can also be very useful when one is examining the abdomens of foals and calves.

In the current market, the cost of rare earth phosphor screens is approximately 2.4 times that of regular calcium tungstate screens. Despite this cost differential, these new products can significantly improve radiographic quality in most radiology departments.

An excellent review of this subject as it applies to medical radiology has recently been published (Skucas and Gorski, 1980).

FLUOROSCOPIC METHODS OF RECORDING MOTION STUDIES

Fluoroscopy. A fluorescent screen may be used instead of film to record an x-ray image. Recording an image on a fluorescent screen has the obvious advantages of instant display and the ability to record dynamic events. Many special radiographic procedures require the use of such equipment.

A conventional fluoroscope screen consists of a fluorescent material mounted on a plastic sheet approximately 3 mm thick, which is covered (on the operator side) by a layer of glass containing lead salts of sufficient quantity to stop x-rays, thereby preventing exposure of the operator to the primary x-ray beam. The fluoroscope screen is placed immediately adjacent to the patient while the x-ray beam is directed through the patient onto the screen. The resultant image is thereby displayed on the screen (Fig. 2–20). Spot film devices may be used to insert an x-ray cassette into the beam, allowing the production of a permanent record when desired for certain phases of a dynamic study.

Fluoroscope screens are essentially the same as intensifying screens. The fluorescent crystals generally used are of zinc cadmium

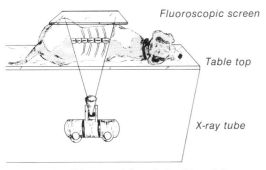

Fluoroscopic screen

Table top

X-ray tube

Figure 2–20. Diagram of the relationships of the x-ray tube, patient and viewing screen using a conventional fluoroscopic table.

sulfide, since these crystals show maximum sensitivity at about 5300 Angstrom units (one Angstrom unit equals 10^{-8} cm), which is very near the peak sensitivity of the rods of the retina (Johns and Cunningham, 1974). Crystals exposed to the x-ray beam fluoresce with an intensity that is directly proportional to the number of x-rays interacting with the fluorescent screen. It is obvious that increased patient thickness requires increased primary exposure to the patient and secondary exposure to the operator. Patient exposure rates of 3 to 300 milliroentgens per minute (mr/min) are needed to produce screen images in the visible range in a darkened room with properly adapted eyes (Chamberlain, 1942). This exposure level produces an image approximately 1/30,000 of the brightness of this page being read under normal conditions (Johns and Cunningham, 1974).

It is obvious that special conditions must be met to allow adequate visualization of the fluoroscopic image. The decreased illumination of the fluoroscopic image requires maximum use of rod vision, which necessitates adapting the eye to dark prior to viewing. Most frequently, dark adaptation is accomplished by wearing red goggles for approximately 15 minutes prior to fluoroscopic viewing. The room must also remain dark during the examination, which produces further disadvantages for the conventional fluoroscopic equipment. Attempts to increase the image brightness to a level of intensity that would allow the use of cone vision have been made, but the amount of patient exposure became prohibitive.

Image Amplifiers. To eliminate the many inherent disadvantages of the conventional low output fluoroscope screen, an electronic device for image amplification was developed. These devices, called image amplifiers, consist of a fluorescent screen that is bonded to a light-sensitive photocathode and incorporated into a suitable vacuum envelope (Fig. 2–21). The light patterns produced by the fluorescent screen are converted into low energy photoelectrons, which are then accelerated toward a fluorescent anode or output viewing screen smaller in diameter than the original input screen. Focusing electrodes are used to maintain image sharpness, thus preserving detail. Increased image brightness is accomplished by decreasing (concentrating)

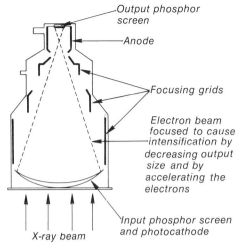

Figure 2–21. Diagram of an image amplifier, which is used to replace the conventional fluoroscopic screen.

the size of the image at the smaller output screen and by accelerating the photoelectrons, which causes them to interact with the output phosphor at markedly increased velocities. In addition, the photoemissive cathode that is applied to the input screen is more sensitive than the human eye to the light radiated from the x-ray–sensitive fluorescent screen.

Image amplification by this method may be viewed directly or after a mirror and lens apparatus angulates the image toward the operator; or the image may be viewed indirectly through a closed circuit television system, consisting of a camera and a monitor. Permanent records of the motion studies may be produced on videotape, or by using a 16 mm or 35 mm cine film, as well as small spot films. Various combinations of these capabilities may be obtained to meet the requirements of the particular radiology department (see Chap. 6).

REFERENCES

Bartels, J. E., and Hoerlein, B. F.: Radiographic examination. *In* Hoerlein, B. F., Canine Neurology: Diagnosis and Treatment. 2nd ed. Philadelphia, W. B. Saunders Co., 1971.

Buchanan, R. A., Finkelstein, S. I., and Wickersheim, K. A.: X-ray exposure reduction using rare-earth oxysulfide intensifying screens. Radiology, *105*:185–190, 1972.

Cahoon, J. B.: Formulating X-Ray Techniques. 7th ed. Durham, N.C., Duke University Press, 1970.

Chamberlain, W. E.: Fluoroscopes and fluoroscopy. Radiology, *38*:382, 1942.

Christensen, E. E., Curry, T. S., III, Dowdey, J. E.: An Introduction to the Physics of Diagnostic Radiology. 2nd ed. Philadelphia, Lea and Febiger, 1978.

Eastman Kodak Company: The Fundamentals of Radiography. 11th ed. Rochester, N.Y., 1980.

Gillette, E. L., Thrall, D. E., and Lebel, J. L.: Carlson's Veterinary Radiology. 3rd ed. Philadelphia, Lea and Febiger, 1977.

Glasser, E., Quimby, E. H., Taylor, L. S., Weatherwax, J. L., and Morgan, R. H.: Physical Foundations of Radiology, 3rd ed. New York, P. B. Hoeber, Inc., 1961.

Hagar, R. A.: Machlett Dynascope X-Ray Image Intensifier Tubes. Part II. Qualitative Theory and Construction. Cathode Press, Springdale, Conn., The Machlett Laboratories, Inc., Vol. 22, No. 3, 1965.

Johns, H. E.: Radiation therapy: depth dose. *In* Glasser, O. (Ed.), Medical Physics, Vol. II. Chicago, Ill., The Year Book Publishers, Inc., 1950.

Johns, H. E., and Cunningham, J. R.: The Physics of Radiology. 3rd ed. Springfield, Ill., Charles C Thomas, Publisher, 1974.

Koblik, P. D., Hornof, W. J., and O'Brien, T. R.: Rare earth intensifying screens for veterinary radiography: an evaluation of two systems. Vet. Radiol., *21*(5):224–232, 1980.

Rossmann, K.: Modulation transfer function of radiographic systems using fluorescent screens. J. Optical Soc. Amer., *52*:774, 1962.

Selman, J.: The Fundamentals of X-Ray and Radium Physics. 5th ed. Springfield, Ill., Charles C Thomas, Publisher, 1977.

Skucas, J., and Gorski, J.: Application of modern intensifying screens in diagnostic radiology. Med. Radiogr. Photogr., *56*(2): 25–36, 1980.

Ticer, J. W.: Production of diagnostic radiographs in veterinary medicine. II. Recording factors. Calif. Vet., *23*:30–32, 1969.

3

Darkroom Theory and Technique

FILM PROCESSING TECHNIQUE

Film processing is an extremely important part of quality radiography. Many correctly positioned and exposed radiographic examinations are spoiled by improper processing methods. Proper processing can only be accomplished routinely in an environment that is conducive to careful film and cassette handling. Knowledge of processing technique alone will not insure against poor results if adequate facilities and equipment are not provided.

DARKROOM AND DARKROOM EQUIPMENT

Darkroom facilities need not be large or elaborate for the average veterinary practice (see Chap. 7) but must be efficiently designed to allow a "dry bench" area for loading and unloading cassettes, an area for proper film storage, and an area for wet tanks or automatic processor. Additional features such as a cassette transfer box between the x-ray room and the darkroom, and a film dryer are desirable but not absolutely necessary (Ticer, 1969). A list of darkroom equipment appears in Table 3–1.

The processing tanks should be placed at a remote position from the dry bench. This separation prevents solutions from being splashed on dry films or intensifying screens. An added precaution against accidental contamination of film and screens by solutions or water is the placement of a towel rack and towel next to the dry bench so that hands may be dried after placing a film in the tanks.

It is desirable to provide a hard-surfaced wall behind the dry bench, rising approximately 20 inches above the bench surface. The hard surface will prevent the wall from being damaged by opened cassette lids.

Multiple electrical outlets should be placed above the hard-surfaced wall in order to provide easily accessible electrical power for the operation of dry bench equipment, such as the flash printer, safelights, view box and timer. By keeping the electric cord lengths short, the bench top may remain clutter-free.

Processor Tanks

The processor tanks should be large enough to accept a 14 × 17 inch film hanger. Developer solution capacity is determined by the caseload in the radiology department, which affects the rate of solution depletion. Generally, the five gallon insert tank is adequate for the average clinic practice (Eastman Kodak Co., 1980). Increased tank size should be obtained for higher caseload practices. The fixer tank should be larger than the developer tank, since the fixer solution tends to deplete at a faster rate than the developer solution because of volatilization of active ingredients.

Covers should be provided for both the developer and fixer tanks. This will decrease the rate of volatilization and evaporation of the solutions. The wash tank need not be covered.

35

Table 3–1. DARKROOM EQUIPMENT

Tanks for developer, fixer and wash
    water*
Film storage bin
Film dryer*
Cassette transfer box
Safelight illuminators
Film hangers*
Timer*
Flash labeler
Labeling cards
Radiographic view box*
Corner cutter*
Thermometer*
Solution stirring paddles*
Exhaust fan

*This equipment is unnecessary with automatic processing.

Stainless steel tanks provide corrosion-free, low maintenance service. In addition, the heat conduction efficiency of these tanks allows more rapid heating and cooling of the solutions by the surrounding wash water (Eastman Kodak Co., 1980).

Stainless steel or rubberized stirring rods are necessary to mix the developer and fixer solutions. A floating thermometer should be provided in the developer tank to monitor solution temperature.

A mixer valve on the hot and cold water lines supplying the wash tank compartment will aid in the maintenance of a standard temperature for the entire tank, including the developer and fixer tanks. A modern shower-bath mixer control may be installed with relatively little expense and allows easy control of the temperature of the water in the wash tank and solution insert tanks (Ticer, 1969). A practical method dealing with excessively warm cold-water temperatures is to use automatic processing film and solutions. The chemistry of this system tolerates the warm temperatures used in automatic processors and allows rapid manual processing (40 seconds developing time at 80° F [27° C]). (See p. 48.) Flow rate for the wash tank water should be sufficient to allow a complete change of water at least 10 times per hour. This rate allows a complete washing of films in approximately 20 minutes.

Periodic cleaning of tank surfaces must be a routine procedure in darkroom maintenance. If spilled solutions are not wiped up at once, they evaporate, leaving a chemical dust that may contaminate and damage film and screens.

Automatic Processors

The interior of the darkroom should contain the input tray for the large automatic processor. The processor may be installed in the wall in such a manner that the output film bin is outside the darkroom.

Small, low capacity processors may be installed on a bench top. Bench top installation allows both the input and output trays of the unit to be inside the darkroom. The room must therefore be large enough to allow easy operation and servicing of the unit. It may be necessary to build a special bench for the processor in order to avoid crowding the dry bench area.

Film Storage

X-ray film is a delicate, sensitive product and must be handled and stored properly to insure maximum usefulness. The product must be protected from light, electromagnetic radiation (x-rays and gamma rays), various gases, heat, moisture and pressure (Eastman Kodak Co., 1980). The film storage area must be designed to minimize the exposure of stored x-ray film to these elements.

Purchasing x-ray film in small amounts decreases the possibility of prolonged exposure to most of the damaging elements (even when the storage method consists of closing the top of the box in which the film was purchased). Additional protection may be provided by storing opened film boxes in a darkened cabinet. This cabinet should be located at a maximum distance from the x-ray machine in order to avoid exposure to scattered radiation.

Ideally, unexposed film should be stored in a room with a temperature between 50 and 70° F (10 and 21° C), and opened film boxes kept at a relative humidity of 30 to 50 per cent (Eastman Kodak Co., 1980). Film should never be stored in a drug room or next to sources of formalin, hydrogen sulfide, hydrogen peroxide, or ammonia vapors (Eastman Kodak Co., 1980). Films should be placed on end, since stacking tends to produce pressure artifacts after exposure and development. The oldest film should always be used first.

Film storage bins that can be installed under the dry bench for easy access are available commercially (see Chap. 7). The increased accessibility of film for cassette loading makes these bins a highly desirable accessory to the darkroom equipment; they should always be considered when new darkrooms are being built or when an old darkroom is being remodeled.

Cassette Transfer Box

For increased efficiency of cassette handling, a cassette transfer box may be installed between the darkroom and the x-ray room (Ticer, 1969). This container is installed in the wall and is accessible from either side. An interlock mechanism prevents inadvertent opening of the box on the light side (x-ray room) while the darkroom is in use. This box provides a convenient and readily accessible storage area for loaded cassettes (Fig. 3–1).

Darkroom Illumination

Either direct or indirect lighting is satisfactory for illuminating darkrooms. White light illumination is necessary to visualize mainte-

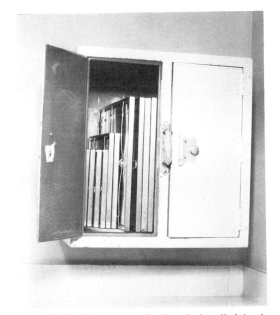

Figure 3–1. Cassette transfer box is installed in the wall between the x-ray room and the darkroom. This box provides a convenient storage place for loaded cassettes that are readily accessible from either room.

nance procedures adequately. Control of these lights should be within the darkroom.

Safelights. Safelight lamps are an indispensable item since they provide light of a quality that will not affect x-ray film during handling and processing. Excessive exposure of film to safelight lamps will, however, result in fog due to activation of silver halide crystals and will cause an overall gray quality (loss of contrast) to the developed radiograph. Careful arrangement of these lamps is therefore an important item to consider when planning a darkroom. Three zones of safelight intensity are desirable: the brightest zone, where the films are washed and put in the dryer; a medium zone, where the films are developed and fixed; and a dim zone over the dry bench, where the cassettes are loaded and unloaded and the film is placed on hangers (Eastman Kodak Co., 1980).

Indirect lighting is suggested for general darkroom illumination (Eastman Kodak Co., 1980). In addition, one or two direct lamps may be located over the processing areas. Proper light color and intensity are essential for high quality radiography. The proper color is provided by filtration on the face of the lamp. Most medical x-ray film has maximum sensitivity to the blue light emitted by the intensifying screen and may be safely handled when this wavelength is filtered from the light source. This is generally accomplished by a Wratten Series 6B filter (Selman, 1977). A red or ruby bulb should never be used as a safelight. The dim illumination emitted from these bulbs is not safe, since the blue light spectrum has not been filtered. Filters should be inspected periodically for cracks that leak unfiltered light.

Green light–sensitive orthochromatic film that is used with some rare earth phosphor screens (see Chapter 2) requires a filter that removes both the blue and green light from the spectrum. The Kodak GS-1 is an example of such a filter. These filters may also be used when processing conventional blue-sensitive film.

The intensity of the safelight illumination should be low but not so dim that lack of illumination interferes with efficient operation. A white frosted 6½ to 10 watt bulb is adequate for most lamp fixtures. These fixtures should be placed 48 inches (122 cm) above the working surface.

Light Leaks. White light leaks around darkroom doors and ventilators and through wall cracks make quality radiography impossible since film exposed to unfiltered light, even of very low intensity, results in a finished radiograph with an overall gray appearance, thus markedly decreasing radiographic contrast. Light seals at the darkroom door margins should fit properly. Closure of the door should not require unnecessary effort, yet the seal should fit tightly enough to eliminate light leaks. Visual examination for light leaks should be made after the eyes are properly adapted to the dark, which requires approximately five minutes in the darkroom. A guillotine-type seal at the bottom of the door is efficient and decreases wear that results from opening and closing the door.

The installation of a cylindrical revolving door should be considered for very busy x-ray departments. Passage through these doors may be accomplished without allowing outside light into the darkroom, thereby increasing efficiency. It is not necessary to delay entry or exit while film is being handled by other personnel.

The darkroom walls should be a color that will reflect the safelight illumination, thus increasing lighting efficiency. Black or dark walls are not necessary or desirable. They only increase the need for light intensity.

Safelight Test. Testing safelight illumination is accomplished by first subjecting film in a cassette to a moderate x-ray exposure. This exposure will increase the sensitivity of the film to fog-producing light (Selman, 1977). Density should be in the gray range, which will allow identification of increased exposure that is produced by light. The proper density can usually be achieved with 1 to 2 mas and 40 to 50 kv exposure.

The test is performed by (1) unloading the film in the darkroom and placing it on the loading bench; (2) covering half of the film with cardboard or black paper and exposing the other half to safelight conditions for slightly longer than is usually required to handle a routinely exposed film; (3) developing the film as usual and examining it for increased density in the light-exposed area. Increased density indicates unsafe conditions. The source of light leak must then be determined.

Radiographic Illumination. A fluorescent radiographic viewing illuminator should be mounted over the washing compartment so that wet films may be examined without contaminating processing solutions. This viewer

is not necessary when automatic processing is used.

Ventilation

Adequate darkroom ventilation provides an environment that is free from volatile chemicals. Proper air circulation also helps control temperature and humidity. A light-tight exhaust fan installed in the ceiling, when accompanied by a light-tight air-intake louver, usually permits sufficient air circulation. Heater exhausts from film dryers and automatic processors should be vented to the exterior of the darkroom. Automatic processor exhausts should not enter the x-ray room since the volatilized chemicals may harm certain electrical equipment.

Hanger Storage and Care

Film hangers should be stored in a readily accessible area above or below the processing bench. They should be segregated by size. Periodic adjustment of film hanger tension will result in bulge-free film placement during processing. Excessive film bulge may allow film-to-film contact and thereby decrease the quality of the developing or fixing process. Proper spring tension is obtained when the distance between the upper clips and the lower clips is approximately ½ inch greater than the length of the film they accommodate (Eastman Kodak Co., 1980). The springs may be bent to provide this distance.

Corner clips should be inspected and cleaned periodically. Gelatin from film emulsion adheres to clip surfaces and provides a medium for solution absorption, thereby increasing the possibility of transporting excessive chemicals from one solution to another. Solution contamination may result in streaks on the corners of a finished radiograph. Excessive gelatin build-up may also result in inefficient gripping of film corners. A solution of trypsin and sodium bicarbonate will dissolve or loosen these contaminants so that they can be brushed away in a water rinse.

A corner cutter should be provided to remove the rough projections on the corners of dried films that have been processed on hangers (Fig. 3–2). These protrusions prevent sliding the films into an envelope with ease. Damage to film surface also occurs when

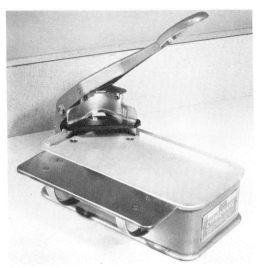

Figure 3–2. Corner cutter used to trim the corners of dried radiographs for the purpose of removing the sharp projections caused by hanger clips.

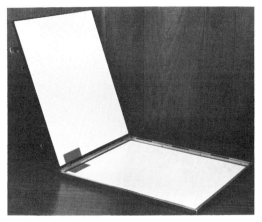

Figure 3–4. An open cassette showing the lead blockers in the upper left-hand corner of the intensifying screens. The lead blockers serve to eliminate both the x-ray and intensifying screen light exposure of the film in the region that they cover. This area is then available to be labeled by a printed card in the light flasher.

these projections are sharp. Corner cutting is not necessary when film is processed automatically.

Film Labeling

Many methods of film labeling are available. Lead numbers and letters placed on the cassette at the time of exposure are reproduced in white on the finished radiograph. This method is relatively inefficient, however, since handling such letters and numbers is time consuming.

Another method of labeling consists of writing the identifying information on a piece of graphite-impregnated tape and placing this on the cassette at the time of exposure. Since various exposures are required for the various radiographic examinations performed, back-up x-ray absorbing materials are necessary to insure a readable density for the resultant label. This requirement decreases the efficiency of this labeling system.

By far, the most satisfactory darkroom labeling method utilizes a light flasher to imprint the desired information on the exposed film (Fig. 3–3). Use of this system requires a small, leaded blocker in the upper left-hand corner of the intensifying screens to prevent exposure of the film in that region to either x-rays or intensifying screen light (Fig. 3–4). Information is imprinted on this unexposed region by placing a card containing the desired information (Fig. 3–5) and the film

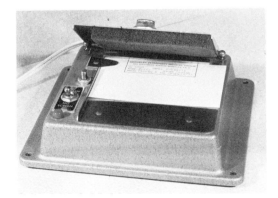

Figure 3–3. Light flasher for labeling radiographs before development.

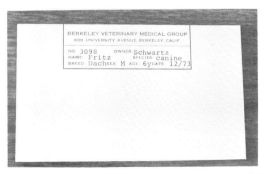

Figure 3–5. A sample label card that is used to imprint identification on an undeveloped radiograph.

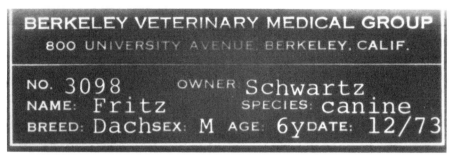

Figure 3–6. The resultant image of the label card imprinted on the edge of a finished radiograph.

in the light flasher, where light is passed through the card and onto the film. The printed material is thereby placed on the film in the form of a latent image and is developed when the radiograph is processed (Fig. 3–6).

The cards used in light-flasher labeling should be of high quality material, since poor quality paper tends to produce a mottled background. These cards, with the desired printed information, may be obtained from any film supplier. The cost of the light flasher is minimal. The lead blockers for the intensifying screens are readily available commercially.

In addition to identification labels, left and right markers and timing indicators for contrast studies should be provided in the form of leaded indicators placed on the cassette at the time of exposure.

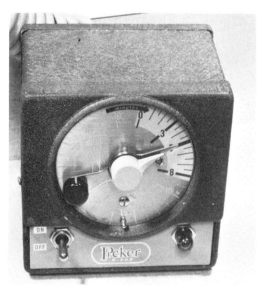

Figure 3–7. A timer is used for accurate timing of the x-ray development process. This model has an automatic re-set feature.

Timers

Since the rate of the chemical reaction involved in developing radiographs is dependent upon temperature, some type of timing apparatus is necessary for accurate, reproducible results. The time of development must be determined by the temperature of the developing solution.

Timers vary in both cost and ease of operation. Although small, wind-up egg timers may be adequate for the radiology department with a light work load (Ticer, 1969), an electrical, pre-set timer is more functional for the busy facility (Fig. 3–7).

HANDLING FILM AND CASSETTES

Film Handling

X-ray film is a delicate product that is sensitive to damage and alteration by many physical factors, including electromagnetic energy (x-rays, gamma rays, light), pressure, heat, moisture and various gases and fumes. Handling and storage methods must, therefore, take these factors into consideration.

When handling a sheet of film, pressure, creasing, buckling and friction must be avoided. Care must be exercised when removing a film from a carton or a cassette in order to avoid rapid film movement across a surface. This action tends to cause static elecrical discharge, which produces a treelike black artifact on the finished radiograph (Fig. 3–8). Excessively low humidity will also predispose film to static discharge artifacts.

Film should be lifted from a box or cassette with the thumb and one finger. Film without interleaving paper should be handled by the corners. Film shipped in containers with paper interleaving wrappers on the individual

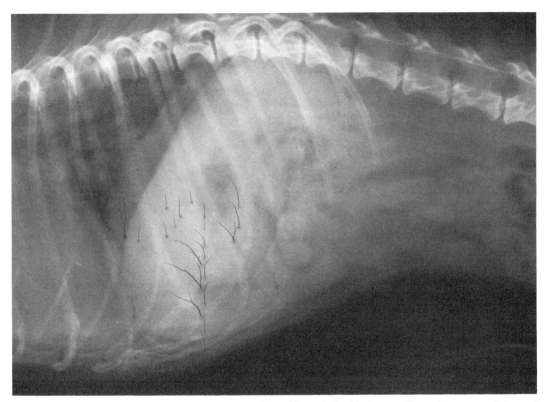

Figure 3–8. Radiograph of an abdomen with superimposition of the black, tree-like artifacts caused by static electrical discharge.

films has much less likelihood of having fingerprints on the film surface. These films should, nevertheless, be handled with care, since bending and folding can cause artifacts on the finished radiographs.

After exposure, the film is removed from the film container (envelope or cassette) and placed on a processing hanger. The hanger is inverted and the film, being held by the thumb and finger at the corner, is attached first to the left clip and then to the right clip. The hanger is inverted and the upper left and right clips are attached in such a manner that the springs on the upper clips provide a taut film that will not bulge during processing.

Care of Screens and Cassettes

Loading and unloading cassettes must be done with extreme care, since physical wear and tear are responsible for shortening the useful life of these rather delicate instruments. To prevent excessive wear on screen surfaces, manufacturers coat the surface areas with a protective layer of thin transpar-

ent material. Since close screen-film contact is necessary for the production of high detail radiographs, this protective layer must be very thin. Care should be taken to avoid contact with abrasive materials. When loading a cassette, the film should be dropped into position and not allowed to slide across the screen surface (Fig. 3–9). This is particularly important when using film with square corners. Rounded corners are obviously preferred.

When removing a film from a cassette, rock the cassette on its hinged end with the lid open. The film will fall free against the fingers and can then be removed. The cassette should not remain open while the film is being developed. Close the lid and reopen when ready to reload.

Always load and unload cassettes on the dry side of the darkroom, away from solutions that may contaminate screen surfaces (Ticer, 1969). The dry bench surface should be wiped clean daily with a moist sponge or cloth.

Since there is a momentary vacuum inside a cassette when it is opened, particles such

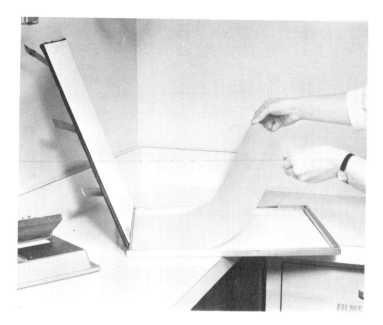

Figure 3–9. Proper cassette loading. The film is held by the edge and dropped into place.

as dust, lint and hair will be drawn into the cassette. Hair or any similar object caught between intensifying screens and film prevents the fluorescent light of the screen from exposing the silver halide crystals of the film. A white artifact of the size and shape of the contaminant will appear on the finished radiograph. White artifacts are also produced by splashes of fixer or developer and by fingerprints on intensifying screens (Fig. 3–10). As a general rule, well-circumscribed white artifacts on a finished radiograph are produced by screen contaminants. Similar artifacts can obviously be produced by defects that remove fluorescent crystals from a screen surface.

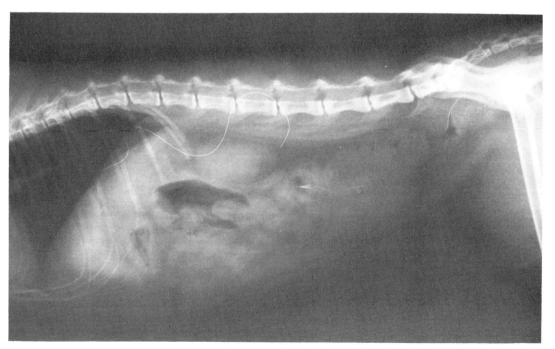

Figure 3–10. An abdominal radiograph showing the imprints of hair and other debris that were present between an intensifying screen and the film.

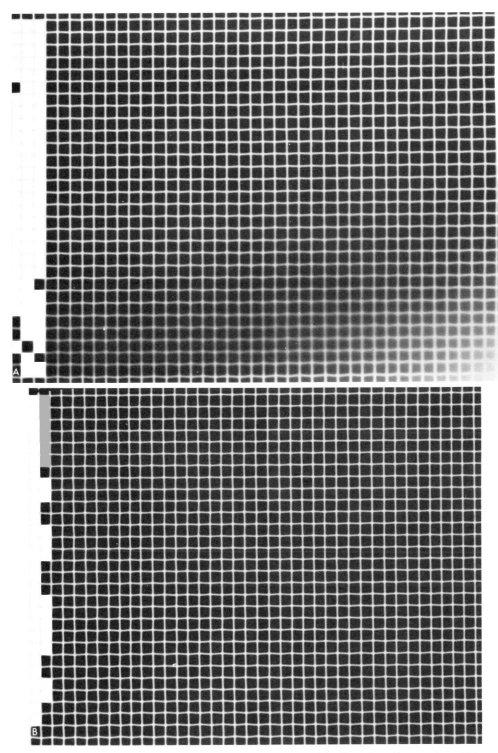

Figure 3–11. *A*, Radiograph of a wire mesh screen showing the loss of detail produced by poor intensifying screen-film contact. *B*, Radiograph of a wire mesh screen showing the increased detail produced by close intensifying screen-film contact.

Other common screen and cassette defects that result in poor quality radiographs are poor film-screen contact, worn lid light seal and loose, broken or bent hinges or latches. Poor screen-film contact results in an excessive divergence of fluorescent light emitted by the screen. This will produce an area of decreased detail, manifested by a fuzzy, poorly defined image. Poor screen-film contact can be caused by a warped cassette front, a sprung or cracked cassette frame, warped screens, a foreign body beneath the surface of a screen, or worn, bent or broken latches.

A simple test of poor screen-film contact may be made by radiographing a wire mesh screen. A copper or brass screen of uniform one-eighth inch mesh is laid over a loaded cassette and exposed at approximately 40 kv and 2 mas, at a 40 inch FFD (see Chap. 4). If the developed radiograph shows areas of fuzzy or blurred outlines, there is poor contact between the screens and the film in that area (Fig. 3–11). A close examination of these areas will show a lack of sharpness or detail of the wire images. It is helpful to stand back a few steps when inspecting the film on an illuminator. The viewing angle should be about 45 degrees.

Trying to determine the cause of the poor screen-film contact without the aid of a qualified representative of the company that produced the cassette is not advisable. When the cause is not obvious, seek help, since these instruments are expensive. Repair of faulty cassettes should be the job of a factory representative.

Routine inspection and cleaning of intensifying screens and cassettes are necessary for the production of diagnostic radiographs and should be done at least once a month—more often in departments with a high caseload or in an area such as an inner city, where soot and other air contaminants are likely to settle on screen surfaces.

Screen cleaning should be done with a commercially available cleaning solution and a soft, lint-free cloth. While drying, opened cassettes should be placed on edge so that the screen surfaces will not become contaminated with dust or lint that may settle on them. Cassettes should not be left open longer than is required for the cleaning solution to dry.

Occasionally, screen (white) artifacts may be detected on finished radiographs between regular cleaning intervals. In this case, it is helpful to be able to find the contaminated cassette so that unloading and cleaning of all cassettes of that particular size may be avoided. A simple method of identification is to record the screen serial number on the outside of the cassette lid. Because this black number, which is located on the edge of most screens, is opaque to fluorescent light, is recorded on each film exposed in the cassette. An alternative method is to write a number (1, 2, 3, etc.) on the edge of the screen with a black ink pen (Magic Marker) and then to record this number on the cassette lid. This number will also be recorded on each film exposed in the cassette.

PRINCIPLES OF PROCESSING

Radiographic Photography

X-ray film consists of a layer of silver halide–containing (mostly bromide) emulsion on each side of a supporting base (see Chap. 2). Each silver halide crystal contains a small impurity of silver sulfide, which serves as a sensitive speck or development center (Selman, 1977). When photons of light or x-rays interact with the silver halide crystals, the valance (outer) electron of the bromide ion (or other halide) is liberated and drifts to the sensitive speck (silver sulfide), to which it imparts a negative charge. The positive silver ion is then attracted to the negatively charged sensitive speck, where it is reduced to a silver atom. This process may be repeated often in a short time interval. The number of susceptible crystals that are affected depends upon the number of photons interacting with a given area of the film.

Crystals in which the sensitive specks have acquired silver atoms during exposure are invisible and constitute the *latent image* (Selman, 1977).

When the latent image is exposed to reducing agents in the developer solution, the process initiated by the photon interaction is continued. The sensitive speck acts as a development center for the entire crystal. Electrons are made available from reducing agents, allowing an increase in the number of reduced silver atoms (metallic silver), which appear as black foci on the finished radiograph. The finished radiograph, therefore, consists of dark areas of metallic silver in a very fine state of subdivision. The amount of metallic silver deposited in a given area is directly proportional to the intensity of the initial x-ray exposure received by that area.

During development, the bromide (and other halide) ions diffuse out of the developed crystals and into the surrounding solution. This process and the gradual exhaustion of the electron supply in the reducing agents result in deterioration of the developer.

The development process is governed by the kinetics of chemistry and therefore proceeds at a greater rate with increasing temperatures. The process is also time-dependent and is subject to increasing intensity with increased time. From these relationships, the so-called time-temperature development process was evolved. This relationship dictates decreased development time when solution temperature is increased and, conversely, increased development time when solution temperature is decreased. Standard manual developing requires from three to five minutes at 68° F (20° C) to obtain optimum film density, depending on the products used. With manual processing, the chemistry of the film and reducing agents in the developer solution provides maximum latitude at 68° F (20° C). Increasing the developing temperature decreases the latitude, which has the practical result of decreasing the magnitude of allowable error in developing time; hence, the films must be removed from the developer with more exact timing. Decreasing developing temperature and increasing developing time have the practical disadvantage of decreasing darkroom efficiency.

Fixer solutions remove the unexposed and unreduced silver salts from the film emulsion. Sodium thiosulfate (hypo) is the chemical used to accomplish this action in powder fixers, whereas ammonium thiosulfate is used in liquid fixers (Eastman Kodak Co., 1980). These chemicals "clear" the film so that the black metallic silver image formed by the reduced silver salts may be visualized. Improperly cleared film contains unexposed silver salt crystals, which darken when reduced by the action of light and tend to obscure the radiographic image. The magnitude of this artifact tends to increase with storage time.

Fixer solutions also contain a hardener (usually salts of aluminum) that is used to prevent excessive swelling and softening of the emulsion during washing, and serves to prevent slippage of the emulsion on the film base. Film hardening also reduces drying time.

Acetic acid or another acidic medium is used for the clearing agent and to neutralize any alkaline developer that may be residual in the film (Selman, 1972). The volatility of acetic acid makes it necessary to provide a cover for the fixer tank to insure long life for the solution.

A finished radiograph is essentially a negative of the structures being examined, since the regions of increased silver reduction are those where increased patient penetration by the x-ray beam occurred—i.e., the soft tissues and air-containing structures. In areas where penetration is decreased (such as under bony structures), there is a decreased degree of silver reduction, and the resultant image is relatively clearer after the fixation process. This image mimics that of a negative in ordinary photography.

Preparation of Solutions

Tank Cleaning. Preparation and maintenance of processing solutions is a very important aspect of high quality diagnostic radiography. Replacement of old solutions should always be preceded by a thorough cleaning of the processing tanks. The cleaning of these tanks may be simplified by using a commercially prepared stainless steel tank cleaner. Generally, a thorough washing with a good detergent followed by rinsing with fresh water is sufficient. Wipe the tank dry with a clean cloth or cellulose sponge. Avoid abrasive cleaning products.

Algae build-up on the walls of the water compartment is a problem in some areas. Filtration of the incoming water supply is an effective method of controlling this problem. Filters with a mean pore opening of not more than 35 micrometers are recommended.

Algae may be removed from the tank walls by several methods. Commercially available algicides may be used. A dilute solution of laundry bleach may also be used effectively. Thorough rinsing with water should precede re-use. In severe problem areas, the water compartment may be allowed to dry over the weekend as an aid to algae control. Ultraviolet irradiation of the drained tank has been ·suggested; however, in most cases, the developer and fixer solution inserts provide a shield for a large number of algae.

Mixing Solutions. Developer and fixer chemicals may be purchased in concentrated liquid form or as a dry powder. Regardless of the type used, the manufacturer's directions should be followed carefully. Mixing and storage containers should be made of corrosion-resistant materials such as enamel, glazed earthenware, polyethylene or polypropylene plastic, glass, hard rubber, or stainless steel with 2 to 3 per cent molybdenum (Eastman Kodak Co., 1980). Never use reactive metals such as tin, copper, zinc, aluminum, or galvanized iron. Tanks or containers that have soldered joints should not be used since chemical reaction between solder and processing solutions may cause chemical fog on film.

Proper dilution of concentrated solutions or dry chemicals depends on knowledge of processing tank capacity. This may be measured by actually filling these tanks with water, using a gallon container, or by calculation, using a constant (231 cubic inches per gallon) to convert cubic inches to gallons:

$$\frac{\text{Width} \times \text{Length} \times \text{Depth (Solution Level)}}{231}$$

$$= \text{Capacity (gal.)}$$

If significant bulge of the tank sides occurs when the tank is filled, it is preferable to actually measure the capacity.

Solution level should be approximately one inch below the height of the tank so that solutions will cover the film hangers.

Preparation of liquid chemicals is a simple matter of diluting the concentrated solution in the processing tanks. It is good practice to partially fill the tank with water, add the concentrated solution and then fill the tank to the desired level. This will prevent inadvertently filling the tank with too much water, leaving insufficient room for the concentrated solution.

Preparation of dry chemicals requires much more attention to detail. Since powdered chemicals are extremely reactive, dust control must be maintained throughout the mixing procedure. In fact, these chemicals are best prepared in a concentrated solution form in a room other than the darkroom. If solutions are prepared from dry chemicals directly in the processing tank, certain precautions must be taken to control chemical dust. Close and store all cassettes, close all windows and

doors and turn off fans. Immediately after mixing the solution, all benches should be wiped with a damp cloth and the floor mopped.

The actual mixing of dry chemicals for processing solutions is accomplished by filling the tank half full with water at approximately 80° F (27° C). Add chemicals slowly while stirring. After the chemicals are in solution, bring the water level to desired height using cold water. Adding cold water will bring the solution toward a desirable processing temperature of about 68° F (20° C). Any scum, lint or dust should be removed prior to processing films. This may be accomplished by drawing an absorbent paper towel across the solution surface.

Replenisher Technique

Developer Solution. The chemical activity of the developer solution diminishes as the reducing agents become exhausted. In addition, a volume loss occurs as the developer solution is physically carried out of the tank on the surface of developed films. Evaporation accounts for minimal losses if the tanks are kept properly covered.

Depletion of the reducing agent concentration and volume loss must be compensated for by a systematic replenisher plan if uniform radiographic quality is to be maintained. Replenisher systems are designed to maintain both the volume and the activity of the developer solution. The most satisfactory method seems to be merely adding a concentrated developer solution to the original solution as volume is needed. A concentrated replenisher solution replaces the depleted developing chemical while adding minimally to the volume. When properly calculated, the replenisher solution concentration may be made to approximate the depleted chemicals and volume simultaneously. These calculations are made on the assumption that approximately 2¾ ounces of solution are carried out of the tank with every 14 × 17 inch film (Eastman Kodak Co., 1980). This means that approximately one gallon of replenisher solution will be used for every fifty 14 × 17 inch films developed. A proportionately smaller amount of solution is carried out on smaller films, and these films deplete the reducing agent at a proportionately decreased rate. Commercially available replenisher solution should be used, thus making it unnecessary to compute the concentration of replenisher needed.

In practice, small amounts of the replenisher solution are added at frequent intervals so that the volume of developer solution is kept nearly constant. The solution should be stirred vigorously after each solution addition.

Replenishment to maintain volume and concentration should not continue indefinitely, since aerial oxidation and the accumulation of gelatin, sludge and mechanical impurities eventually make it necessary to replace the entire developer solution with new materials. This replacement should be done every two to three months with average usage, more often with heavy usage (Eastman Kodak Co., 1980; Selman, 1977).

Fixer Solution. Fixer solution also diminishes in chemical activity with usage, and increased fixing time is then required to adequately fix and harden films. Maintenance of the fixer solution concentration increases the efficiency of the film processing operation. A simplified method of maintaining fixer concentration is to remove a small amount of old fixer solution and add a like amount of fresh, normally concentrated fixer solution. Removal of some old solution is necessary, since water is carried into the fixer tank on each film processed. The volume of fixer solution to be discarded can be calculated based on the number of films processed, but the variables of acetic acid volatilization and water evaporation make this calculation unnecessarily complex. In practice, discarding old solution and adding fresh solution in a volume equal to the developer volume being replenished maintains adequate fixation and hardening activity.

Manual Method of Time-Temperature Processing

X-ray processing solutions interact with film at rates governed by the kinetics of chemistry. Thus, increased processing temperature results in faster reaction rates which, in turn, reach the same end point in a shorter period of time. The end point of the developing process is consistent, reproducible radiographic density and contrast. It follows that for a given radiographic density, increased developer temperature requires re-

moval of the film from the developer solution after a shorter period of time than would be necessary with solutions of lower temperatures. This concept has resulted in the so-called "time-temperature" method of processing x-ray films.

Processing solution temperatures below 60° F (16° C) result in inadequate development and fixation owing to the sluggish activity of the chemical reactions. Temperatures above 75° F (24° C) may soften film emulsion and may cause excessive chemical fog when conventional hand processing film is used. In areas where cold water temperature exceeds 75° F (24° C), automatic processing film and chemicals should be used. A temperature of 68° F (20° C) produces optimum radiographic quality while providing a maximum latitude of error. That is, noticeable differences in radiographic quality will not exist if moderate over- or under-developing time has occurred inadvertently. By keeping processing temperature constant, standardized processing time may be maintained for the developing and fixing reactions.

When it is necessary to process film at temperatures other than 68° F (20° C), adjustment in the processing time must be made. Higher temperatures require shorter processing times and lower temperatures require longer processing times. Variations from the optimal 68° F (20° C), five-minute development time are given in Table 3–2. Standardization of three-minute development time may be desired to decrease darkroom time; however, the five-minute procedure is preferable since maximum radiographic contrast is obtained (Selman, 1977).

To increase darkroom efficiency and decrease the cost of film (see Chapter 2), the use of automatic processor film and solutions is recommended. This rapid film may be processed in the same way as hand processed film with conventional solutions, using 68° F

Table 3–2. TIME-TEMPERATURE GUIDE FOR DEVELOPING X-RAY FILMS

Solution Temperature (°F)	Development Time (minutes)
75 (24° C)	3¼
70 (21° C)	4½
68 (20° C)	5
65 (18° C)	6
60 (16° C)	8½

(20° C) for five minutes; however, since the emulsion on these films is heat tolerant, rapid processing at high temperatures in hand tanks may be used. The solution temperatures should be at 80° F (27° C) and the film developed for 40 seconds, rinsed briefly and fixed for 80 seconds. Washing requires an additional three to five minutes. The time-temperature relationship for developing requires the addition of 15 seconds for each degree Fahrenheit of temperature below, and the subtraction of 15 seconds for each degree Fahrenheit of temperature above, 80° F (27° C). This relationship holds for about two degrees on either side of 80° F (27° C). Prompt removal of the film from the developer solution when the required development time has elapsed is absolutely essential. Latitude of error is nonexistent with this method.

Standard Developing Procedure. Solutions should be thoroughly stirred before processing film. This should be done if an interval of three to four hours has elapsed since the last film was processed. Preferably, different stirring paddles or plungers should be used for the developer and fixer. If these are not available, the stirrer should be thoroughly rinsed prior to stirring a different solution, in order to minimize cross contamination.

The solution temperature must be noted and the time pre-set. The film or films are placed on hangers and then immersed in the developer solution. Agitate the hangers vertically several times to remove all air bubbles that may be in contact with the film surfaces.

Air bubbles cause underdevelopment of the film, since contact with solution is not obtained. These artifacts appear as small, round, clear spots on the finished radiograph because the unreduced silver salts in these regions are dissolved and washed away during the fixation process (Eastman Kodak Co., 1980).

Film hangers should be separated by approximately 1 inch in the processing tanks. Care should be taken to prevent the film from touching the tank wall since such contact will also cause localized underdevelopment. These underdeveloped areas, wherein only one side of the emulsion is developed, are produced by film contact with the sides of the tank or with other film and are called "kiss marks."

The timer must be set for the predetermined amount of time dictated by solution temperature. At the end of development time, remove the hangers and allow drainage back into the tank for a maximum of 2 seconds. The final drippings contain badly oxidized developer and tend only to weaken and contaminate the remaining solution. Excessive drainage may also result in streaks or chemical fog.

Rinse the films by immersing in clean, fresh water, with vigorous agitation for 15 to 45 seconds (Eastman Kodak Co., 1980). Minimal rinsing time is required if the temperature is at 68° F (20° C) and the films are agitated vigorously. With rapid, 80° F (27° C) hand processing, rinsing should require no more than 10 seconds. Without thorough rinsing, fixation may occur unevenly and cause streaking of the finished radiograph (Selman, 1977). Be sure the tops of the hangers are rinsed well to avoid contamination of the fixer solution by the alkaline developer. Lift the hangers from the rinse water and allow to drain completely before placing films in the fixer solution. This will prevent dilution of the fixer solution.

Films should be placed in the fixer solution and agitated in the same manner used in the developing procedure. Agitation insures that fresh, nonstagnated solution will come in contact with the film surface. Fixing time should generally be twice the clearing time. During clearing, the milky appearance of the film disappears as the unreduced silver salts are dissolved. After clearing, time must be allowed for these salts to diffuse from the film. Hardening of the film also occurs during this time. Adequate emulsion hardening decreases drying time and insures preservation of the finished radiograph. Generally, this total time is five minutes. Approximately twice this time is required to properly fix and harden nonscreen films because of the increased emulsion thickness (Eastman Kodak Co., 1980).

Films should never be viewed with white light until fixation has occurred for at least one minute. Films should not be allowed to dry during preliminary viewing and should be agitated well upon return to the fixer solution for the completion of fixation.

Removal of film from the fixer solution should be done more rapidly than from the developer solution in order to decrease contamination of the fixer solution in the tank with the used solution that is in close

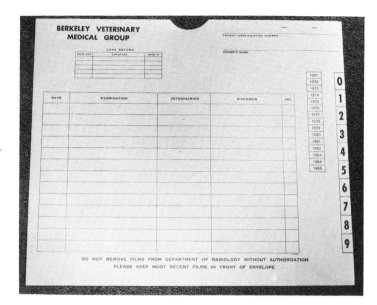

Figure 3–12. A re-usable radiographic storage envelope.

contact with the film surface and to prevent volume build-up. These films may then be immediately immersed in the wash water.

Washing films requires approximately 20 minutes in fresh, running water. There should be a flow rate that results in a complete change of water at least 10 times per hour. Hanger tops should be below the surface of the water to insure removal of all solutions, thus preventing contamination of the developer solution when the hangers are used again. Nonscreen films require approximately 40 minutes to wash adequately (Eastman Kodak Co., 1980; Selman, 1977). Exact timing is not necessary; however, care should be taken to avoid lengthy washing, since prolonged exposure to water tends to cause excessive emulsion swelling and increases the drying time required.

Drying of washed radiographs may be accomplished by suspending the hangers at room temperature. This method is to be discouraged in all but departments with very low caseloads, since the hangers are not available for re-use until drying is complete, and a shortage of hangers usually results. Film dryers using temperatures below 120° F (49° C) enhance the drying process markedly and make the operation of the radiology department more efficient. After drying is completed, films should be removed promptly, since prolonged exposure to high temperatures may result in brittle, cracked finished radiographs.

After removal of the radiographs from the hangers, sharp corners should be removed so that handling and storage may be accomplished with minimum danger of scratching the finished surface. Sorting and filing of the radiographs in properly labeled storage envelopes should be performed immediately to avoid misplacement of valuable diagnostic information. Figure 3–12 shows an adequate storage envelope, which provides easy identification of the radiograph and a summary of important facts that may be needed in radiographic interpretation. A summary of manual processing technique is given in Table 3–3.

A summary of common darkroom causes of unsatisfactory radiographs is given in Table 3–4.

Automatic Processing

Automatic x-ray film processing has minimized the traditional bottleneck created by the time and effort that is required for manual processing in many radiology departments. The savings in labor and time required to produce a finished radiograph and the consistent radiographic quality produced by an automatic processor make it a highly desirable instrument for all but the small radiology department.

Basically, an automatic processor mechanically transports a film through the developer,

Table 3–3. SUMMARY OF MANUAL PROCESSING TECHNIQUE

Stir solutions.
  Use separate paddles for developer and fixer solutions.

Check developer temperature.
  Adjust to 68° F (20° C) if possible

Load film on hanger.

Set timer.
  Time is determined by time-temperature relationship (see Table 3–2).

Immerse film in developer.
  Agitate vertically several times.

Rinse hands, dry and reload cassettes.

Remove film from developer after proper time interval.
  Do not allow drainage back into developer solution for more than 2 seconds.

Rinse 15 seconds.
  Agitate film vertically. Drain well.

Immerse in fixer solution.
  Agitate vertically several times. Leave in fixer for 5 minutes (10 minutes for nonscreen film).

Remove film from fixer.
  Do not allow drainage back into fixer solution.

Immerse in running wash water for 20 minutes (40 minutes for nonscreen film).

Remove from wash water and drain.

Dry on racks or in warm air dryer.
  Keep films separated.

Remove from hanger and trim corners to remove sharp clip marks.

Store in well-identified envelopes.

fixer, wash and dryer at a uniform rate, which results in a finished (dry) radiograph within as little as 90 seconds (Fig. 3–13). Specially formulated chemicals and film are necessary to accomplish this high-speed, high-temperature process.

Solution replenisher rates are governed by the length of the films being processed. Generally, these devices are adjusted to correspond to the short side of the film; hence, films should be placed in the processor sideways to avoid overreplenishment.

Automatic processors are complex mechanical devices and should be maintained by professional service personnel where such service is available. Only in rare instances should veterinarians depend on their staff to perform this function.

A summary of common causes of unsatisfactory processing technique with automatic processing is given in Table 3–5.

Silver Recovery

Metallic silver may be recovered from used fixer solution and from old radiographs that are purged from files. Fixer solution may be sold to commercial solution service companies for silver recovery; however, these services usually offer less money for the raw solution than for recovered metallic silver. Methods of silver recovery from fixer solutions include a metallic replacement process, electrolytic recovery and chemical precipitation. Metallic replacement techniques use other metals, usually iron, to replace the

Text continued on page 53

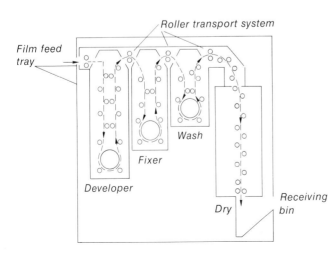

Roller transport system

Film feed tray

Wash

Fixer

Developer

Dry

Receiving bin

Figure 3–13. Diagram of the essential features of an automatic x-ray film processor. The roller assembly is designed to transport the film through the developer, fixer and wash tanks, and finally to the dryer at a fixed rate, to ensure constant, predictable radiographic quality.

Table 3–4. COMMON DARKROOM CAUSES OF UNSATISFACTORY RADIOGRAPHS

Low Density
I. UNDERDEVELOPMENT
  A. Improper development
    1. Time too short
    2. Temperature too low
    3. Combination of both
    4. Inaccurate thermometer
  B. Exhausted developer
    1. Chemical activity depleted
    2. Activity destroyed by contamination
  C. Diluted developer
    1. Water added to raise level instead of adding fresh developer
    2. Melted ice from cooling attempt
    3. Water overflow from wash tank
    4. Insufficient chemicals mixed originally (tank actually larger than judged)
    5. Improper developer additions
  D. Incorrectly mixed developer
    1. Exact capacity of tank unknown
    2. Mixing ingredients in wrong sequence
    3. Omission of ingredients
    4. Unbalanced formula composition

High Density
I. IMPROPER DEVELOPMENT
  A. Time too long
  B. Temperature too high
  C. Combination of both
  D. Inaccurate thermometer
  E. Insufficient dilution of concentrated developer
  F. Omission of bromide when mixing

Fog
I. UNSAFE LIGHT
  A. Light leaks into the processing room
    1. Leaks through doors, windows, etc.
    2. Poorly designed labyrinth entrance
      a. Bright light at outer entrance
      b. Reflection from white uniforms of persons passing through
    3. Sparking of motors
      a. Ventilating fans
      b. Dryer fans
    4. Light leaks from cassette transfer box
  B. Safelights
    1. Bulb too bright
    2. Improper filter
      a. Not dense enough
      b. Cracked
      c. Bleached
      d. Shrunken
  C. Turning on light before fixation is complete
  D. Luminous clock and watch faces
  E. Lighting matches in darkroom

II. RADIATION
  A. Insufficient protection
    1. During delivery or transportation
    2. Film storage bin
    3. Loaded cassette racks
    4. Not enough protection for loading darkroom
  B. Improper storage
    1. Radium or other isotopes nearby with improper shielding
    2. X-ray machine

III. CHEMICAL
  A. Prolonged development
  B. Developer contaminated
    1. Foreign matter of any kind (metals, etc.)

IV. DETERIORATION OF FILM
  A. Age (use oldest film first)
  B. Storage conditions
    1. Too high temperatures
      a. Hot room
      b. Cool room but near radiator or hot pipe
    2. Too high humidity
      a. Damp room
      b. Moist air
    3. Ammonia or other fumes present in darkroom or other working areas
  C. Delivery conditions
    1. Moisture precipitation when cold box of film is opened in hot, humid room
    2. Fresh boxes should be stored overnight at room temperature before opening

Table 3–4 continued on the following page

Table 3–4. COMMON DARKROOM CAUSES OF UNSATISFACTORY RADIOGRAPHS (*Continued*)

V. EXCESSIVE PRESSURE ON EMULSIONS OF UN-PROCESSED FILM
    A. During storage
    B. During manipulation in darkroom

VI. LOADED CASSETTES STORED NEAR HEAT, SUNLIGHT OR RADIATION

Strains on Radiographs
    I. YELLOW
        A. Exhausted, oxidized developer
            1. Old developer
            2. Covers left off
            3. Scum on developer surface
                a. Oil from pipelines
                b. Impure water used when mixing
                c. Dust
        B. Prolonged development
        C. Insufficient rinsing
        D. Exhausted fixing bath

    II. DICHROIC (doubly refracting crystals exhibiting different colors when viewed in different directions)
        A. Old, exhausted developer
            1. Colloidal metallic silver
        B. Nearly exhausted fixer
        C. Developer containing small amounts of fixer
        D. Films partially fixed in weak fixer, exposed to light and refixed
        E. Prolonged intermediate rinse in contaminated rinse water

    III. GREEN TINTED
        A. Insufficient washing

Deposits on Radiographs
    I. METALLIC
        A. Oxidized products from developer
        B. Silver salts reacting with hydrogen sulfide in air to form silver sulfide
        C. Improper solder used in repair of hinges
        D. Silver loaded fixer

    II. WHITE OR CRYSTALLINE
        A. Milky fixer
            1. Acid portion added too fast while mixing
            2. Acid portion added when too hot
            3. Excessive acidity
            4. Glacial acetic acid mistaken for 28 per cent acetic acid

        5. Developer splashed into fixer
        6. Insufficient rinsing
        B. Prolonged washing
    III. GRIT

Marks on Emulsion Surfaces
    I. RUNS
        A. Insufficient fixing
            1. Weakened fixer
            2. Unbalanced formula
            3. Exhausted ingredients
            4. Low acid content
                a. Deficient when fresh
                b. Diluted from rinse water
                c. Neutralized by developer because of insufficient or no rinsing
        B. Drying temperature too high
        C. Contact with hot viewing box

    II. BLISTERS
        A. Formation of gas bubbles in gelatin
            1. Carbonate of developer reacting with acid of fixer
            2. Unbalanced processing temperatures
                a. Combination of hot fixer and cool developer
                b. Combination of cool fixer and hot developer
            3. Excessive acidity of fixer
            4. No agitation of film when first placed in fixer

    III. RETICULATION
        A. Nonuniform processing temperatures
            1. Developer (hot)
            2. Rinse
            3. Fixer (cool)
            4. Wash
        B. Weakened fixer with little hardening action

    IV. FRILLING
        A. Weakened fixer with little hardening action
        B. Hot processing solutions
            1. Developer
            2. Rinse
            3. Fixer
            4. Wash
        C. Prolonged washing

    V. AIR BELLS
        A. Air bubbles trapped on film surfaces preventing development

Table 3–4 continued on the opposite page

Table 3–4. COMMON DARKROOM CAUSES OF UNSATISFACTORY RADIOGRAPHS (*Continued*)

B. Dropping film into developer without agitation as soon as immersed

VI. DRYING MARKS FROM UNEVEN DRYING OF GELATIN
  A. Excessive drying temperatures
  B. Extremely low humidity
  C. Puddles (buckshot marks)
    1. Drops of water striking semi-dried emulsion surface
  D. Streaks
    1. Drops of water running down semi-dried emulsion surface
      a. Water trapped on hanger frames
      b. Water splashes
      c. Dirty hangers
      d. Drying air flow too rapid

VII. WHITE SPOTS
  A. Screens pitted
  B. Grit or dust present on film or screens, or other contaminants
  C. Chemical dust settling on film or screens (particles of certain chemical dusts will also cause black spots)

VIII. ARTIFACTS
  A. Crescents—rough handling
  B. Smudge marks—fingerprints or fingernail abrasions
  C. Bands in marginal areas—usually due to screen mounting medium
  D. Kiss marks—films were touching each other or side of tank during development

Slow Drying
I. WATERLOGGED FILMS
  A. Insufficient hardening in fixer
    1. Too short fixing period
    2. Weakened fixer from splashing wash water
    3. Exhausted fixer
    4. Insufficient acidity in fixer
  B. Prolonged washing
  C. Wash water too warm

II. AIR TOO HUMID

III. AIR TOO COLD

IV. DRYER AIR VELOCITY TOO LOW

Brittleness of Finished Radiographs
I. EXCESSIVE DRYING TEMPERATURE

II. EXCESSIVE DRYING TIME

III. EXCESSIVE HARDENING IN FIXER
  A. Excessive fixation
  B. Excessive acidity

Streaks on Radiographs
I. INSUFFICIENT AGITATION WHILE PROCESSING

II. FOG (RADIATION, CHEMICAL OR PRESSURE)

III. CHEMICALLY ACTIVE DEPOSITS (DRIED CHEMICALS ON HANGERS)

IV. SCRATCHES
  A. Careless handling
  B. Grit present in air, in cassettes, or on illuminator

V. EXPOSURE TO WHITE LIGHT BEFORE COMPLETE FIXING

VI. UNEVEN DRYING DUE TO HIGH TEMPERATURE AND LOW HUMIDITY

Static
I. LOW HUMIDITY

II. IMPROPER HANDLING IN:
  A. Removal from box
  B. Removal from interleaving paper
  C. Loading cassette
  D. Unloading cassette
  E. Loading hanger
  F. Films stacked before processing

silver in solution. This process is accomplished in a container with a recovery cartridge at the bottom to collect the precipitate. This system features low initial cost and ease of maintenance. Approximately 99 per cent of the silver is recovered by this method; however, the purity of the precipitate is less than that obtained with electrolytic methods. Electrolytic recovery is accomplished by passing a current through the solution between

Table 3–5. COMMON CAUSES OF UNSATISFACTORY PROCESSING TECHNIQUE WITH AUTOMATIC PROCESSORS

Decreased Density
  Under-replenishment
  Developer temperature low
  Exhausted developer. Drain and clean tanks every six months or after processing 50,000 films, whichever occurs first
  Developer improperly mixed

Increased Density
  Over-replenishment
  Developer temperature high
  Contamination of developer with fixer
  Developer improperly mixed
  Light leaks in processor cover or darkroom door

Failure of Film to Transport
  Chemicals improperly mixed
  Chemicals contaminated or diluted
  Chemical temperature too high
  Incorrect replenishment rates
  Dirty racks, turnarounds, or crossovers
  Racks or crossovers not seated properly or warped
  Dirty wash water
  Overlapped films
  Tacky films in dryer section
  Incorrect dryer temperature
  Dryer air tubes incorrectly located or seated
  Hesitation in drive assembly which causes film to pause in transit
  Film not tracking through the processor on a straight course

Scratches
  Guide shoe out of line or dirty
  Dryer air tubes not seated properly

Processing Streaks
  Rollers and crossovers encrusted with chemical deposits
  Dirty wash water
  Film not hardened properly by chemicals

Drying Streaks
  Dirty air tubes
  Film not hardened properly by chemicals

"Pi-Lines"*
  Deposits on rollers in the developer tank

Insufficient Drying
  Temperature too low
  Thermostatic control or heater inoperative
  High humidity in dryer section indicating one of the following:
  1. Insufficient air venting resulting in back pressure
  2. Damper in exhaust line not open far enough
  3. Exhausting into an existing line carrying a higher pressure than that coming from the processor
  4. Lack of or insufficient air conditioning
  Film not hardened properly by chemicals

*"Pi-lines" are thin black longitudinal lines running across the film. They are most often seen in new machines, and will usually disappear after about 500 films have been processed.

two electrodes (anode and cathode). The silver plates out on the cathode. Solutions may be directly supplied from the fixer tank of an automatic processor. Chemical precipitation results in a silver sulfide sludge, which is recovered by filtration. Consult with a film supplier for advice on the system best suited for your radiology department.

REFERENCES

Gillette, E L., Thrall, D. E., and Lebel, J. L.: Carlson's Veterinary Radiology, 3rd ed. Philadelphia, Lea and Febiger, 1977.

Carlson, W. D., and Corley, E. A.: Radiographic equipment and supplies. *In* Felson, B., Ed., Roentgen Techniques in Laboratory Animals. Philadelphia, W. B. Saunders Co., 1968.

Eastman Kodak Company: The Fundamentals of Radiography. 11th ed. Rochester, N.Y., 1980.

Fuchs, A. W.: Principles of Radiographic Exposure and Processing. 2nd ed. Springfield, Ill., Charles C Thomas, Publisher, 1961.

Johns, H. E., and Cunningham, J. R.: The Physics of Radiology. 3rd ed. Springfield, Ill., Charles C Thomas, Publisher, 1974.

Selman, J.: The Fundamentals of X-ray and Radium Physics. 5th ed. Springfield, Ill., Charles C Thomas, Publisher, 1977.

Ticer, J. W.: Production of diagnostic radiographs in veterinary practice. III. Processing factors. Calif. Vet., 23:19–21, 1969.

4

Exposure Factors

Milliamperage, length of exposure, kilovoltage, focal-film distance, grid ratio, and film and intensifying screen type are readily adjustable variables that affect the number and quality of x-rays produced in an x-ray machine. Proper selection of these variable factors results in radiographs of diagnostic quality. After their initial selection, focal-film distance, film type, intensifying screen type and grid ratio generally become fixed; variations of milliamperage, length of exposure, and kilovoltage are then used as variables to produce adequate exposure. An understanding of these factors is necessary for the production of high quality diagnostic radiographs.

Milliamperage

The number of electrons moving from cathode to anode (current flow) within the x-ray tube is the principal factor controlling the number of x-rays generated (see Chapter 1). Decreasing the electron flow results in a decreased x-ray output, and conversely, increasing the electron flow results in an increased x-ray output.

The measure of current flow is the ampere (1 coulomb/sec or 6.3×10^{18} electrons/sec). Since the current flow through an x-ray tube is small, the standard measure is the milliampere (0.001 ampere). Most diagnostic x-ray tubes used in veterinary radiography are operated with current flows of 20 to 300 milliamperes (ma). Some high capacity units may utilize up to 2000 ma current flow for certain specialized procedures.

Adjustment of the milliamperage control

on an x-ray machine permits selection of the number of x-rays desired per unit time. Increased radiographic density may be obtained by increasing the milliamperage, and decreased radiographic density may be obtained by decreasing the milliamperage (Selman, 1977).

Length of Exposure

By varying the time that the current is allowed to flow from cathode to anode, the total number of x-rays generated in each exposure may be controlled. The total number of x-rays reaching the recording surface ultimately determines the density of the resultant radiograph.

Milliampere-second Concept

Variation of both the milliamperage (controlling the number of x-rays generated per unit time) and the time of exposure results in a variation of the radiographic density. An increase in milliamperage allows shortening of the exposure time, and conversely, a decreased milliamperage requires lengthening of the exposure time to maintain adequate radiographic density.

These relationships between milliamperage and exposure time have resulted in the concept of the milliampere-second (mas), which is the product of the milliamperes of current flow and the time (in seconds) that the current is allowed to flow. Thus, an exposure made with 100 ma for 1/10 sec has an mas factor of 10. Likewise, an exposure made at 200 ma for 1/20 sec has an mas factor of 10.

Both exposures generate the same number of x-rays and will produce the same radiographic density.

The radiograph produced at 1/20 sec is preferable in veterinary radiography, where patient motion is likely to cause a loss of detail due to blurring of the radiographic image. Consequently, x-ray equipment with high milliamperage capabilities is needed for examinations of uncooperative patients and for regions such as the abdomen and thorax, where imperceptible motion is likely to occur.

Kilovoltage

Voltage applied between the cathode and anode of the x-ray tube is used to accelerate electrons toward a collision interaction with the x-ray tube target. Higher voltages cause increased electron speed, thereby increasing the collision force. This results in a higher mean energy of the x-ray beam and ultimately causes increased penetrability of the x-rays (see Chapter 1).

Voltages commonly used in veterinary radiography range from 40,000 to 110,000 volts (40 to 110 kilovolts [kv]). Increasing kilovoltage increases radiographic density because a greater number of the x-rays penetrate the patient and expose the film. Generally, increased kilovolt values are used for thicker body parts, since greater penetration is necessary to produce adequate radiographic density.

Higher kilovoltage and greater patient penetration increases the scale of contrast on the radiograph, which will have more tones of gray that represent subtle differences in tissue density and thickness (see Chapter 2). For this reason, high kilovoltage radiographic technique is used for soft tissue examination where the small differences in tissue densities need to be illustrated radiographically. Conversely, bone examinations require the recording of relatively fewer tissue density differences, and a lower kilovoltage technique may be used.

The kv variation necessary to increase or decrease radiographic density varies with the original kilovoltage. Adequate radiographic density may be maintained by adding 2 kv for each centimeter increase in patient thickness when the original kv value is below 80. In the range from 80 to 100 kv, the addition

of 3 kv for each centimeter increase in patient thickness is necessary. Above 100 kv, the addition of 4 kv per cm is necessary. Decreased kilovoltage values may also be used to compensate for decreasing patient thickness.

Relatively large increases or decreases in radiographic density may also be accomplished by altering the kv value. The amount of kilovoltage change necessary to effectively double or halve the technique also varies with the original kv value (Table 4–1). These kilovoltage alterations are used to change radiographic density approximately the same as would be obtained by doubling or halving the mas. As a general rule, the addition or subtraction of 15 per cent of original kv value will be equivalent to doubling or halving the mas value.

Large alterations in kilovoltage may be used to increase or decrease the scale of radiographic contrast. For example, when soft tissue examinations require a long scale of contrast, the kilovoltage may be increased by an amount indicated in Table 4–1. Approximately the same radiographic density may be maintained by simultaneously halving the mas value.

High kv technique has the additional advantage of increasing the latitude of the exposure. Latitude is a measure of allowable error in technique that will result in a diagnostic radiograph (see Chapter 2). In the range of 46 to 55 kv, an error in the x-ray machine setting of plus or minus 2 kv will result in an adequate radiographic density, whereas in the range of 86 to 95 kv, an error of 10 kv is allowable (Gillette et al., 1977).

Table 4–1. CHANGES IN Kv VALUES THAT RESULT IN RADIOGRAPHIC DENSITY CHANGE EQUIVALENT TO HALVING OR DOUBLING MAS

Kv Range	Kv Value[1]
41–50	8
51–60	10
61–70	12
71–80	14
81–90	16
91–100	18
101–110	20

[1]Amount to be subtracted for density change equal to halving mas or to be added for density change equal to doubling mas.

Focal-Film Distance

The focal-film distance (FFD) is the distance from the x-ray tube target to the recording surface. Increasing the FFD decreases the total number of x-rays available to penetrate the patient and expose the film.

This relationship follows the inverse square law: the intensity of the x-ray beam at a point is inversely proportional to the square of the distance from the x-ray source (Matthews and Barnhard, 1968). Simply expressed, this relationship means that doubling the distance between x-ray tube target and the film will result in one-fourth the number of x-rays being available to produce radiographic density, because, when the distance is doubled, the same radiation field is spread over an area four times as great.

The following simple calculations may be made to determine new mas requirements for maintaining proper radiographic density when the FFD is changed:

$$\text{old mas} \times \frac{[\text{new FFD}]^2}{[\text{old FFD}]^2} = \frac{\text{new mas}}{\text{requirement}}$$

For example, if a satisfactory radiograph were produced with 10 mas at 20 inches FFD and the new FFD were 40 inches:

$$10 \text{ mas} \times \frac{40^2}{20^2} = \frac{16000}{400} = 40 \text{ mas}$$

The new value to maintain radiographic density would be 40 mas.

Grids

A grid improves radiographic contrast by preventing scattered radiation from exposing film (see Chap. 2). The efficiency of scatter radiation removal depends mainly on grid ratio and the number of lead strips per linear inch (Selman, 1977). Grids with increased ratio are more efficient at removing scatter radiation. Increasing the number of lead strips per inch decreases the efficiency, since these strips must be thinner and consequently will absorb less angular (scattered) radiation, especially during high kv operation. With grids of equal ratio, the one with fewer strips per inch has greater efficiency. Therefore, as the number of lead strips per inch increases, the grid ratio must also be increased to maintain the same efficiency of scatter radiation

removal (Selman, 1977). Visibility of grid lines on the finished radiograph makes the use of grids with relatively fewer lines per inch objectionable except when moving grids are used.

Grids with increased ratio require increased exposure to maintain adequate radiographic density (Selman, 1977). It is obvious, then, that there must be a compromise between the need for scatter radiation removal and the magnitude of exposure required. The need for scatter radiation removal varies with the thickness and average density of the part being examined. Radiography of structures that have a high percentage of bone (such as the skull) requires the use of a grid for parts of relatively less thickness when compared with less dense structures such as the thorax (Ticer and Evans, 1969).

Generally, patient parts with a thickness of 10 cm or more require the use of a grid to remove scatter radiation (Gillette et al., 1977). Non-obese patients that have relatively nonpathological thoracic cavities (up to 15 cm in thickness) may be radiographed without the use of a grid. Relatively dense skulls less than 10 cm thick (as with brachycephalic dogs) may require the use of a grid.

Choice of grid ratios depends, in large part, upon the requirements for scatter removal and on the capabilities of the x-ray machine. Practices that radiograph a large number of relatively large dogs or thick parts of large animals require the use of grids with ratios of at least 8:1, preferably 12:1. Since increased grid ratios require increased exposure, the choice of a grid must be tempered by the ability of the x-ray machine to generate sufficient mas with relatively short exposure times to produce adequate radiographic density.

X-ray machines with a 100 ma maximum output dictate the use of grids with an 8:1 ratio or less. These grids require two or three times the exposure needed for the non-grid technique. This means that exposure time must be doubled or tripled to maintain radiographic density. Grids should not be used that require increased exposure of such a magnitude that radiographic detail will be lost as a result of patient motion, which may be perceptible with increased exposure times.

X-ray machines that have capabilities of generating 300 or 400 ma allow the use of grids with ratios of 12:1. Requirements for grids with ratios of greater than 12:1 are not

Table 4–2. SUGGESTED EXPOSURE INCREASES WHEN USING GRIDS

Grid Ratio	Increase Exposure by a Factor of
5:1	2
8:1	3
12:1	4
16:1	4.5

found in most veterinary radiography because techniques using a kilovoltage above 100 kv are not often used. Efficiency requirements for grids with 16:1 ratios are needed only with high kv technique, where the production of scatter radiation is increased (Selman, 1977). These situations may be found during examination of large animal abdomens and a large animal thorax with severe pleural fluid accumulation or severe pulmonary infiltrate.

Increased exposure requirements vary with the grid ratio. The magnitude of the increased exposure should be determined by trial since other factors (such as the type of body part being radiographed) affect the proportion of primary to secondary (scatter) radiation emerging from the patient. Table 4–2 provides a guide for the start of a trial exposure technique.

For example, if a radiograph of a Boston terrier skull 9 cm thick has adequate density when exposed at 100 ma, $\frac{1}{20}$ sec (5 mas) and 70 kv, but lacks detail because of scatter radiation, the use of a grid is indicated. If a grid with a 5:1 ratio is used, the exposure must be increased by a factor of 2. This is accomplished by increasing either mas or kv. Increases in mas usually provide the practical method of increasing exposure. Since most techniques utilize the maximum x-ray machine milliamperage, increased exposure time is used to increase mas. In practice, increasing the exposure by a factor of 2 is accomplished by doubling the time of exposure to $\frac{1}{10}$ sec. This effectively increases the mas to 10 (100 ma × $\frac{1}{10}$ sec).

Film Type

Several film types are available to the medical radiographer. The choice of film type is governed by the speed, detail and latitude requirements. High-speed film requires approximately one half the exposure needed by par-speed film to produce a given radio-graphic density (Eastman Kodak Co., 1980). High-speed film, on the other hand, produces radiographs with a granular appearance that results in a loss of detail. For this reason, high-speed film is only recommended for use with x-ray machines that have maximum capabilities of less than 60 ma.

Par-speed film usually produces radiographic detail that is satisfactory for average diagnostic use. Detail or slow-speed film may be desirable for certain specialized uses where fine structure is being examined, such as cat skulls, birds or peripheral appendicular skeletons. This film requires approximately twice as much exposure as par-speed film.

Alternatively, high-detail examinations may be made using par-speed film and detail screens. This technique has decreased exposure requirements and results in a radiograph with a shorter scale of contrast and is therefore preferred for radiology departments that have a relatively high case load of this type of examination.

High-detail radiography may be performed with nonscreen film. This film type has approximately one fifth the speed of par-speed film and therefore requires five times the exposure to produce the same radiographic density (Carlson and Corley, 1968; Matthews and Barnhard, 1968). This film may be used when examining peripheral skeletal structures or feline skulls of 5 cm or less in thickness.

Latitude film (see Chapter 2) is preferred for examinations of large animal distal extremities, since soft tissue and periarticular and periosteal reactions can be seen on radiographs of the relatively dense bones.

Intensifying Screen Type

Intensifying screen speed, like film speed, varies the exposure requirements. Increasing the screen speed decreases the exposure requirements needed to produce similar radiographic density (see Chapter 2). Par-speed screens require approximately twice the exposure to produce the same density as high-speed screens. The difference in radiographic detail is not as marked between par- and high-speed screens as it is between par- and high-speed film. The use of high-speed intensifying screens is therefore recommended for most veterinary radiology departments because of the decreased exposure requirements (one half the exposure time).

Certain examinations may require fast detail or detail screens that require two and four times the exposure, respectively, that is required for par-speed screens. Owing to the expense involved in purchasing these items, nonscreen film is usually recommended for high-detail examination in low–case load radiology departments.

Exposure requirements may be markedly decreased by using rare earth phosphor screens (see Chap. 2). Combinations of these screens and film of various speeds may reduce exposure requirements by a factor of twelve when compared to par-speed screens and film; however, mottle becomes objectionable at these speeds. It is therefore recommended that rare earth screen-film combinations that result in speed increases no higher than a factor of eight be used for routine examinations. Detail rare earth phosphor screens are useful with low ma x-ray machines, since they require approximately the same exposure as par-speed calcium tungstate screens and result in marked improvement in radiographic detail.

TECHNIQUE CHARTS

Usable radiographic technique charts provide a convenient and reliable source of information about exposure factors that are needed for the production of diagnostic radiographs. Such charts should be formulated for each x-ray machine. Even x-ray machines of the same make and model vary in both quantity and quality of output, owing to variations in input voltage, calibration, and condition of component parts, especially the x-ray tube target. Charts constructed for one x-ray machine should not be used for another machine, since these variables are often unique.

Although the art of quality radiography can only be achieved after extensive training and experience, an adequate compromise between poor quality and excellent quality can be obtained if good technique charts are constructed and followed.

Small Animal Technique Charts

Variable Kilovoltage Technique Chart

A basic variable kilovoltage technique chart may be constructed from data obtained during a series of trial exposures. A normal, nonobese, mature dog with a lateral abdominal measurement of 8 to 9 cm should be used as a test subject. Three test radiographs are made of the lateral recumbent projection. These test exposures may be made using one 14 × 17 inch film that is blocked off by lead sheets or by a folded lead apron over the areas not being exposed (Fig. 4–1). X-ray machine settings for the trial exposures vary with the film and intensifying screen type and with the capabilities of the x-ray machine. The following list of exposure factors is presented as a starting point:

1. Focal-Film Distance (FFD) = 36 inches.
2. Par- (average-) speed film. High-speed film requires half the mas requirements and should only be used for x-ray machines with less than 60 ma capabilities.
3. High-speed calcium tungstate intensifying screens.
4. Kilovoltage = 65 kv.
5. Milliampere-seconds = 1.66 mas for the first exposure, 2.5 mas for the second, and 5 mas for the third in a series of trial exposures. Variables 1 through 4 are not changed.
6. Standard film processing (manual, manual rapid processing or automatic processing; see Chapter 3).

When determining the milliamperage and time settings to obtain the desired mas factors of 1.66, 2.5, and 5, the highest ma and the shortest time should be chosen. For example, if the maximum ma output of a machine is 100, the exposure time to be used may be calculated by rearranging the following mas formula:

$$mas = ma \times t \text{ in seconds}$$
$$t = \frac{mas}{ma}$$

The desired time then becomes:

$$t = \frac{1.66}{100} = \frac{1}{60} \text{ sec}$$

Solving the time requirement for 2.5 and 5 mas, the values of $\frac{1}{40}$ and $\frac{1}{20}$ sec, respectively, are obtained.

The fastest exposure time available is always used when determining x-ray machine settings for a given mas requirement. If the fastest time available, in combination with the highest ma, exceeds the desired mas, the milliamperage should be decreased. For example, if the x-ray machine has a 300 ma capability with a minimum of ⅟₆₀ second timing, mas values of less than 5 may be calculated. The formula for mas (mas = ma × t in seconds) may be rearranged as:

$$ma = \frac{mas}{t}$$

The desired mas (in this case, 1.66) and minimal time factors are then substituted, and the milliamperage to be used is determined as follows:

$$ma = \frac{1.66}{1/60} = 100 \ ma$$

Solving the ma requirement for 2.5 mas, the value of 150 ma is obtained. Therefore, the three trial exposures for this 300 ma machine would be produced using ⅟₆₀ sec timing and 100, 150 and 300 ma.

After development of the trial exposures using standard processing, the most "diagnostic" radiograph is selected. Variations of radiographic density should be observed on the three radiographs. If inadequate density is obtained on the 5 mas radiographs, make another exposure at 10 mas. On the other hand, if the 1.66 mas radiograph has excessive density, another exposure should be made using approximately 0.83 mas.

For the purpose of illustration, assume that adequate radiographic density was obtained on the trial radiograph of an 8 cm canine abdomen using 5.0 mas. Insert those factors into a variable kilovoltage technique chart as illustrated in Table 4–3.

For this example, an x-ray machine of 100 ma, 100 kv, and ⅟₆₀ sec timing capabilities will be used. The same calculation principle exists with any x-ray machine. Only the variables of milliamperage and time need to be adjusted to arrive at the proper mas value, and the shortest time possible should be used in order to decrease the probability of recording imperceptible patient motion.

The variable kilovoltage chart is then completed by subtracting 2 kv for each decreased cm of thickness and adding 2 kv for each

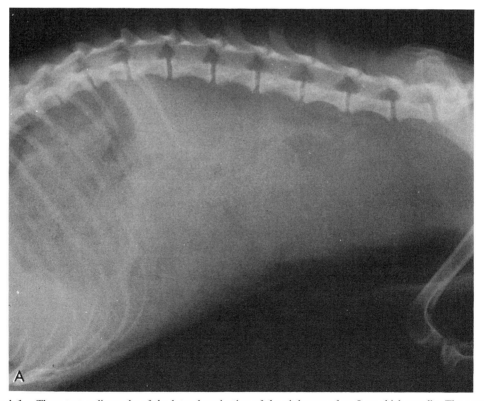

Figure 4–1. Three test radiographs of the lateral projection of the abdomen of an 8 cm thick poodle. The exposure factors of par-speed film, high-speed screens, 36 in. FFD and 65 KV were constant. *A* was produced at 1.66 mas, *B* at 2.5 mas, and *C* at 5 mas. The most desirable radiographic density was produced at 2.5 mas. In this case, the 2.5 mas factor would be used as the starting point for constructing a technique chart.

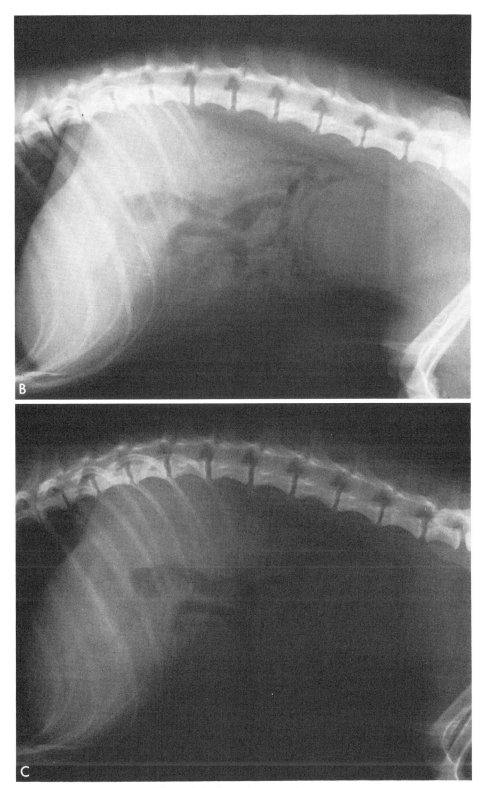

Figure 4–1 *Legend on opposite page.*

Table 4–3. VARIABLE Kv TECHNIQUE CHART FOR AN X-RAY MACHINE WITH 100 Ma, 100 Kv, $\frac{1}{60}$ SEC CAPABILITIES

Thickness (cm)	Kv	Ma	Time (Seconds)	Mas	FFD (Inches)	Grid (5:1 ratio)
1	51	100	1/20	5	36	No
2	53	100	1/20	5	36	No
3	55	100	1/20	5	36	No
4	57	100	1/20	5	36	No
5	59	100	1/20	5	36	No
6	61	100	1/20	5	36	No
7	63	100	1/20	5	36	No
8[1]	65	100	1/20	5	36	No
9	67	100	1/20	5	36	No
10[2]	69	100	1/10	10	36	Yes
11	71	100	1/10	10	36	Yes
12	73	100	1/10	10	36	Yes
13	75	100	1/10	10	36	Yes
14	77	100	1/10	10	36	Yes
15	79	100	1/10	10	36	Yes
16	81	100	1/10	10	36	Yes
17[3]	84	100	1/10	10	36	Yes
18	87	100	1/10	10	36	Yes
19	90	100	1/10	10	36	Yes
20	93	100	1/10	10	36	Yes
21	96	100	1/10	10	36	Yes
22	99	100	1/10	10	36	Yes
23[4]	82	100	1/5	20	36	Yes
24	85	100	1/5	20	36	Yes
25	88	100	1/5	20	36	Yes

[1] Trial radiograph with adequate density using these exposure factors.

[2] Grid added for thickness of 10 cm or greater. A 5:1 ratio grid requires twice the exposure (double mas by exposing at $\frac{1}{10}$ sec) to maintain adequate radiographic density (Table 4–2).

[3] 3 Kv per cm of increased thickness is added above 80 kv.

[4] The kilovoltage requirements for 23 cm thickness would have been 102 kv, which is not within this x-ray machine's capabilities. Subtracting 20 kv resulted in halving the exposure, thereby bringing the kv setting down to 82. To compensate for this decrease, the mas was doubled, thereby maintaining radiographic denisty.

increased cm of thickness. After 80 kv is reached (at 16 cm on this chart), 3 kv are added for each cm increase in thickness up to the limits of the machine (100 kv).

Patient parts in excess of 9 cm should be radiographed with the aid of a grid in order to control fog-producing scatter radiation. In this example, a 5:1 ratio grid is used. Increased exposure is then required to maintain adequate radiographic density. Addition of a 5:1 ratio grid usually requires doubling the exposure (Table 4–2), which, in this case, was accomplished by doubling the mas from 5 to 10. Since the 100 ma used for the chart represents the maximum value for the machine, mas was doubled by doubling the exposure time from $\frac{1}{20}$ to $\frac{1}{10}$ sec.

At the 23 cm thickness line on the chart, the required kilovoltage is 102, which exceeds the limits of this x-ray machine. By substract-

ing 20 kv (Table 4–1) from the needed 102 kv value, the exposure may be effectively halved. The new value of 82 kv is then inserted on the 23 cm thickness line. To compensate for the decreased radiographic density that would occur, the mas value is then doubled from 10 to 20 by doubling the exposure time from $\frac{1}{10}$ to $\frac{1}{5}$ sec. The variable technique chart is then completed by adding 3 kv per cm thickness to the remaining lines.

Table 4–4 is a variable kv technique chart constructed for a 300 ma, 125 kv, $\frac{1}{60}$ sec capability x-ray machine, using the same starting point as was used for Table 4–3 (8 cm thick abdomen, 65 kv, 5 mas). The chart was constructed using the same method of increasing and decreasing kilovoltage. Calculation of the exposure time using 300 ma yielded $\frac{1}{60}$ sec ($t = \dfrac{5 \text{ mas}}{300 \text{ ma}} = \frac{1}{60}$ sec).

Table 4–4. VARIABLE Kv TECHNIQUE CHART FOR AN X-RAY MACHINE WITH 300 Ma, 125 Kv, $\frac{1}{60}$ SEC CAPABILITIES

Thickness (cm)	Kv	Ma	Time (Seconds)	Mas	FFD (Inches)	Grid (8:1 ratio)
1	51	300	1/60	5	36	No
2	53	300	1/60	5	36	No
3	55	300	1/60	5	36	No
4	57	300	1/60	5	36	No
5	59	300	1/60	5	36	No
6	61	300	1/60	5	36	No
7	63	300	1/60	5	36	No
8	65	300	1/60	5	36	No
9	67	300	1/60	5	36	No
10[1]	69	300	1/20	15	36	Yes
11	71	300	1/20	15	36	Yes
12	73	300	1/20	15	36	Yes
13	75	300	1/20	15	36	Yes
14	77	300	1/20	15	36	Yes
15	79	300	1/20	15	36	Yes
16	81	300	1/20	15	36	Yes
17[2]	84	300	1/20	15	36	Yes
18	87	300	1/20	15	36	Yes
19	90	300	1/20	15	36	Yes
20	93	300	1/20	15	36	Yes
21	96	300	1/20	15	36	Yes
22	99	300	1/20	15	36	Yes
23	102	300	1/20	15	36	Yes
24[3]	106	300	1/20	15	36	Yes
25	110	300	1/20	15	36	Yes

[1]Grid added for thickness of 10 cm or greater. An 8:1 ratio grid requires three times the exposure (triple the mas by exposing at $\frac{1}{20}$ sec) to maintain adequate radiographic density (Table 4–2).
[2]3 Kv per cm thickness increase is added above 80 kv.
[3]4 Kv per cm thickness increase is added above 100 kv.

An 8:1 ratio grid was used to increase the radiographic detail for parts greater than 9 cm thick, which required three times the exposure (Table 4–2). This was accomplished by tripling the exposure time.

Since the upper kilovoltage limit of this x-ray machine is 125 kv, the kv-mas alteration was not necessary at the 23 cm thickness line. Note that 4 kv per cm of increased thickness was added above 100 kv. If a shorter scale of contrast is desired, the kv values may be kept in a range below 90 by decreasing the kilovoltage at the 20 cm line from 93 to 75 kv (Table 4–2) and doubling the mas to 30 by doubling the time to $\frac{1}{10}$ sec.

Thorax Technique Chart

The thorax has less x-ray absorbing tissues than other parts of the anatomy and therefore requires fewer x-rays to produce a given radiographic density on the film. As a rule, thoracic radiography has 50 to 75 per cent the mas requirements of other body parts of similar thickness. A considerable amount of experience is necessary to be able to estimate the variation in thoracic tissue density that must be penetrated by the x-ray beam.

Generally, thorax examinations for normal, nonobese small animal patients require 50 per cent of the mas needed for other body parts (Gillette et al., 1977). Patients that are somewhat obese or those that have pathological states such as pleural effusion, pulmonary infiltrate, or massive cardiomegaly require approximately 75 per cent of the mas needed for the abdomen.

A usable technique chart for thoracic radiography (Table 4–5) may be constructed by modifying the variable kv chart shown in Table 4–3. This modification is accomplished by decreasing the mas factor by halving the exposure time. In thoracic radiography, a

Table 4–5. VARIABLE Kv TECHNIQUE CHART FOR THE THORAX (MODIFIED FROM TABLE 4–3)

Thickness (cm)	Kv	Ma	Time (Seconds)	Mas	FFD (Inches)	Grid (5:1 ratio)
5[1]	59	100	1/40	2.5	36	No
6	61	100	1/40	2.5	36	No
7	63	100	1/40	2.5	36	No
8	65	100	1/40	2.5	36	No
9	67	100	1/40	2.5	36	No
10	69	100	1/40	2.5	36	No
11	71	100	1/40	2.5	36	No
12	73	100	1/40	2.5	36	No
13	75	100	1/40	2.5	36	No
14	77	100	1/40	2.5	36	No
15[2]	79	100	1/20	5	36	Yes
16	81	100	1/20	5	36	Yes
17	84	100	1/20	5	36	Yes
18	87	100	1/20	5	36	Yes
19	90	100	1/20	5	36	Yes
20	93	100	1/20	5	36	Yes
21	96	100	1/20	5	36	Yes
22	99	100	1/20	5	36	Yes
23	82	100	1/10	10	36	Yes
24	85	100	1/10	10	36	Yes
25	88	100	1/10	10	36	Yes

[1]Started at 5 cm thickness because thorax measurements are usually greater than 5 cm.

[2]Grid added for thickness of 15 cm or greater. A 5:1 ratio grid requires twice the exposure (double mas by exposing at 1/20 sec) to maintain adequate radiographic density.

grid is usually needed only for thicknesses of 15 cm or more.

When radiographing patients that have an increased ratio of soft tissue (fat or fluid) to air-filled lungs, the kv or mas values of the chart should be increased. Increasing the kv value is the method of choice for increasing the exposure factors in these cases, since short exposure times may be maintained. Increased kilovoltage values from 10 to 15 per cent, depending on the patient type and pathological state, will usually produce adequate radiographic density.

Increased Mas Base for Extremities, Pelvis, Skull and Spine

Utilizing a variable kilovoltage technique chart using a lateral view of the abdomen as reference point usually results in satisfactory radiographs for the abdomen, and other soft tissue structures, such as those in the cervical region. By halving the mas value, a usable thoracic chart may be constructed. Some veterinarians, however, prefer a shorter scale of contrast when examining extremities, pelvis, skull and spine. This may be accom-

plished by doubling the mas factor of the original values and decreasing the kilovoltage and appropriate amount depending upon the original kilovoltage range (see Table 4–1). This technique results in a shorter scale of contrast and tends to present a more pleasing representation of dense, thick bony structures.

Variable Mas Technique Chart

A variable kilovoltage technique chart may not be practical for all x-ray machines. Certain older machines do not allow for kilovoltage variation in steps of 1 or 2 kv that are necessary for an accurate use of a variable kilovoltage chart. Unfortunately, the timing interval of most x-ray machines does not permit the accurate use of a variable mas technique chart.

A compromise between a variable kilovoltage and a variable mas chart works best for equipment that does not have short kilovoltage selection intervals. For example, if kilovoltage settings may be made only in 10 kv intervals, increased radiographic density may be attained for each cm of increased patient

Table 4–6. EXAMPLE OF A VARIABLE Mas METHOD TO COMPENSATE FOR AN X-RAY MACHINE WITH Kv SETTING INTERVALS OF 10 (MODIFIED FROM TABLE 4–3)

Thickness (cm)	Kv	Ma	Time (Seconds)	Mas	FFD (Inches)	Grid
1	50	100	1/20	5	36	No
2	50	100	1/15	6.66	36	No
3	50	75	1/10	7.5	36	No
4	50	100	1/12	8.3	36	No
5	50	100	1/10	10	36	No
6	60	100	1/20	5	36	No

thickness by adding small amounts of mas to the exposure technique.

In order to modify the variable kilovoltage chart in Table 4–3 for use with an x-ray machine with a 10 kv interval limitation, a chart was constructed (Table 4–6) that allows adjustment of both kilovoltage and mas in alternate intervals. From Table 4–1, the approximate mas change that has the equivalence of the 10 kv change can be determined. In this case, the kilovoltage interval of 10 (for kilovoltage in the range of 51 to 60) is approximately equal to doubling the mas. Therefore, if the mas is raised from 5 to 10 for the thickness interval of 1 to 5 cm the inability to raise kilovoltage will be compensated for. The value of 10 mas is then used for the 5 cm thickness line. The mas values for the 2, 3 and 4 cm thickness lines are estimated according to the milliamperage and timer setting combinations available on the x-ray machine. The remaining lines may be calculated in a similar manner.

A major disadvantage of the variable mas method of calculating exposure is the necessity of using relatively long exposure times to obtain some needed mas values.

High Kilovoltage Technique Charts

Certain radiographic examinations require the use of relatively high kilovoltage technique to demonstrate subtle differences in soft tissue densities or to radiograph structures having marked variation in radiodensity, such as the dorsoventral view of a thorax. In order to penetrate the thoracic vertebrae through the dense cardiac silhouette without overexposing the radiolucent lungs, a relatively low mas, high kilovoltage technique should be used (Douglas and Williamson, 1972).

Practical application of this technique is possible by modification of the exposure values on the variable kilovoltage chart (Table 4–5). The kilovoltage and mas values are determined from the chart after measurement of the thorax. The kilovoltage is then increased by a factor indicated in Table 4–1, depending on the kilovoltage range, and the mas value is halved to maintain radiographic density.

For example, examination of a 14 cm thick abdomen using a high kilovoltage technique may be accomplished by determining the exposure factors from the variable kilovoltage chart (Table 4–3). The 77 kv, 10 mas technique may be altered by increasing the kilovoltage by 14 (from Table 4–1) and halving the mas. The new, high kilovoltage exposure factors would then be 91 kv and 5 mas (100 ma at 1/20 sec).

This method is also useful for decreasing exposure times while maintaining radiographic density when examining patients with rapid respiratory movements.

Nonscreen Film Technique Chart

Medical nonscreen film may be used to examine bony parts (such as peripheral limbs and small skulls) when increased radiographic detail is needed. Table 4–7 is an example of a technique chart constructed for use with nonscreen film. The factors should be deter-

Table 4–7. NONSCREEN FILM TECHNIQUE CHART FOR USE ON PERIPHERAL LIMBS

Thickness (cm)	Kv	Ma	Time (Seconds)	Mas	FFD (Inches)
1	50	100	3/20	15	36
2	52	100	3/20	15	36
3	54	100	3/20	15	36
4	56	100	3/20	15	36
5	58	100	3/20	15	36

mined for each x-ray machine using the trial exposure method.

Large Animal Technique Charts

There is considerable variation in equipment requirements for large animal radiography, depending upon the anatomical regions to be examined. For distal extremities, and in some cases the skull and cervical regions, low milliamperage portable equipment is usually employed. The shoulder, hip joints, pelvis and thorax of mature large animals require the use of mobile or fixed equipment with 300 to 1000 ma capabilities.

The availability of rare earth phosphor intensifying screens has reduced the milliamperage requirement considerably; however, the small portable units that are usually available for distal extremity examinations remain inadequate for examinations of these thick areas.

Portable X-ray Machine Technique Chart

Examination of the distal extremities is usually performed with portable x-ray machines with 15 to 25 ma and 90 kv maximum capabilities. Timing capabilities vary considerably. Examination of the carpus and tarsus

Table 4–8. PORTABLE X-RAY MACHINE TECHNIQUE CHART FOR LARGE ANIMALS*

Anatomical Region	Kv	Ma	Time (seconds)	Mas	FFD (inches)	Grid
Elbow						
Lateromedial (without grid)	85	20	0.2–0.3	4–6	30	NO
(with grid)	90–100	20	0.4–0.5	8–10	30	6:1 ratio
Craniocaudal (without grid)	90	20	0.3–0.4	6–8	30	NO
(with grid)	100	20	0.5–0.6	10–12	30	6:1 ratio
Carpus						
Dorsopalmar, lateromedial or oblique	85	20	0.2	4	30	NO
Lateromedial† (flexed)	100	20	0.1	2	30	NO
Stifle						
Lateromedial	100	20	0.4–0.5	8–10		6:1 ratio
Caudocranial	100	20	0.6–0.8	12–16		6:1 ratio
Tarsus						
Lateromedial or oblique	85	20	0.2	4	30	NO
Dorsoplantar	90–100	20	0.25–0.3	5–7	30	NO
Metacarpus or Metatarsus						
Dorsopalmar or dorsoplantar	85–90	20	0.2	4	30	NO
Lateromedial or oblique	85–90	20	0.16	3.2	30	NO
Fetlock						
All views except flexed	80–85	20	0.1–0.15	2 3	30	NO
Flexed†	100	20	0.05–0.1	1–2	30	NO
Phalanges						
All views	80–85	20	0.1–0.15	2–3	30	NO
3rd Phalanx						
Dorsopalmar or dorsoplantar	75	20	0.05–0.1	1–2	30	NO
Navicular						
Dorsopalmar or dorsoplantar	80–85	20	0.2–0.25	4–5	24‡	6:1 ratio
Proximodistal (skyline of flexor surface)	90	20	0.25	5	24‡	6:1 ratio
Dental Exams						
Left or right lateral	85–90	20	0.3–0.4	6–8	30	NO
Oblique	100	20	0.5–0.6	10–12	30	6:1 ratio

*Example for a machine with 20 ma, 100 kv, 0.04 sec. minimum time capabilities used for equine examinations. Kodak regular screens and Par-Speed Latitude film (XL–1).

†Since flexing the carpus or fetlock joints increases the probability of motion, the kv is increased and the time of the exposure is decreased to decrease the likelihood of motion unsharpness.

‡The FFD was decreased for exposures of the navicular bone in order to decrease the mas requirement due to the use of a grid.

and distal structures is usually performed without a grid, using high-speed intensifying screens and par-speed latitude film. Factors of milliampere-seconds and kilovoltage should be determined for each anatomical region using a fixed FFD. The use of latitude film allows a greater margin of error in selecting these exposure factors, especially the FFD. FFD is very difficult to accurately reproduce during each examination when portable equipment is used.

Use the factors listed in Table 4–8 as a reference for the first trial radiographs. Individual x-ray machines vary considerably in x-ray output for a given set of variable factors, thus requiring the establishment of a specific chart for each machine. After trial radiographs of each region are produced, adjustment of the exposure factors can then be made to establish a chart that is unique

for each machine. If excessive radiographic density is obtained on a radiograph, halve the mas by halving the exposure time and repeat the test. Likewise, insufficient radiographic density requires doubling the mas prior to repeating the trial exposure.

Grids are usually required for the examination of the elbow and stifle joint of mature large animals. A 6:1 ratio grid is recommended for use with low-ma portable units.

Skull, cervical vertebrae and shoulder joints may be examined with low-ma portable equipment if combinations of rare earth phosphor screens and par-speed film are used. A $6\times$ or $8\times$ system is recommended (see Chapter 2). An additional exposure advantage for examination of thick parts may be obtained by eliminating the use of a grid and making the exposure through the back (lid) of the cassette. The relatively nonpenetrating scat-

Table 4–9. MOBILE OR STATIONARY X-RAY MACHINE TECHNIQUE CHART FOR LARGE ANIMALS*

Anatomical Region	Kv	Ma	Time (seconds)	Mas	FFD (inches)	Grid
Thorax						
Left-to-right or right-to-left lateral field 1 (caudodorsal)	80–90	300	1/12–1/10	25–30	72	10:1 ratio
Field 2 (craniodorsal)	95–100	300	1/12–1/10	25–30	72	10:1 ratio
Field 3 (cranioventral)	95–100	300	1/8–1/6	37.5–50	72	10:1 ratio
Field 4 (caudoventral)	95–100	300	1/8–1/6	37.5–50	72	10:1 ratio
Cervical Spine						
C1, C2, C3	75–80	300	1/15–1/12	20–25	72	10:1 ratio
C4, C5, C6	80–85	300	1/15–1/12	20–25	72	10:1 ratio
C7, T1	90–100	300	1/6–1/5	50–60	72	10:1 ratio
Skull						
Left-to-right or right-to-left lateral	80–85	300	1/15–1/12	20–25	72	10:1 ratio
Ventrodorsal	80–90	300	1/12–1/10	25–30	72	10:1 ratio
Pelvis						
Left-to-right or right-to-left lateral	125	300	1⅔–2	500–600†	48	2 10:1 ratio grids crossed‡
Ventrodorsal	110–115	300	1–1⅓	300–400†	48	2 10:1 ratio grids crossed
Stifle						
Lateromedial	75–80	300	1/20–1/15	15–20	48	10:1 ratio
Caudocranial	85	300	1/10	30	48	10:1 ratio
Shoulder						
Mediolateral	85	300	1/10	30	48	10:1 ratio
Tarsus						
Lateromedial	65–70	300	1/60–1/40	5–7.5	48	NO
Craniocaudal	75–80	300	1/40–1/30	7.5–10	48	NO

*Example for a machine with 300 ma, 125 kv, 1/60 sec. minimum time capabilities to be used for equine examinations. $8\times$ system using Quanta III screens (DuPont) and Par-Speed Latitude film, XL-1 (Kodak).

†May exceed limits of the tube. Consult the tube rating chart.

‡Use lead sheet under the cassette to reduce back scatter.

Table 4–10. COMMON EXPOSURE CAUSES OF UNSATISFACTORY RADIOGRAPHS

Low Density
  I. UNDEREXPOSURE
     A. Wrong Exposure Factors
        1. Too low kilovoltage
        2. Too low milliamperage
        3. Too short exposure
        4. Too great focal-film distance
     B. Meters out of calibration
     C. Timer out of calibration
     D. Inaccurate setting of meters or timer
     E. Drop in incoming line voltage
        1. Furnaces and blowers on same circuit
        2. Insufficient size of power line or transformers
     F. Central ray of x-ray tube not directed on film
     G. FFD not correct for grid used
     H. One or more rectifiers not functioning

High Density
  I. OVEREXPOSURE
     A. Wrong exposure factors
        1. Too high kilovoltage
        2. Too high milliamperage
        3. Too long exposure
        4. Too short focal-film distance
     B. Meters out of calibration
     C. Timer out of calibration
     D. Inaccurate setting of meters or timer
     E. Surge in incoming line voltage

Low Contrast
  I. OVERPENETRATION FROM TOO HIGH KILOVOLTAGE
     A. Overmeasurement of part to be examined
     B. Incorrect estimate of material or tissue density
     C. Meters out of calibration
     D. Meters inaccurately set
     E. Drop in incoming line voltage
     F. Overmeasurement of focal-film distance
  II. TOO LONG EXPOSURE
     A. Timer out of calibration
     B. Timer inaccurately set

Lack of Detail or Fuzziness
  I. MOTION (TUBE, FILM, SUBJECT)
     A. Inadequate immobilization
     B. Too long exposure
     C. Vibration of floor
     D. Failure to arrest tube vibration after positioning before making exposure
  II. POOR CONTACT OF INTENSIFYING SCREENS
  III. IMPROPER DISTANCE RELATIONSHIP
     A. Object-film distance too great
     B. Target-film distance too short
  IV. IMPROPER FOCAL SPOT
     A. Too large
     B. Damaged (cracked or pitted)

ter radiation will be absorbed in the metal of the cassette back and will result in better detail than that of radiographs produced without a grid that are exposed through the front of the cassette (Spencer, 1982). This technique requires less exposure increase than that required with a 6:1 ratio grid and thus allows shorter exposure times. The efficiency of scatter removal is not as great as with the use of a grid; however, the decreased exposure requirements make it a method worth considering if low-ma equipment is used. Cassettes used for this technique must be free of strap-type latches that might be superimposed on the radiograph.

As with the distal extremities, trial exposures should be followed by definitive adjustment of exposure factors in order to establish a workable technique chart.

Mobile or Stationary X-ray Machine Technique Chart

The increased ma capabilities of mobile and stationary x-ray machines allow their use in the examination of the thorax, pelvis, skull and cervical region of large animals. Rare earth phosphor intensifying screens and par-speed latitude film should be used. An 8:1 or 10:1 ratio grid is also necessary. Table 4–9 lists exposure factors that will serve as a starting place for trial exposures. Adjustments of exposure factors are then followed by repeat trials, if necessary, prior to the establishment of a finished technique chart.

The mas for the thorax may be decreased by 50 per cent for the examination of 400- to 500-lb foals and by 75 per cent for the newborn foal (Farrow, 1981).

Common Exposure Causes of Unsatisfactory Radiographs

Periodic readjustment of technique charts is necessary due to the instability of some variable factors and the decreased efficiency of certain x-ray machine components, especially in x-ray tube target. Common exposure causes of unsatisfactory radiographs are listed in Table 4–10. Consulting this table may aid in differentiating the cause of poor radiographs and in determining if technique chart readjustment is necessary.

REFERENCES

Gillette, E. L., Thrall, D. E., and Lebel, J. L.: Carlson's Veterinary Radiology, 3rd ed. Philadelphia, Lea and Febiger, 1977.

Carlson, W. D., and Corley, E. A.: Radiographic equipment and supplies. *In* Felson, B., Roentgen Techniques in Laboratory Animals. Philadelphia, W. B. Saunders Co., 1968.

Douglas, S. W., and Williamson, H. D.: Principles of Veterinary Radiography. 3rd ed. Baltimore, Williams and Wilkins Co., 1980.

Eastman Kodak Company: The Fundamentals of Radiography. 11th ed. Rochester, N. Y., 1980.

Farrow, C. S.: Equine Thoracic Radiology. J.A.V.M.A. *179*:776–781, 1981.

Matthews, H. G., and Barnhard, H. J.: Radiographic technique. *In* Felson, B., Roentgen Technique in Laboratory Animals. Philadelphia, W. B. Saunders Co., 1968.

Morgan, J. P., Silverman, S., and Zontine, W. J.: Techniques of Veterinary Radiography, 2nd ed. Davis, Ca., Veterinary Radiology Associates, 1977.

Selman, J.: The Fundamentals of X-ray and Radium Physics, 5th ed. Springfield, Ill., Charles C Thomas, 1977.

Spencer, C. P.: Personal Communications, 1982.

Ticer, J. W., and Evans, J. W.: Production of diagnostic radiographs in veterinary practice. IV. Technique chart for small animal radiography. Calif. Vet. *32*:29, 1969.

5

LOUIS A. CORWIN, JR.

Radiation Protection

This chapter will discuss the hazards of radiation from diagnostic x-rays, the approximate levels of exposure that are considered safe, and the means that the veterinarian and veterinary personnel can employ to minimize exposure. A brief discussion of the regulatory control of veterinary radiology is included.

HAZARDS

In this atomic age, the hazards from ionizing radiation are well defined and the effects of excessive exposure to diagnostic radiation on the older physician and veterinarian have been well publicized. Particularly, indiscriminate use of the fluoroscope with ungloved hands in the fluoroscopic x-ray beam has been shown to produce severe skin damage, including carcinoma, to the exposed areas (Messife et al., 1957). At present, there is also great concern about the more subtle long-term effects from continued exposure to *low levels of* radiation. Possible results of accumulative radiation exposure, besides the long-term skin effects, are increases in cancer and inheritable genetic mutations, induction of cataracts, and shortening of life span. Protection of the veterinarian, veterinary personnel, and the general public can only be accomplished if the practicing veterinarian is aware of the recommended limits of radiation exposure (maximum permissible doses), the probable dose ranges experienced in radiographic procedures, and the ways of minimizing the exposure hazards.

MAXIMUM PERMISSIBLE DOSES (MPD)

Table 5–1 is a summary of the maximum permissible dose levels for radiation workers, which include veterinarians and employees involved in producing radiographic examinations. Dose equivalent units are given in terms of *r*oentgen-*e*quivalents–*m*an (rem), which is the unit used to express human biologic doses resulting from exposure to ionizing radiation. For practical purposes, the measured exposure in roentgens of diagnostic x-rays is equivalent to rem. In this discussion, the measured exposure in milliroentgens (mr, or 1/1000 of a roentgen) will be used as equivalent to the millirem unit. The limiting factor in determining the MPD is the radiation exposure to particularly vulnerable or "critical" organs. Since the gonads, the bone marrow and the lenses of the eyes are especially sensitive, particular care should be taken to shield these areas during radiographic procedures. The lenses of the eyes are vulnerable, since they are not ordinarily shielded by the usual protective gloves and aprons. The MPD for the whole body (including gonads, bone marrow and lenses) is 100 millirems (mrem) per week or 5000 mrem per year for occupationally exposed persons.

Table 5–1. MAXIMUM PERMISSIBLE DOSE (MPD) FOR VETERINARIAN OR ANY EMPLOYEE INVOLVED IN RADIOGRAPHIC PROCEDURES*

	Week	Year
Whole body: Gonads, bone marrow, lens of eyes	100 mrem†	5,000 mrem
Hands, forearms, feet	1,500 mrem	75,000 mrem

*Recommendations of the International Commission on Radiological Protection. (General Public MPD = 1/10 of stated doses.)
†For X ray, milliroentgens (mr) = millirem (mrem).

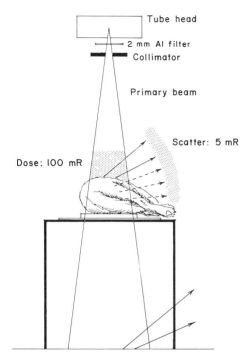

Figure 5–1. Exposure levels in the primary x-ray beam at the top of a dog (32 inches from the x-ray tube) and scattered x-rays at the edge of the table. X-ray machine factors were 80 kv and 10 mas. (after O'Riordan, 1970.)

It should be understood that these are maximum permissible doses. Under proper conditions of practice, these dose levels should never be approached.

EXPOSURE LEVELS

Typical exposure levels in diagnostic radiographic procedures have been calculated (McCullogh and Cameron, 1970; O'Riordan,

1970; Corwin et al., unpublished). Figure 5–1 depicts the situation in which a lateral radiograph of the pelvis of the dog is being produced. The tube head is 40 inches from the table top and the machine factors are 80 kv, 100 ma and 1/10 second or 10 mas. In this situation, a hand exposed to the primary beam on top of the dog would receive about 100 mr per radiograph. At the side of the table, the scatter to the body of the operator, if standing close, could be approximately 5 mr per radiograph. Since radiation intensity decreases to one fourth if the distance between the source (patient's body) and the operator is doubled, further decreased exposure levels may be attained by standing at a maximum distance from the patient (see Chap. 4). There would also be scatter from the floor if the sides of the table are unshielded. If the 2 mm of aluminum filtration were removed, the exposure levels could be three to four times as high. Without proper collimation and filtration or protective apparel, and with careless technique, the operator could possibly receive the weekly MPD to the whole body from a single radiographic procedure.

Figure 5–2 depicts a typical fluoroscopic situation. The exposure level in the primary x-ray beam between the body of the dog and the screen could be of the order of 5000 mr per minute and the scatter from the side of the animal up to 100 mr per minute. Obviously, a few minutes of fluoroscopy exposes the veterinarian to much more radiation than the taking of a single diagnostic radiograph. There is shielding intrinsic to the fluoroscope screen, which protects the operator's face, and there should be a lead drape to the side of the screen to protect the operator's body.

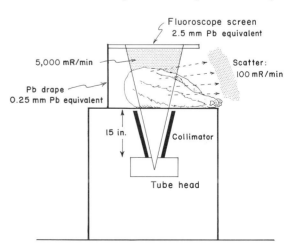

Figure 5–2. Exposure levels in the primary x-ray beam and scattered x-rays from a typical fluoroscopic procedure.

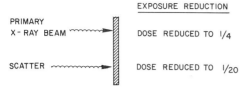

PERSONNEL SHIELDING

0.5 mm LEAD APRONS AND GLOVES

EXPOSURE REDUCTION

PRIMARY
X - RAY BEAM ⟶ DOSE REDUCED TO 1/4

SCATTER ⟶ DOSE REDUCED TO 1/20

Figure 5–3. Approximate exposure reduction provided by protective apparel.

It is assumed that protective apparel such as leaded gloves and aprons would be used in the two procedures depicted. However, veterinarians should understand the limitations of this type of shielding. Protective apparel is designed to protect against scatter radiation, which has lower energy than the primary x-ray beam. The lead shielding material in these gloves and aprons usually will reduce the dose of scatter radiation well below one twentieth of the scatter radiation exposure dose. However, the higher energy of the primary x-ray beam may be only attenuated to one fourth by the gloves (Fig. 5–3). Thus, in the typical diagnostic exposure situation, gloved hands in the primary beam could still receive approximately 25 mr from a single radiographic exposure.

Figure 5–3 schematically illustrates the amount of exposure reduction by gloves and aprons from the primary x-ray beam or scatter radiation. It is assumed that the apron and gloves would have a minimum of 0.5 mm of lead equivalency, which would reduce the primary x-ray intensity to approximately one fourth and that of the scatter radiation to a negligible amount.

Published reports on veterinary personnel exposure and surveys of veterinary radiographic installations have shown that normal exposure to the whole body beneath the protective apron is below measurable levels (Kangstrom and Kilibus, 1972; Unwin, 1970). The dose equivalent to the unprotected areas (head, neck, and elbows) can range between 15 mrem to approximately 100 mrem per week, depending on the work load and the amount of manual restraint performed (Kangstrom and Kilibus, 1972; O'Riordan, 1968; Corwin et al., unpublished). While these exposure levels are still below the MPD levels for the respective body regions, strict radiation safety practices must be maintained to reduce the hazards to as low as reasonably achievable (Jacobsen and van Farowe, 1964).

It should be emphasized that the foregoing MPD levels were established for radiation workers who are working under controlled conditions and wear monitoring devices. The MPD for the general public and for personnel in noncontrolled areas is one tenth of that listed for the radiation worker.

REGULATORY CONTROL

Legal requirements for the use of diagnostic x-ray machines are under the control of the respective states. These requirements are available from the appropriate state agency, usually the State Health Department. The requirements will vary from state to state but usually have the elements shown in Table 5–2. Most states require registration of a diagnostic x-ray machine and will usually survey the machine and the facility after the initial registration. At that time, specific recommendations may be made regarding the equipment and the operative procedures to aid the veterinarian in following proper radiation safety practices. The National Council on Radiation Protection and most present state health codes would permit occupationally exposed persons (i.e., veterinarians and their employees) to manually restrain and position animal patients for radiography when it is absolutely necessary. However, there are

Table 5–2. SUMMARY OF RADIATION PROTECTION RECOMMENDATIONS

Machine:	Properly shielded tube head.
	2 mm aluminum added filtration.
	Rectangular, adjustable collimator and aiming device.
Table:	Permanently mounted fluoroscope screen with shield.
	Shielded table sides.
Personnel:	Lead gloves and apron (0.5 mm lead equivalent).
	Minimum manual restraint.
	Film badge monitoring with monthly report.
	No person under 18 years of age or pregnant female.
Accessories:	Fastest speed screens and film for the procedure.
	Proper radiographic technique and procedures.
Records:	Log to record exposure factors and personnel performing the examination.

state codes in effect that prohibit manual restraint of animals during the production of diagnostic radiographs by occupationally exposed personnel. This would imply that the animal owner or other staff personnel not routinely involved in radiographic procedures would have to be used for this purpose. The present federal regulations concerning performance standards for diagnostic x-ray systems are concerned with diagnostic x-ray machines for use on humans and, at the present time, these regulations are usually interpreted as not applying to veterinary medicine (Federal Register, 1972).

RADIATION PROTECTION FACTORS

Equipment

The radiation produced by a diagnostic x-ray machine must be controlled whether the machine is stationary or portable.

Tube Head. Since the x-ray tube emits radiation in all directions, it is important that the tube head be well shielded. Normally, a properly manufactured tube head can be considered safe. If the machine is old or if there is a question of radiation leakage, the tube head should be checked by a health physicist or by the radiation safety unit of the State Health Department.

Filtration. At least 2 mm of aluminum filtration equivalent should be added to the primary x-ray beam, usually between the tube window and the collimator, to absorb the softer x-rays, which do not contribute to the diagnostic radiograph but do increase exposure to the operator and patient. Without filtration, the exposure doses may be increased three to four times.

Collimator. The collimator should be an adjustable rectangular type, which can restrict the primary beam to within the size of the cassette. A light source that both acts as an aiming device and indicates the limits of the x-ray beam is particularly desirable. With the addition of this type of collimator, the total equivalent aluminum filtration of the primary beam exceeds the recommended total of 2.5 mm of aluminum filtration. To improve the diagnostic quality of the film as well as reduce the scatter radiation exposure to personnel, the collimator should restrict the beam to the area of clinical interest.

Fluoroscope. Hand-held fluoroscopes should never be used. The fluoroscopic unit should be constructed so that the x-ray beam is restricted to the leaded glass screen or the image intensification device. The leaded glass should be at least the equivalent of 1.5 mm of lead with a 0.25 mm lead equivalent drape between the patient and operator. The tube head should be at least 15 inches below the table top, with at least 2.5 mm of aluminum filtration in the primary x-ray beam. If there is a slot for a bucky tray below the table top, it should similarly be shielded by a lead drape.

Portable X-Ray Machines

The foregoing discussion applies to all diagnostic x-ray equipment; however, there are special considerations for portable x-ray machines and their use in large animal radiography. The machines should have a fixed tube stand (Fig. 5–4). It is extremely hazardous for the operator to hold a machine by hand, and some states have regulations that specifically prohibit this (Zontine, 1980). The machine should have an exposure control cord of such a length that the operator can be a minimum of six feet from the tube housing and the exposed part of the animal at the time the exposure is made. To avoid exposure to the primary beam, a cassette holding device should always be used in large animal radiography (Rendano and Watrous, 1980). A cassette holder with a handle must be used for radiography of the extremities (Fig. 5–5).

A wooden block with grooves for the cassette may be used for some radiographic views of the lower extremities (Fig. 5–6). These devices permit the individuals assisting in the procedure to stay out of the primary beam, and they increase the distance from the exposed part of the animal, which is the source of the secondary scatter.

Personnel

Neither persons under 18 years of age nor pregnant women should be involved in radiographic procedures. No individuals other than the operator and those necessarily involved in the procedure should be in the x-ray room when exposures are being made. All persons in the room should wear protec-

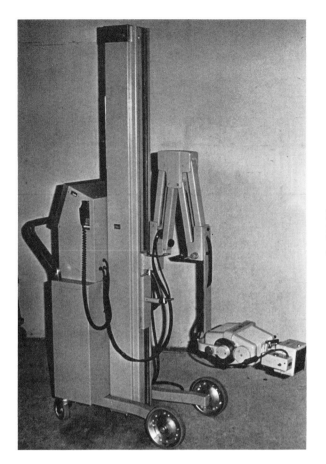

Figure 5–4. A mobile x-ray machine modified for large animal use. Note the fixed tube stand, the adjustable rectangular columnator with light aiming device and the six foot exposure cord.

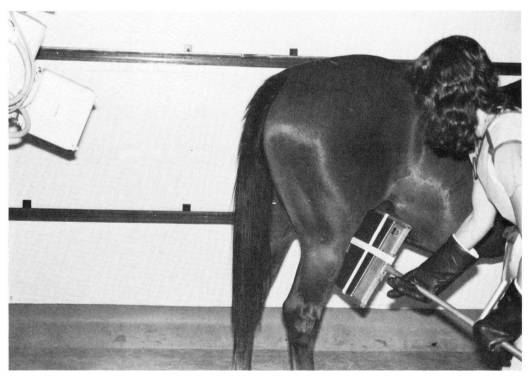

Figure 5–5. A cassette-holding device with handle being used to take the radiograph of the equine stifle. Note that the assistant is out of the primary beam and further from the secondary scatter than he would be if he were holding the cassette by hand.

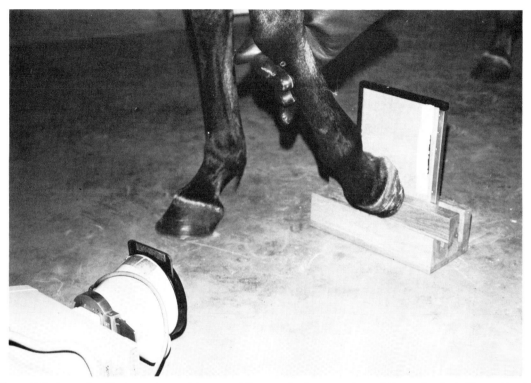

Figure 5–6. A wooden block may be used to support the cassette for some views of the equine foot. The assistant's gloved hands are out of the primary beam and the body is protected from the secondary scatter by the lead apron.

tive apparel. Ideally, the gloves and aprons should have a 0.5 mm lead equivalent. Animals should not be manually restrained for radiography. Chemical restraint, such as short-acting anesthetics or tranquilizers, combined with supporting and restraining devices, should be employed as much as possible. If in the judgment of the clinician, the animal cannot tolerate pharmaceutical restraint, personnel wearing protective gloves and aprons may do so. However, they should position themselves as far away from the primary x-ray beam and the patient as possible. The operator's body should not be exposed to the primary x-ray beam even if shielded, since the type of shielding used usually will not adequately protect against the more penetrating energy of the primary x-ray beam.

Ideally, the animal would be restrained adequately by supporting devices. The operator should be in a shielded booth or behind a shielding screen or at least 6 feet from the x-ray table when the exposure is made (Fig. 5–7).

Fluoroscopic procedures should be performed in a similar manner, with the operator taking particular care not to expose any part of the body or hands to the primary x-ray beam even though wearing protective gloves and apron. Since fluoroscopy is extremely hazardous, because of the potentially high exposures, it should be performed only by qualified personnel and then only when needed to obtain specific diagnostic information. Fluoroscopy should never be used as a substitute for a non-motion radiographic examination. Fluoroscopic procedures should be carefully planned in advance so that the fluoroscope is turned on only for brief periods and the total time kept to an absolute minimum.

Personnel monitoring devices should be worn at all times by any individuals who may be involved in the radiographic procedures. Ideally, two film badges should be worn, one under the protective apparel at the belt level, to monitor whole body exposure, and the other above the protective apparel at the neckline, to estimate the exposure to the skin

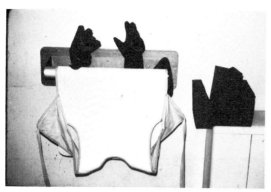

Figure 5–7. Wall rack for proper storage of gloves and aprons in diagnostic x-ray room. Note also foam cushions which aid in positioning to minimize manual restraint.

of the head and neck and the lenses of the eyes. If there is a fairly heavy workload, the use of protective glasses or face shields might be considered. Even ordinary glass eyeglasses will provide protection from the scatter radiation.

Film badges or thermoluminescent dosimeters can be obtained from commercial firms that provide this service for a nominal cost. For the average veterinary practice, the personnel monitors should be exchanged once a month. For practices with a low radiology workload, replacement of the monitors once every three months is probably adequate.

Accessory Equipment

The use of the highest speed screen and fastest film compatible with the radiographic detail requirements will reduce the amount of radiation needed to produce a diagnostic radiograph and, therefore, reduce the exposure to the personnel involved. The recently developed rare earth phosphor screen systems can produce a radiograph equivalent in quality to that made with conventional calcium tungstate screens at one half to one fourth the exposure (Koblik et al., 1980). Proper radiographic technique and darkroom procedures will ensure a quality radiograph and reduce the number of repeat studies, thereby reducing the amount of exposure per examination.

Protective aprons should never be folded flat, since the lead shielding material tends to separate after repeated bendings. A rack should be provided in the diagnostic x-ray

room for proper storage of the aprons (Fig. 5–7). Gloves may be placed on the rack or stored with open-ended cans placed in the gauntlet to permit drying and prevent cracking of the material (Fig. 5–8). All protective apparel should be inspected periodically for defects.

Records

A permanent log should be maintained for each radiographic examination. The date, names of the patient and personnel involved, and the milliamperage, kilovoltage, and exposure time should be recorded. Besides providing useful information that may be used as a check against the technique chart, this record provides an indication of the workload and the amount of radiation to which individuals are exposed. It also provides a guide to permit distributing the workload among all the personnel available so that no one individual is exposed excessively.

Installation

The diagnostic x-ray room should be located away from the traffic flow and in particular away from areas where clients or the general public might be inadvertently exposed. Radiology workload in the average veterinary hospital usually does not require extensive shielding; however, there should be some provision for a primary barrier (Fig. 5–9). This may be any wall or surface through which the primary beam can be directed. A satisfactory amount of shielding is provided

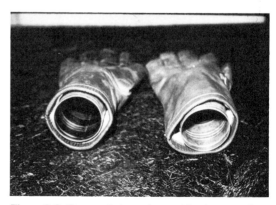

Figure 5–8. Open-ended cans inserted in gloves to allow drying and prevent cracking of shielding material.

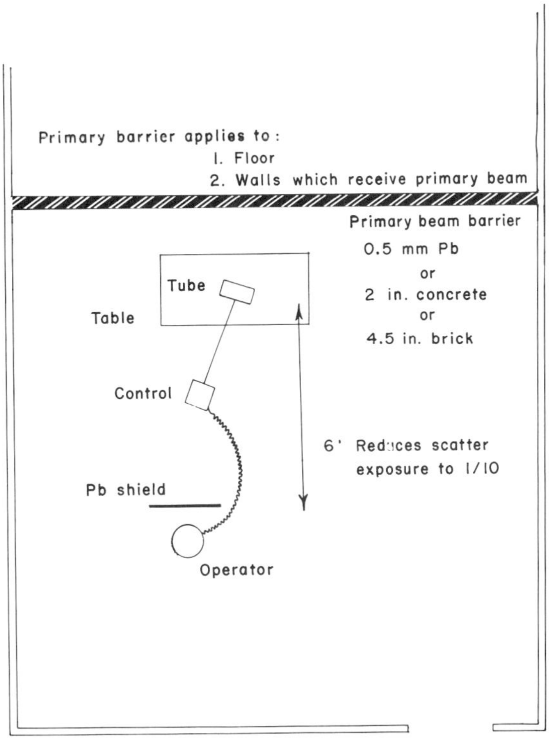

Figure 5–9. Diagram of a typical veterinary diagnostic x-ray room. Ideally the control panel should be located in a shielded booth or behind a barrier. The heavy wall at the top is the primary barrier when producing horizontal beam radiographs. (After O'Riordan, 1970).

by lead and some usual building materials. No barrier wall is necessary if horizontal x-ray beams are directed toward an outside wall. It is recommended that the exposure control be located so that the operator is at least 6 feet from the table at the time the exposure is made, and preferably behind a screen barrier.

REFERENCES

Corwin, L. A., Jr., Lee, P. K., and Larsen, S. J.: Exposure dose to dog gonads in radiography for canine hip dysplasia. Unpublished data, 1975.

Corwin, L. A., Jr., and Lee, P. K.: Exposure levels to personnel in veterinary diagnostic radiography. Unpublished data, 1975.

Council of State Governments: Suggested State Regulations for Control of Radiation. Council of State Governments, 1313 E. 60th St., Chicago, Ill.

Jacobsen, G. A., and van Farowe, D. E.: Survey of x-ray protection practice among Michigan veterinarians. J.A.V.M.A., 145:783, 1964.

Kangstrom, L. E., and Kilibus, A.: Radiation safety in small animal radiography. Acta Radiol. Suppl., 319:147, 1972.

Koblik, P. D., Hornof, W. J., O'Brien, T. R.: Rare earth intensifying screens for veterinary radiography: an evaluation of two systems. Vet. Radiol., 21:224, 1980.

McCullough, C. E., and Cameron, J. R.: Exposure rates from diagnostic x-ray units. Brit. J. Radiol., 43:448, 1970.

Messife, J., Troisi, F. M., and Kleinfield, M.: Radiological hazards due to x-radiation in veterinarians. Amer. Med. Ass. Archiv. Industr. Hlth., 16:48, 1957.

National Council on Radiation Protection and Measurements: Radiation Protection in Veterinary Medicine. Report No. 36, NCRP Publications, Washington, D.C., 1970.

O'Riordan, M. C.: Occupational exposure to x-rays in veterinary practices. Vet. Rec., 82:22, 1968.

O'Riordan, M. C.: Examinations of a veterinary practice for radiation hazards. J. Small Anim. Pract., 11:515, 1970.

Regulations for the Administration and Enforcement of the Radiation Control for Health and Safety Act of 1968. Title 42, Part 78. Federal Register, Vol. 37, No. 158, August 15, 1972.

Rendano, V. T., and Watrous, B. J.: Radiation safety. Mod. Vet. Prac., 61:730, 1980.

Unwin, D. D.: Radiation protection in a veterinary practice. J. Small Anim. Pract., 11:523, 1970.

Zontine, W. J.: Role of radiation safety in equine practice. Proc. Am. Assoc. of Eq. Pract., 26:449, 1980.

6

NEIL KOOYMAN
JAMES W. TICER

Equipping Your Radiology Department

X-RAY EQUIPMENT

Radiographic equipment requirements for veterinary practice vary considerably, depending on caseload, prevalent patient type, and degree of sophistication desired. An outpatient-type of practice that stresses general patient care does not have the same requirements as a larger practice performing more comprehensive care in a hospital environment. Likewise, a practice serving clientele that have predominantly large breeds of dogs as pets does not have the same equipment requirements as a practice serving a population of cat and small dog owners.

Equipment for large animal practices requires mobility for producing radiographs of extremities. This equipment must usually be portable so that it may be transported to the patient. High milliamperage, stationary equipment is usually needed to examine the thorax, pelvis and proximal femur and is desirable for examining the head, neck, and proximal thoracic limb.

Unfortunately, requirements based on need must also be tempered by economics. Generally, the higher the milliamperage and the shorter the timing capabilities of the equipment, the greater will be the costs. A balance of requirements and costs must therefore be attained during the planning stage of any construction or upgrading program.

Basic Equipment

Basic radiographic equipment that is necessary to perform routine radiographic examinations includes the x-ray generating system (consisting of controls, high voltage transformer, and x-ray tubes), the x-ray beam localizing system (collimator), the grid, and the handling devices (which include the table, tubestand, and positioning aids).

Controls. The x-ray control system contains all of the circuitry necessary to vary independently the x-ray tube current (ma), the voltage applied across the tube (kv), and the time of exposure. The degree of independence and reproducibility or accuracy of these three parameters and the magnitude of the power to be controlled determine the size and complexity of the components and circuitry. Standard items in the control system are an x-ray tube starter and power circuits for locks, Bucky motor, lights, and other auxiliary equipment. Optional equipment in the control system includes circuits for tube protection, fluoroscopy, spot film device, and photo-timing. The physical size of the control, then, is determined by the space needed to house all the circuits in such a way that they are serviceable. Solid state circuitry has enabled manufacturers to reduce the physical size and weight of the controls, which, in turn, makes installation, servicing, and space-planning less of a problem than in the past.

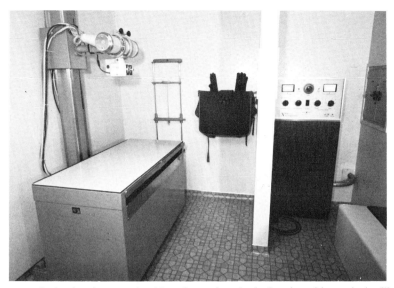

Figure 6–1. An x-ray unit showing the control, table, tubestand, and tube housing with attached collimator. Courtesy of Drs. R. L. Maahs and Robert Conness, San Carlos, California.

A typical 300 ma, 125 kv, 1/60 sec time control is shown in Figure 6–1.

For the modern, nonspecialty small animal practice, a single phase control rated for 200 to 300 ma at 125 kv, with at least 1/60 sec timing, will provide the necessary range of exposure capabilities for most routine examinations. Some of the features found in this size control which are not usually found in the smaller 30 to 100 ma controls are preset ma stations activated by dial or pushbutton, space charge compensation, accurate kilovoltage selection in small increments (1 to 2 kv) over the whole kilovoltage range, electronic timing, line voltage compensation, tube protection circuits, ma stabilization, and, in some controls, electronic contacting. With a control of this type, the unpredictable results caused by smaller, less expensive controls is replaced with greater predictability.

Outpatient practices with a preponderance of the caseload consisting of small dogs and cats may find 100 ma control systems to be adequate. This is particularly true when a well-equipped hospital facility is available for referral of larger patients or those requiring complicated special radiographic procedures. A minimal timing capability of 1/60 sec is highly recommended with a 100 ma unit, since quality radiography of rapidly breathing patients requires short exposure times. The recently available rare earth phosphor intensifying screens, with their increased speed, allow utilization of faster exposure times,

since the mas requirements are decreased. With their use, 1/120 sec exposures may become routine.

Central hospital facilities and specialty practices usually find minimal ma requirements to be in the 300 to 500 ma range. In this milliamperage range, 1/120 sec timing is practical and desirable. Solid state or electronic contacting makes the 1/120 sec timer reliable.

High Voltage Transformer. The high voltage transformer is electrically matched to the control system and is contained in a separate metal enclosure. This enclosure contains the core and windings of the high voltage transformer, the filament transformers for the x-ray tubes, the cable socket changeover switch if more than one tube is to be used, the cable sockets for the high voltage cables, the rectification circuit, and the insulating coil. The size of the enclosure has been reduced recently to about one half its former size and weight owing to the use of solid state rectifiers and smaller transformer cores. Along with this reduction in size, the efficiency and reproducibility of output have been improved.

X-Ray Tube. The x-ray tube used with high milliamperage controls is commonly a double focus rotating anode tube. Recent improvements in this type of tube have been in the radiation shielding of the housing. The rhenium-tungsten-copper anode is the most common type in use presently and it differs from the solid tungsten-copper anode in its improved ability to dissipate heat. The improved shielding reduces leakage of radiation below the amount allowed by law.

X-Ray Localizing System. The collimation system (Fig. 6–1) aligns and modifies the conical x-ray beam so that it conforms to the size of the film being used or patient part being examined. Manually operated, multi-leaved collimators that provide a light field coincident with the x-ray beam have replaced cones as the means of accomplishing beam shaping. With these collimators, exposures can be reduced to the desired rectangular (or circular in some cases) shape, thereby reducing scatter radiation to the point where split film techniques can be performed without additional lead shielding.

It is a common practice when using a Bucky mechanism or stationary grid cabinet to have the central x-ray beam centered to the cassette by coupling the tubestand to the Bucky or grid cabinet. With the cassette secured in a cassette tray inside the Bucky or grid cabinet under the table, it is difficult to know the exact longitudinal and transverse settings of the collimator that will coincide with film size. To remedy this, the Federal regulations (in effect after 1974) require that sensing devices be used to determine the size of the film in the cabinet tray and to automatically set the collimator opening to this size before an exposure can be made. Although these regulations apply only to medical radiography, the benefits of automatically limiting beam size and thus reducing scatter radiation are desirable in veterinary practice as well.

The use of a Bucky mechanism or stationary grid is necessary in medium-to-thick body part examination. Good clean-up of scatter radiation is obtained with either an 8:1, 80 line per inch stationary grid or a par speed 8:1, 80 line per inch Bucky device. Stationary grids with increased lines per inch improve the quality of radiographs by decreasing visibility of grid lines. The motion and noise of the older model Bucky mechanism usually do not produce patient excitement while the film is being made since the maximum sound is emitted by this device when the grid travel is terminated, which is after an exposure has been made. Modern reciprocating or reciprocatic Bucky mechanisms are relatively quiet and produce no patient excitement problem.

Handling Devices. Handling devices such as the table, tubestand, and positioning aids deserve special consideration when designing an x-ray department. Equipment construction should allow for the following: easy placement of the x-ray tube and film holder in line with the part of the body to be examined; positioning of the patient so that personnel can be in a protected area when the exposure is made (this area usually requires the most improvement); and adequate size to accommodate all patients. A table-tubestand combination such as the one shown in Figure 6–1 fulfills essential construction requirements. The tubestand should move the entire length of the table, hold the x-ray tube so that the central x-ray beam is centered to the table and Bucky cabinet, allow the tube to be moved vertically to 40 inches from the table top, and allow the tube to be rotated for horizontal exposures. The tubestand should be attached to the Bucky or grid cabinet so that the central x-ray beam is always centered on the cassette tray for routine exposure technique. Alternatively, a light beam emitted from the collimator may be used to assist in proper location of the cabinet. This type of table-tubestand combination is made by a number of manufacturers and usually measures about 3 feet in width (including the tubestand) and about 5 feet in

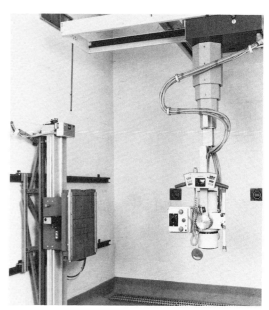

Figure 6–2. An x-ray unit designed for producing horizontal beam radiographs of standing large animal patients. The tube head may be rotated and used to produce vertical beam radiographs of recumbent patients. Courtesy of Dr. Crispen Spencer, University of Florida.

length. For veterinary use, this device should be free of dirt-catching edges.

A ceiling-mounted tube stand and wall mounted grid cabinet make an ideal arrangement for examining the thorax, head, neck and proximal limbs of large animals (Fig. 6–2). The tube head should rotate so that it may be used for producing vertical beam radiographs when the patient is recumbent. The grid should have a focal range of up to 72 inches for thoracic radiography. The wall mounted grid cabinet may contain a Bucky mechanism.

Some available positioning and restraining devices are shown in Figure 6–3. (See Atlas section for further illustration of these devices.) These devices assist in positioning the patient and permit the operator to make exposures from a protected area. The need for a complete restraining-positioning device which will accommodate all patients is obvious.

Special Purpose Equipment

Special purpose radiographic equipment is being used with increased frequency by teaching institutions, specialty practices, and some group practices. Requirements for special equipment used in motion studies and body section examinations vary considerably with caseload and degree of sophistication desired. Generally, a system for image intensification fluoroscopy is needed in specialty practices and teaching institutions where motion studies are a routine part of internal medical examinations. A method of recording the fluoroscopic image for future detailed study should also be provided. This may be accomplished with cine photographic filming, videotape or disc recordings, or by the use of a spot filming device. Cine filming and videotaping provide recordings of motion, whereas a spot filming device records a series of single radiographic images.

Rapid sequential filming is usually accomplished with a rapid film changer. This equipment is used to provide a detailed record of dynamic studies.

Body section equipment may be desirable for specialized studies where the details of structure may be obscured by overlying body parts.

The generator used for special procedure equipment is generally more complex and contains more protective devices than those used for basic radiographic equipment. Capabilities as high as 1000 ma, single or three phase, may be required for the extremely

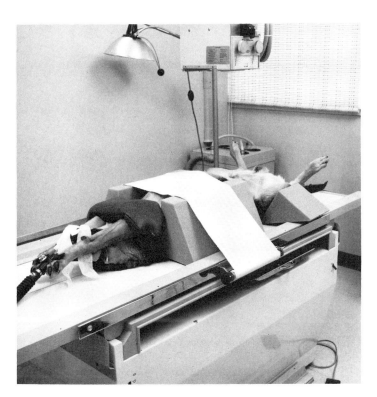

Figure 6–3. Positioning aids. Sponge blocks, sand bags, and compression band shown in use during the examination of an abdomen.

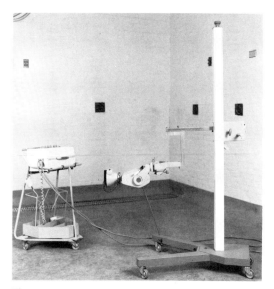

Figure 6–4. A portable x-ray machine with 20 ma, 100 kv and 1/10 sec timing capabilities. Note the tube stand for supporting the tube housing. The control stand may be detached so that bulk and weight of the unit may be decreased for greater mobility. Courtesy of Dr. Crispen Spencer, University of Florida.

short exposure times needed in some rapid film changer studies.

Special tables with four-way moving tops, with space underneath to house either an x-ray tube or imaging system, are normally used for special radiographic procedures. The tubestand or tubestands should be ceiling-mounted to allow freedom of movement on all sides of the table and to save valuable floor space for the ancillary equipment that is often needed.

Image Amplifier Systems. Most dynamic special examinations are not possible without an image amplifier system. Basically, the image amplifier converts the fluoroscopic image at its input surface to an image 3000 to 10,000 times the intensity of a fluoroscopic screen. The image at the output side is then viewed directly by a mirror optical system or by a closed circuit television camera, or is recorded on 16, 35, 70, or 100 mm photographic film. If a video system is used, videotape or core recorders may be used to preserve the dynamic portions of an examination for future review and study. Slow motion and still frame techniques increase the usefulness of the video recording methods.

Rapid Film Changers. Rapid film changers are used to record dynamic studies radiographically. They find extensive use in cardiovascular studies where radiographic detail is needed. Cassette changers have exposure rates of up to 2 per second and the cut film changers have exposure rates up to 12 exposures per second.

Mobile X-Ray Equipment. Mobile x-ray equipment may be desirable for mixed practices or large animal practices in which examinations of the head, neck, shoulder and stifle joint are routinely performed. Two types of mobile equipment are available: the conventional high voltage, single-phase transformer type and the capacitor discharge type. The conventional type is a mobile version of the basic generator and varies in size from a 30 ma, self-contained x-ray tube machine to a 300 ma, 125 kv machine. Increased ma capacity requires that high ampere power sources be available where the machine is operated, thus requiring extensive hospital wiring for great mobility. A capacitor dis-

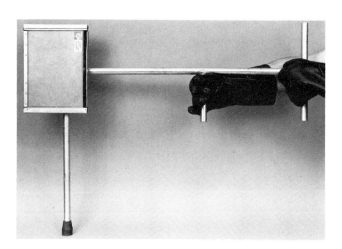

Figure 6–5. A cassette holding device with a long handle that allows the person holding the cassette to stand remote from the primary x-ray beam. Also note the extension "foot" that aids in stabilizing the cassette when it is resting on the floor. Courtesy of Dr. Crispen Spencer, University of Florida.

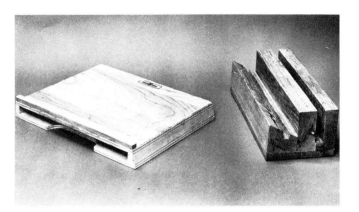

Figure 6–6. A cassette tunnel and a slotted wooden positioning block for examining the phalanges and navicular bone.

charge unit alleviates the wiring problem, since high voltage applied across the x-ray tube is built up over a Villard-type voltage doubling circuit, thus eliminating the high voltage transformer. When the charge is sufficient, an exposure can be made. Power input may be provided by conventional 110 volt electrical outlets.

Portable X-Ray Equipment. Most large animal extremity examinations are made with portable equipment. The capacity is usually between 10 and 25 ma, 90 to 100 kv with timing minimums of 1/20 second. The tube and control may be contained in the same housing; if the tube housing is separated, however, the size and weight may be decreased, making mobility easier (Fig. 6–4). The tube should be mounted on a tube stand so that it need not be held by hand.

The use of portable and mobile x-ray equipment requires special devices that allow the person holding the cassette to stand outside the range of the primary x-ray beam. This is usually best accomplished with the use of a cassette holding device with a long handle (Fig. 6–5). The use of an extendable "foot" aides the operator in steadily supporting the cassette. This device may be as simple as a metal tube that slides through a sleeve and is fixed in position with a thumb screw.

Cassette support for examining large animal phalanges may be provided by a slotted wooden positioning block or the cassette may be inserted into a wooden tunnel when the patient must stand on the cassette (Fig. 6–6). Figure 6–7 shows the positioning block in use for examining the navicular bone.

A grid with metal channels attached makes a convenient method of holding a cassette adjacent to the grid surface while performing examinations with portable equipment (Figure 6–8). A wall-mounted grid cabinet is very

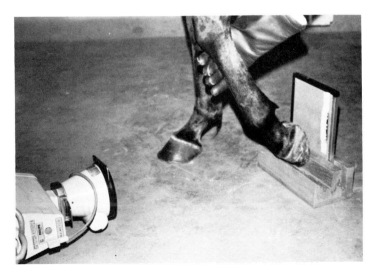

Figure 6–7. A slotted wooden positioning block being used to support the foot and cassette while examining navicular bone.

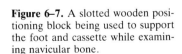

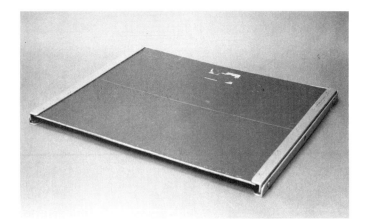

Figure 6–8. A grid with metal channels attached for holding a cassette adjacent to the surface.

helpful when examining thick large animal parts in the standing position. This is especially true for thoracic examinations when it is difficult to align the grid and cassette with the central x-ray beam with the patient placed between the two objects. In this case, alignment of the cassette and x-ray tube may be accomplished before the patient is moved into position. In some cases, radiographic detail may be improved while examining a thick part such as the skull or neck by making the exposure through the metal back of a cassette instead of using a grid. These cassettes must not have strap-type fastening devices that will interfere with the image formation. The thin metal sheet in the back of cassettes is designed to prevent the relatively nonpenetrating back scatter from producing fog on the film. When an exposure is made through the back of the cassette, a significant portion of the scatter radiation produced by a thick patient part may also be removed (Spencer, 1982). This method works well when low ma portable equipment is used, since the increase exposure requirements are not as great as when using a grid.

Automatic Film Processors. Automatic film processors are now available in a price range such that a busy practice should seriously consider their use. The large processors, initially used only in major hospitals, have decreased in cost and physical size. Small processors may fit into existing darkrooms and thus require minimal installation effort and expense (Fig. 6–9). Automatic film processing not only provides consistent results, but also, and more importantly, the availability of a readable, diagnostic radiograph with minimal time and effort encourages the use of radiographic examinations.

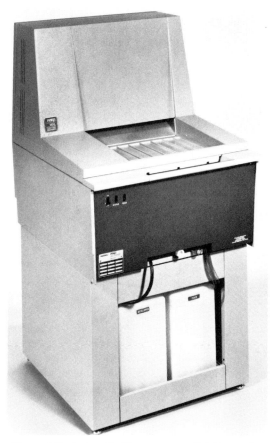

Figure 6–9. Automatic film processor. Solution replenisher tanks are located under the stand.

REFERENCES

Jaundrell-Thompson, F., and Ashworth, W.J.: X-ray Physics and Equipment. 2nd ed. Philadelphia. F.A. Davis Co., 1965.

Spencer, C.P.: personal communications, 1982.

NEIL KOOYMAN

7

Planning Your X-ray Department

LAYOUT AND PLANNING

The layout and planning of your x-ray department should start by integrating the location of the department into the overall traffic-flow plan of the clinic or hospital. In general, the department should be adjacent to the patient preparation area and near the surgery area. There should be sufficient isolation so that each area can be used simultaneously. Once the general area is defined, a representative of the company providing the x-ray equipment should be consulted to determine the floor space needed, and a preliminary drawing locating the equipment should be made. Given this preliminary drawing, along with electrical requirements, junction box locations and plumbing requirements, the architect and contractor should be able to integrate the department's location into the total hospital plan.

FLOOR PLANS

Floor plans and photographs of existing effectively functional veterinary radiology departments which were economical to build in terms of time and cost of construction are shown in Figures 7–1, 7–4, and 7–6. Department size and equipment capabilities were chosen to illustrate the needs of a small practice, a group practice, and a specialty

practice. Dimensions are included only as guidelines for space required.

Generally, two or three junction boxes and a circuit breaker are needed in each x-ray room. Table 7–1 lists the minimum power supply requirements needed for various types of x-ray machines.

Accessory equipment should be located on the drawing during the planning stage. This equipment should include safelights, film bins, cassette transfer box, film dryer, view boxes (both wet and dry), imprinter for labeling film, apron and glove racks, wall cassette holder, and cassette storage cabinets.

In order to enhance visualization of the collimator light field, the lighting in the x-ray room should not create a glare on the table top.

The darkroom should be adjacent to the x-ray room so that a cassette transfer box may be used to good advantage. This box may also be used to store cassettes.

An exhaust fan and light-tight louvered door vent are desirable darkroom items, especially when the work load is heavy. These items improve working conditions especially during warm weather or when a film dryer or automatic processor adds heat to the room.

Finally, you should provide a place to sit down and review the finished radiographic study (Fig. 7–10). At least two view boxes are needed so that the multiple view studies

Text continued on page 93

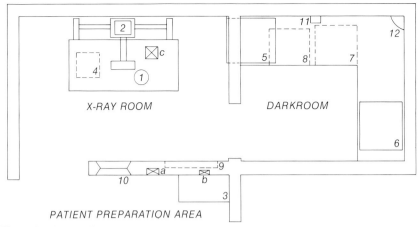

Figure 7–1. Floor plan for a radiology department suitable for a one- or two-person small animal practice. *1,* X-ray table; *2,* tubestand; *3,* x-ray control; *4,* high voltage transformer; *5,* cassette transfer cabinet; *6,* developing tank; *7,* film dryer; *8,* film bin; *9,* illuminator; *10,* leaded window; *11,* imprinter; *12,* safelight; *a,* circuit breaker; *b,* junction box; *c,* floor junction box.

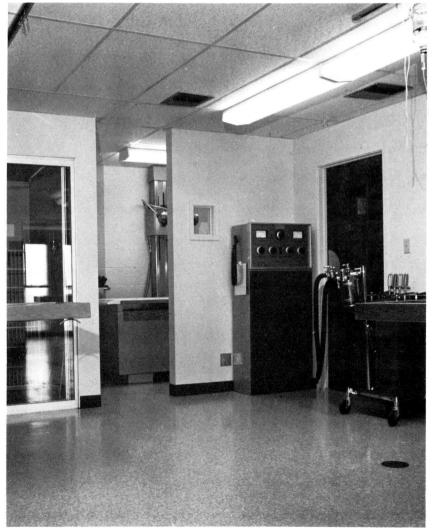

Figure 7–2. View of the x-ray control, leaded window, and door into the x-ray room from the preparation room. Floor plan is as shown in Figure 7–1. Courtesy of Dr. J. E. Rieger, Concord, California.

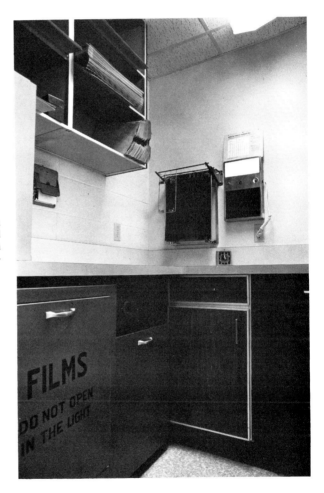

Figure 7–3. View of the darkroom dry bench from the x-ray room. Note the film storage bin and dryer under the bench. Floor plan is as shown in Figure 7–1. Courtesy of Dr. J. E. Rieger, Concord, California.

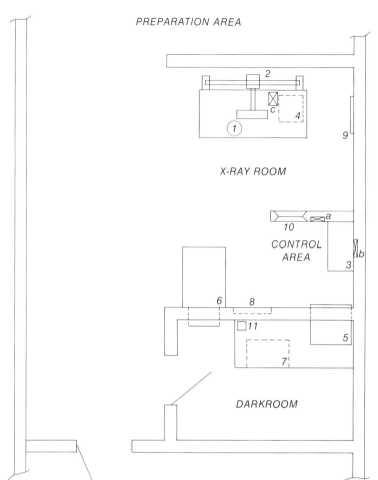

PREPARATION AREA

X-RAY ROOM

CONTROL
AREA

DARKROOM

Figure 7–4. Floor plan for a radiology department suitable for a group practice. *1,* X-ray table; *2,* tubestand; *3,* x-ray control; *4,* high voltage transformer; *5,* cassette transfer cabinet; *6,* automatic processor; *7,* film bin; *8, 9,* illuminator; *10,* leaded window; *11,* imprinter; *a,* circuit breaker; *b,* junction box; *c,* floor junction box.

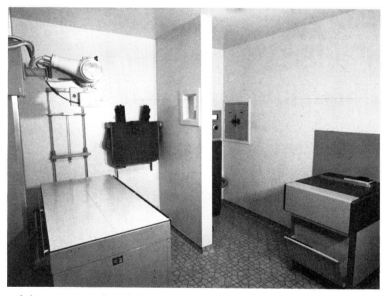

Figure 7–5. View of the x-ray room from hallway. The control is located behind a leaded barrier with a leaded window. The cassette transfer cabinet is located in the wall beside the control. The output of a small automatic processor is installed in the darkroom wall. Floor plan is as shown in Figure 7–4. Courtesy of Drs. R. L. Maahs and Robert Conness, San Carlos, California.

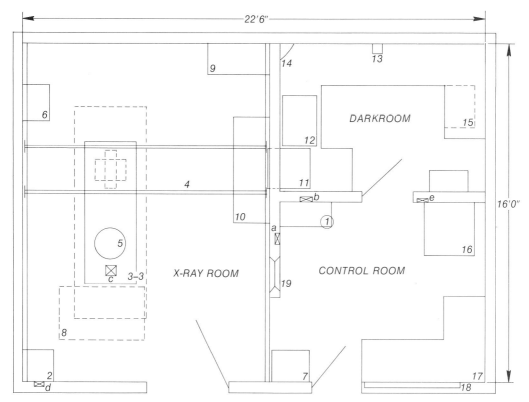

Figure 7–6. Floor plan for a radiology department suitable for a specialty practice. *1,* 300–600 ma x-ray control; *2,* high voltage transformer; *3,* four-way floating table; *4,* overhead tubestand; *5,* image amplifier and television camera under table; *6,* television monitor mounted on wall tracks or cart; *7,* videotape and remote TV monitor; *8,* floor area for film changer; *9,* cardiac monitoring equipment; *10,* sink and storage area; *11,* cassette transfer cabinet; *12,* developing tank covered by hinged counter top; *13,* film imprinter; *14,* safelight; *15,* film bin; *16,* automatic film processor; *17,* film sorting and viewing area; *18,* illuminators; *19,* leaded window; *a,* 70–100 amp circuit breaker, single phase, 220 volt; *b,* wall junction box; *c,* floor junction box; *d,* wall junction box; *e,* 40 amp circuit breaker.

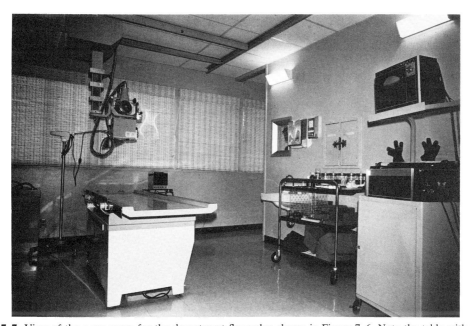

Figure 7–7. View of the x-ray room for the department floor plan shown in Figure 7–6. Note the table with a four-way moving top which contains image intensification and video systems. The TV monitors are seen behind the table and on the right. The large monitor is placed on a cart above a videotape recorder. Note also that the x-ray tube is suspended on a ceiling mounted tubestand. Courtesy of the Berkeley Veterinary Medical Group, Berkeley, California.

89

Table 7-1. XR4-10 MINIMUM POWER SUPPLY REQUIREMENTS COMING TO X-RAY MACHINES

Classification	Rated Ma. @	Output KvP.	Nominal Line Voltage (see Note IV)	Recommended Distrib. Transformer Capacity (KVA)	Wire Size (AWG) from Distrib. Transformer to Disconnecting Means (See Note III) 50'	100'	200'	Wire Size (AWG) from Disconnecting Means to X-Ray Control for Approx. Length of 15'	Grounding Wire Size (AWG)	X-ray Disconnecting Means — Alternate 1 Switch & Fuse: Switch Rating (AMP)	Fuse Rating (AMP)	Alternate 2 Circuit Breaker Rating (AMP)
SELF-RECTIFIED X-RAY MACHINES For Radiography and Fluoroscopy (including dental, portable, mobile, and stationary types)	10	70	120	*1.5		10		12	14	(15)30	15	15
	15	90–100	120	*1.5		8		10	14	(15)30	20	20
	15	90–100	240	*1.5		12		12	14	(15)30	15	15
	30	85	120	5	8	6	3	10	14	(20)30	30**	30
	30	85	240	5	10	8	6	14	14	30	15**	15
	50–60	85	240	10	8	6	3	8	10	60	50	50
	100	100	240	15	4	2	00	8	10	60	60	60
FULL WAVE RECTIFIED X-RAY MACHINES For Radiography and Fluoroscopy (including mobile and stationary types)	50	100	120	5	6	4	1	10	12	60	40	40
	100	100	240	7.5	8	6	3	10	12	60	40	40
	200	125	240	15	4	2	00	8	10	60	60	60
	200	125	240	25	4	2	00	8	10	60	60	60
	300	125	240	25	2	00	250 MCM	6	8	100	70	70
	300	150	240	37.5	2	00	250 MCM	6	8	100	100	100
	400	125	240	37.5	2	00	250 MCM	4	8	100	100	100
	500	125	240	50	1	000	300 MCM	4	6	200	125	125
	500	150	240	50	0	0000	350 MCM	2	6	200	150	150
	600	125	240	50	0	0000	350 MCM	2	6	200	150	150
	600	150	480	75	6	4	1	6	8	100	100	100
	800	125	480	75	4	2	00	6	6	200	110	110
	1000	100	480	75	4	2	00	6	6	200	110	110

Machine type												
THREE-PHASE X-RAY MACHINES For Radiography and Fluoroscopy (stationary types)	500	100	240	45	3	0	0000	2	8	100	80	100
	700	100	240	75	3	0	0000	0	6	200	110	125
	1000	100	240	112.5	1	000	300 MCM	00	6	200	175	175
	1000	100	480	112.5	6	4	1	6	8	100	80	100
	1250	100	480	150.0	6	3	0	6	6	200	110	125
	1500	100	480	150.0	4	2	00	4	6	200	125	125
HALF-WAVE RECTIFIED X-RAY MACHINES	50	60	240	5	10	8	6	12	14	30	25	30
	10	120	120	3	10	8	6	10	14	30	25	30
	10	120	240	3	14	12	8	14	14	30	15	15
	10	140	120	3	10	8	6	10	14	30	25	30
	10	140	240	3	14	12	8	14	14	30	15	15
	30	150	240	7.5	6	4	1	8	10	60	40	40

*Any line with 3 per cent regulation will be suitable.

**Use time lag fuses.

( )Suitable attachment plug receptacles of rating indicated may be utilized.

NOTE I   The above specifications are the minimum requirements for a single X-Ray machine of the rating specified.

NOTE II   The maximum recommended daily line voltage variation, due to causes other than the X-Ray equipment load, should not exceed ±2¹/₂ per cent from the nominal circuit voltage.

NOTE III   The wire sizes "Size Wire (AWG) from Distribution Transformer to X-Ray Disconnecting Means" are based on runs of 50, 100, and 200 feet. If the run is over 200 feet, the manufacturer should be consulted.

NOTE IV   If more than one X-Ray machine is to be used, or additional load is contemplated for the future, larger wire and Transformer size must be specified for satisfactory operation.

NOTE V   The power supply requirements for radiographic and fluoroscopic X-Ray machines are based on an overall line voltage regulation not exceeding 5 per cent as measured at the X-Ray Control at maximum rated output.

NOTE VI   Should the supply line voltage be 208 volts rather than 240 volts, it is recommended that the wire size from the distribution transformer to the disconnect switch be increased to the next larger size.

(From Fischer X-Ray Manual, H. G. Fischer, Inc., Franklin Park, Ill.)

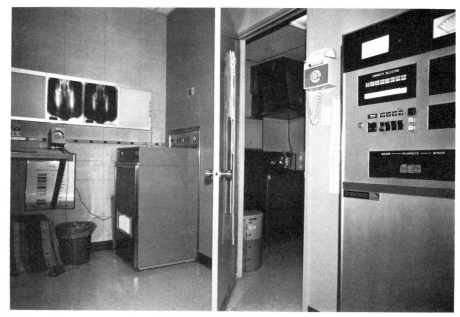

Figure 7–8. View of the control room from the x-ray room for the department shown in Figure 7–6. Note the control on the right and the automatic processor on the left. Processing tanks and dryer mounted overhead are seen through the darkroom door. At times, manual capabilities are desirable for emergency use and for processing some nonscreen film. Courtesy of the Berkeley Veterinary Medical Group, Berkeley, California.

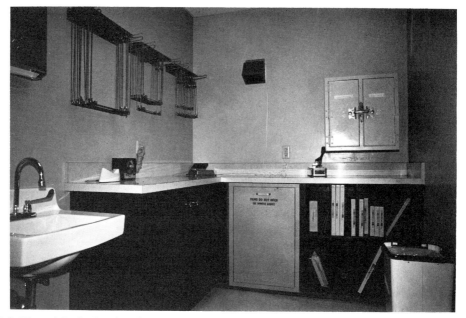

Figure 7–9. View of the dry bench and cassette transfer cabinet for the department shown in Figure 7–6. Courtesy of the Berkeley Veterinary Medical Group, Berkeley, California.

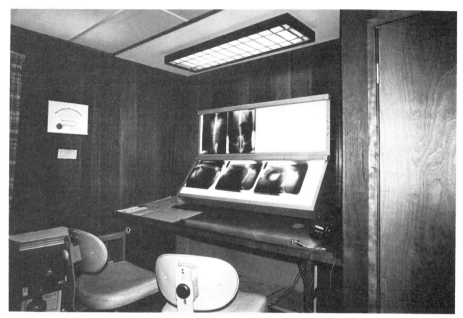

Figure 7–10. View boxes arranged so that multiple-view radiographic studies may be reviewed. This mobile bank of view boxes is surrounded by a slotted table that may be removed to allow transport to a conference room. Courtesy of the Berkeley Veterinary Medical Group, Berkeley, California.

may be examined simultaneously. Multiple view box banks are highly desirable, especially for practices in which multiple view special examinations are performed.

REFERENCE

Scott, W. G., Ed.: Planning Guide for Radiologic Installations. 2nd ed. Baltimore, Williams and Wilkins, 1966.

8

ROBERT E. LEWIS

Setting Fees for Survey Radiographs

Many methods have been used for determining fees for veterinary service, most of which have not been based on cost accounting procedures. For a number of years it was common practice to have close agreement between veterinarians on the fee for a particular procedure. This philosophy ignored the fact that different practices had different costs associated with certain procedures and therefore required a different fee.

When the fee is the same for different practices but the costs are different, the practice with the least costs has the potential for a greater "profit." The practice with the greater costs (larger capacity equipment; newer, more efficient screens; automatic processing; and so forth) will probably not make a "profit" and may actually lose money ("lost leader") on providing radiology service.

The cost accounting technique that is the most accurate for establishing fees is the break-even concept. In this technique the fixed costs (those that do not vary with number of the procedures) and variable costs (those that vary with the number of the procedures) are determined. When the number of procedures is known, a fee for each procedure can be calculated that will pay for all of the fixed and variable costs (Fig. 8–1).

The two most common fixed costs are facilities and equipment. Three types of variable costs are personnel, expendable supplies, and administrative.

For this illustration, the fixed costs will be established by determining the value of facilities (Table 8–1) and equipment (Table 8–2)

94

and calculating a return on investment based on a moderate risk (18 per cent). The building is assessed according to the number of square feet that produce income, i.e., examination rooms, surgery, laboratory, pharmacy, wards. Examples of non–income-producing areas are the reception area, the veterinarian's office, rest rooms, hallways and storage areas. In most veterinary hospitals, the income-producing areas constitute 55 to 65 per cent of the total space.

Equipment is usually classified as items expected to last over one year and costing over $50.00.

The total annual cost of facilities and equipment must also include any maintenance, taxes, and insurance (Tables 8–1 and 8–2).

The assumptions for personnel cost are shown in Table 8–3. The hourly personnel costs are calculated assuming the veterinarian and technician are carrying out income-producing procedures (procedures or service for which the client pays) 60 per cent of the total number of hours employed.

The costs for expendable items are shown in Table 8–4. The items listed represent those required for a radiographic examination of one anatomical part using two views. The value of the expendables is assumed to be an investment of dollars (in inventory, ready to use) and is therefore entitled to return on investment.

The administrative cost includes those items not listed previously and not easily identified with a single procedure or service. These include receptionist's salary; accoun-

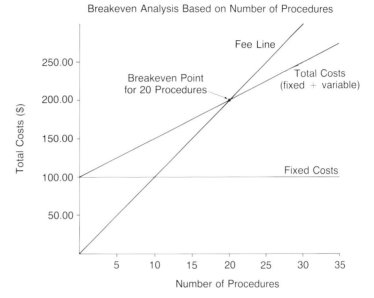

Figure 8–1. Graph showing break-even concept. The horizontal axis represents the number of procedures; the vertical axis represents dollars. The fixed costs are $100. The variable cost per procedure is $5. It is assumed that 20 procedures will be performed. A fee of $10 thus generates $200 when 20 procedures are performed, which will equal the fixed costs of $100 + variable costs ($5 × 20) of $100.

Table 8–1. COST OF FACILITIES

Land	$ 30,000.00
Building—1700 sq. ft @ $50/sq. ft.	85,000.00
Land Improvement	15,000.00
Total Investments	$130,000.00
Return on Investment (annual cost of 18%)	$ 23,400.00
Insurance	1,000.00
Taxes	1,500.00
Maintenance	1,100.00
Annual Cost of Hospital Facilities	$ 27,000.00
Annual Cost Per Income-Producing Square Footage (assuming 1,100 sq. ft.)	$ 24.55
Assume 110 Square Feet Used for Radiology; Thus, Annual Cost of Radiology Facilities	$ 2,700.50

Table 8–2. COST OF EQUIPMENT

X-ray machine	$ 10,000
Developing Tanks	500
Darkroom Equipment (timer, safelights, hangers, photoprinters, film storage cabinet)	450
Cassettes (4)	800
Gloves (2) and Aprons (2)	400
Viewers (4)	350
File Cabinets	200
Total Investment	$ 12,700
Return on investment (annual cost of 18%)	$ 2,286
Maintenance	214
Annual Cost of Equipment	$ 2,500

Table 8–3. COST OF PERSONNEL

	Veterinarian	Technician
Salary	$30,000.00	$10,000.00
Benefits	6,000.00	1,500.00
Total Cost of Benefits	$36,000.00	11,500.00
Assumed Total Income-Producing Hours	1,500.00	1,248.00
Cost per Income-Producing Hour	$ 24.00	$ 9.21

tant and lawyer fees; telephone, utilities, and bank charges; office supplies; continuing education; licenses; and so forth. In most practices this will amount to about 20 per cent of the total cost.

The summary of these data, assuming the foregoing costs and a radiographic case load of 150 per year, is listed in Table 8–5.

Table 8–4. COST OF EXPENDABLE SUPPLIES

Film (@ $2.50 × 2)	$5.00
Developing Chemical (@ 50¢ per film)	1.00
Identification Costs	.10
Envelope for Film	.15
Cost of Items	$6.25
Return on Investment (18% Annually)	$1.13
Cost of Expendables for One Anatomical Area (2 Views)	$7.38

The veterinarian is given 15 minutes to interpret the radiographs and explain the results to the owner. The procedure requires 45 minutes of technician time (two people × 15 minutes to expose the two radiographs, plus one person × 15 minutes to process, dry, code and file the radiographs).

The total cost is probably more than that charged by most practices. If your costs are similar, then radiology is a lost leader in the practice. In this case other areas such as vaccinations and pharmacy must generate more income than expenses to pay for the loss in radiology.

Consideration must also be given if the numbers of cases radiographed per year is different. If the number of cases is less than the 150 used in the illustration the cost will be higher than that given in Table 8–5. If the number is greater because one veterinarian is radiographing a higher percentage of cases or because more than one veterinarian is using the same facility and equipment, there

Table 8–5. COST OF ONE RADIOGRAPHIC EXAMINATION (BASED ON 150 CASES PER YEAR)

	Cost per Procedure
I. **Facilities:** Annual Cost ÷ Number of Cases $2,700 ÷ 150	$18.00
II. **Equipment:** Annual Cost ÷ Number of Cases $2,500 ÷ 150	16.67

III. **Personnel:**
A. Veterinarian:
   Hourly Rate × 0.25 (15 minutes)
      $24.00 × 0.25
	6.00

B. Technician:
   Hourly Rate × 0.75 (45 minutes)
      $9.21 × 0.75
	6.91

IV. **Expendables**	7.38
Total Cost of Facilities, Equipment, Personnel, Expendables	$54.96
V. **Administrative Cost** (20% of the above total)	10.99
Total Cost of 2 Radiographs of One Anatomical Part	$65.96

will be a reduction in the fixed costs (facilities and equipment).

If one veterinarian radiographed 450 cases or 3 veterinarians in the same practice radiographed 450 cases (150 each), the cost would be reduced (Table 8–6). In this example the cost of producing radiographs in a low case load facility is over 70 percent more expensive than that in a high case load.

All of these data are used for illustration purposes. Each practice must determine its cost and number of cases radiographed and calculate the fee for a break-even point.

Table 8–6. COST OF ONE RADIOGRAPHIC EXAMINATION (BASED ON 450 CASES PER YEAR)

	Cost Per Procedure
I. **Facilities:** Annual Cost ÷ Number of Cases $2,700 ÷ 450	$ 6.00
II. **Equipment:** Annual Cost ÷ Number of Cases $2,500 ÷ 450	5.56

III. **Personnel:**
A. Veterinarian:
   Hourly Rate × 0.25 (15 minutes)
      $24.00 × 0.25
	6.00

B. Technician: Hourly Rate × 0.75 (45 minutes)	6.91
IV. **Expendables**	7.38
Total Cost of Facilities, Equipment, Personnel and Expendables	$31.85
V. **Administrative Costs** (20% of the above total)	$ 6.37
Total Cost of 2 Radiographs of One Anatomical Part	$38.22

9

Copying Radiographs and Making Slides for Projection

FULL SIZED RADIOGRAPHIC COPIES

Duplication of radiographs is often necessary when a copy is needed by a client, for consultation with organizations such as the Orthopedic Foundation for Animals or to accompany a patient that has been referred. Radiographic duplicating film is readily available for this purpose. Duplicating film has a solarized emulsion on one side of a blue-tinted polyester base. During the manufacture of this film, the emulsion is exposed to light or treated chemically in such a manner that the maximum film density has been surpassed to the point that a density decrease has occurred. The phenomenon responsible for this decreased denisty with very high exposures is called solarization (Christensen et al., 1978). When the film is exposed to light during the duplicating process, the greater light exposure causes a decreased density; likewise, less exposure causes increased density. This is the opposite of what happens with standard photographic exposures.

The use of duplicating film is relatively simple. The emulsion side of the film is placed next to the radiograph to be copied and subsequently exposed (in the darkroom) to an ultraviolet light source, such as a BLB

ultraviolet, fluorescent lamp. These lamps can be mounted in a 14 × 17 inch radiograph illuminator. A good method of holding the two films in direct contact is to mount them in a glass-front cassette. Exposure time is variable and a few trials are necessary to determine the proper technique for the system. An exposure of 6 seconds with the view box about 2 feet from the cassette provides a good starting place. The exposed film is then processed in a routine manner, either automatically or manually. Fortunately, copy film has a wide latitude of exposure, thereby allowing for some errors. If copies are produced regularly in a practice, a commercially available printer should be purchased (Fig. 9–1).

Remember that excessive density of the duplicate indicates too little exposure. The repeat copy should therefore be exposed for a longer time. If the duplicate is too light, less exposure is necessary.

35-mm SLIDES FOR PROJECTION

35-mm slides of radiographs are often desired when case presentations are made to large groups, such as at meetings, clinical rounds, and so forth. There are several satisfactory ways to produce these slides. Some

98

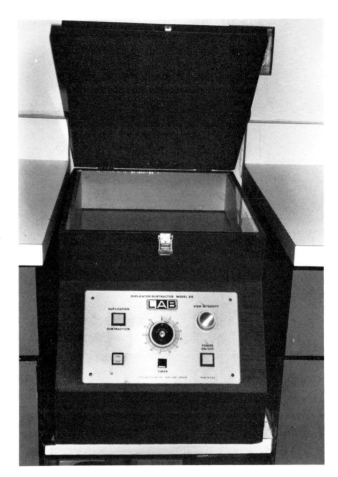

Figure 9–1. A commercially available radiographic copy printer.

methods are less convenient or more expensive than others.

A good balance between expense and convenience is provided by Kodak Rapid Processing Copy Film (Eastman Kodak Co.) or Cronex DP 35 mm Black and White film (E. I. duPont De Nemours & Co., Inc.). Both films are direct positive, fine grain film and are available in 36-exposure magazines. The exposure latitude is great and a few trial exposures will allow the development of a usable technique. Almost any single-lens reflex camera may be used. Extension tubes or a close-up lens may be required for photographing close-up areas or 8 × 10 inch radiographs. Radiographs to be photographed are placed on a standard radiographic view box, and exposures between 10 and 30 seconds at f/3.5 are made at 10-second intervals to produce a trial set of slides (Christensen et al., 1978). A copy stand with camera support and view box makes a convenient place to pro-

duce these slides (Fig. 9–2). The correct exposure time may then be determined. By replacing the white light fluorescent lamps with a high intensity blue lamp T8/B, exposure times may be decreased by about a factor of 4 (Tech Talk Section, Medical Radiography and Photography, 1979). The efficiency of slide production may be increased considerably by using these lamps. They are available from most electrical supply houses.

The film may be processed in an automatic x-ray processor or may be developed manually. For automatic processing, the end of the film strip is taped to a lead film (a discarded 8 × 10 radiograph) with the emulsion side up. A satisfactory tape for this process is Scotch Brand Electrical Tape No. 3 (Morgan et al., 1977). The strip is then fed into the processor while a slight tension is applied to the distal end to ensure smooth transport.

Alternatively, the film strip may be proc-

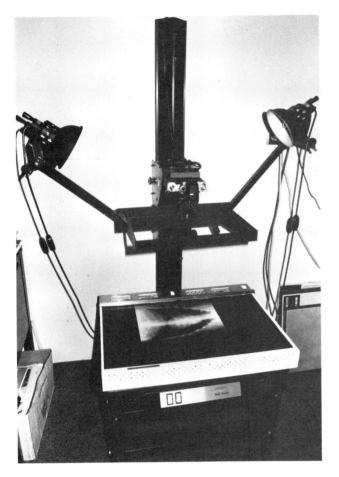

Figure 9–2. A camera stand that is useful for producing slides for projection.

essed using conventional black-and-white chemicals and processor. Your photographic dealer can provide convenient kits for this purpose if you process your own film manually. The strips are then cut and inserted in cardboard, plastic or glass mounts that are readily available at most photographic supply stores.

Project the slides to determine which exposure you prefer. Remember that, just as with solarized radiographic copy film, this 35-mm film requires less exposure if the slide is too light and more exposure if the slide is too dark.

REFERENCES

Christensen, E. F., Curry, T. S., and Dowdey, J. E.: An Introduction to the Physics of Diagnostic Radiology. 2nd ed. Philadelphia, Lea & Febiger, 1978.

Morgan, J. P., Silverman, S., and Zontine, W. J.: Techniques of Veterinary Radiography. 2nd ed. Davis, CA, Veterinary Radiology Associates, 1977.

Faster slides from radiographs: Tech Talk Section. Med. Radiogr. Photogr., 55:77, 1979.

SECTION II

An Atlas of Radiographic Positioning and Technique

10

General Principles

Positioning small animal patients for radiography is a complex and often exacting task that requires the proper means of restraint (chemical and physical), knowledge of anatomy and clinical disease, and a great deal of ingenuity. Proper positioning alone, however, will not guarantee the production of diagnostic radiographs. Careful attention to proper exposure factors as they apply to the specific patient is also necessary.

TECHNIQUE CHART

A usable technique chart should be established for every x-ray machine (Chap. 4). This chart should be easy to use and require minimal alteration in exposure factors for the production of specific radiographs. Alteration of exposure factors to compensate for the changes in contrast and density caused by specific pathologic, physiologic or extraneous factors should be made prior to positioning the patient for radiographic examination.

The proper use of a technique chart demands measurement of each part being radiographed with a caliper that is graduated in centimeters. The thickest region on the part being examined should always be measured (e.g., caudal rib cage for thoracic or cranial abdomen examinations).

Generally, increased exposure is required for examining patients that have an increased amount of x-ray absorbing tissue for a given thickness. For example, patients with pulmonary edema, hemorrhage or contusion, pneumonia, pleural effusion, severe cardiomegaly or diaphragmatic hernia require greater exposure than a patient with a normally aerated thoracic cavity of a given thick-

ness. The increased exposure can be obtained by increasing either the milliampere-seconds (mas) or kilovoltage (kv). Since short exposure times are desirable (especially when radiographing dyspneic patients), increasing the kv is the preferred method. The magnitude of the kv increase depends upon the severity of the pathologic process and the original kv value. An increase of from 10 to 15 per cent is usually sufficient. If the pathologic state is severe and the thorax is over 10 cm thick, a grid should be used.

Pathologic states such as pneumothorax or emphysema require decreased exposure. Either decreasing the mas by decreasing the time of exposure or decreasing the kv will accomplish this. A decrease of approximately one half the mas or 10 to 15 per cent of the original kv value is usually sufficient.

In abdominal examinations, the presence of peritoneal fluid necessitates increased exposure. Increased exposure is also necessary for examining patients with severe obesity or marked enlargement of an abdominal organ, such as the uterus (with pyometra or normal pregnancy). An increase of from 10 to 15 per cent of the original kv value is usually sufficient.

When examining patients that have a positive contrast agent in an organ system (as in such studies as esophagram, the G.I. series, the urogram or the angiogram), the exposure should be increased slightly. The addition of 10 per cent of the original kv value or mas increases of one half (for example, from 5 to 7.5) will usually increase contrast and allow better visualization of structures.

Negative contrast studies, such as pneumoperitoneography and pneumocystography, require decreased exposure to maintain adequate radiographic density. This is usually accomplished by subtracting 10 per cent of the original kv value indicated on the technique chart.

When radiographing structures with an increased amount of x-ray–absorbing bone per centimeter of thickness, such as the skull of brachycephalic dogs, increased exposure is needed for adequate radiographic density. This is usually accomplished by adding 10 per cent to the kv value indicated on the technique chart for a given centimeter of thickness or by increasing the mas value by one half.

Radiographs of patients with a decreased amount of bone per centimeter of thickness, such as immature cats or patients with osteoporotic states, require a decreased exposure. This is usually accomplished by decreasing the kv by 5 per cent of the value indicated on the technique chart for a given centimeter of thickness.

The superimposition of radiodense materials (such as a plaster cast) on the part being examined requires increased exposure. The average dry plaster cast requires doubling the mas or adding 15 per cent of the kv value indicated on the technique chart. Wood, plastic, or aluminum splints and dry bandage material usually do not require increased exposure values when the thickness of the part being examined is measured to include these materials. Bulky cotton dressings such as a Robert Jones bandage does not require increased exposure. The technique for the unbandaged extremity should be used.

Table 10–1 lists some common alterations in exposure technique used to compensate for various pathologic, physiologic or extraneous factors.

NORMAL ANATOMY AND TERMINOLOGY

Knowledge of the normal anatomy and descriptive terminology is necessary for proper patient positioning. Descriptions of various positional relationships of structures being radiographed are illustrated in this atlas section. The positional terminology is that recommended by the Nomenclature Committee of the American College of Veterinary Radiology (Shively et al., 1982) based on two rules:

1. Radiographic projections should be

Table 10–1. COMMON ALTERATIONS IN TECHNIQUE CHART VALUES USED TO COMPENSATE FOR VARIOUS PATHOLOGICAL, PHYSIOLOGICAL, OR EXTRANEOUS FACTORS

Conditions Requiring Exposure Alterations	Method of Altering Exposure
A. Increased Exposure	
1. Increased amount of bone per centimeter of thickness, such as brachycephalic dog skulls.	Add 10% kv or increase mas by one half.
2. Pleural fluid, pulmonary hemorrhage, contusion, edema, pneumonia, severe cardiomegaly, or diaphragmatic hernia.	Add 10 to 15% kv. If thorax is over 10 cm thick, a grid should be used.
3. Peritoneal fluid, severe obesity, or marked organ enlargement, such as of the uterus.	Add 10 to 15% kv.
4. Positive contrast medium in organ system or vasculature.	Add 10% kv.
5. Plaster cast.	Double mas or add 15% kv.
B. Decreased Exposure	
1. Decreased amount of bone per centimeter of thickness, such as in immature cats or in osteoporotic states.	Subtract 5% kv.
2. Pneumothorax or emphysema.	Subtract 10 to 15% kv.
3. Pneumoperitonography, pneumocystography, and other negative contrast examinations.	Subtract 10% kv.

named using only proper veterinary anatomic directional terms as listed in the Nomina Anatomica Veterinaria (International Committee on Veterinary Anatomical Nomenclature, 1973). Any abbreviations used should correspond to those terms (Table 10–2).

2. Radiographic projections should be described by the direction that the central ray

Table 10–2. TERMS AND THEIR ABBREVIATIONS USED TO DESCRIBE RADIOGRAPHIC VIEWS

Left (Le)	Medial (M)
Right (Rt)	Lateral (L)
Dorsal (D)	Proximal (Pr)
Ventral (V)	Distal (Di)
Cranial (Cr)	Palmar (Pa)
Caudal (Cd)	Plantar (Pl)
Rostral(R)	Oblique (O)

of the primary beam penetrates the body part of interest, from the point of entrance to the point of exit.

Using this system, a radiographer should be able to produce the required radiographic view with only the name of the projection.

The directional terms *cranial* and *caudal* apply to the neck, trunk and limbs proximal to the antebrachiocarpal and the tarsocrural (hock) joints. The term cranial is replaced by *rostral* for the head. *Superior* and *inferior* are used for the upper and lower dental arches.

The term *dorsal* refers to the top of the head, neck, trunk and tail. This term replaces cranial on the distal limbs. Caudal is replaced by *palmar* on the distal thoracic limb, and by *plantar* on the distal pelvic limb (distal to the antibrachiocarpal and the tarsocrural joints). *Ventral* is used to describe the bottom of the head, neck, trunk and tail. Positional and directional terms are listed in Table 10–3.

The second rule requires that a radiographic projection describe direction of the primary x-ray beam from the point of entry to the point of exit. Thus, the terms ventrodorsal (VD) and lateromedial (LM) projection fulfill this requirement. Oblique views should also designate anatomically the point of entrance and the point of exit. Additionally, the angle of obliquity may be described. This is accomplished by beginning with the degree of angularity from the first term and progressing toward the second term. For example, Figure 10–1 illustrates a 60-degree angle of central ray direction from the dorsal aspect progressing toward the lateral aspect in the dorsolateral-palmaromedial oblique view (D60°L-PaMO) and 60 degrees toward

Table 10–3. DIRECTIONAL AND POSITIONAL TERMS FOR RADIOGRAPHIC VIEWS OF VARIOUS PARTS OF THE BODY

Head	Neck, Trunk, and Tail	Limbs
rostral	cranial	proximal
caudal	caudal	distal
dorsal	dorsal	medial
ventral	ventral	lateral
left	left	cranial (dorsal*)
right	right	caudal (palmar,* plantar)

*On the limbs, cranial and caudal are used proximal to the carpus and tarsus. Dorsal and palmar and dorsal and plantar are used distal to these joints in the thoracic and pelvic limbs respectively.

the medial aspect in the dorsomedial-palmarolateral oblique (D60°M-PaLO) view.

Angles of obliquity for abdominal or thoracic radiographs are similarly designated. For example a right dorsal-left ventral projection made with the central ray 45 degrees toward the dorsum from the right side would be designated as R45° D-LeVO (Fig. 10–2); other examples are illustrated in the Atlas.

The angular designation of the central x-ray beam usually refers to a plane within the anatomical region; however, the description of angularity of the central beam for oblique views of the equine distal extremity is best accomplished using the supporting surface as a reference, since the normal angulation of the fetlock joint does not allow accurate translation of angles of the x-ray tube, which is oriented to the supporting surface. Additionally there are conforma-

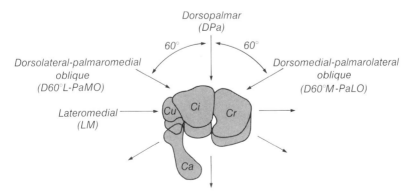

Figure 10–1. Radiographic projections for the examination of the equine carpus to illustrate terminology using the direction of the primary x-ray beam from the point of entrance to the point of exit. Angular notation is used to describe oblique views using the angle from the first term progressing toward the second term. (After Shively et al., 1982.)

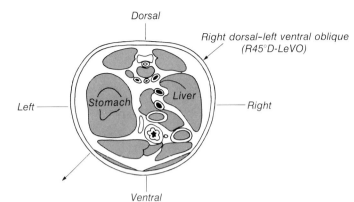

Figure 10–2. Radiographic projection of the cranial abdomen of the canine to illustrate terminology using the direction of the primary x-ray beam from point of entrance to point of exit. Angular notation is used to describe an oblique view of 45 degrees from the right (first term) dorsally (second term). (After Shively et al., 1982.)

tional variations in the angle of fetlock joint extension between different animals. An example is the dorsoproximal-palmarodistal oblique view of the equine distal sesamoid bone (navicular) made at 65 degrees proximal to the supporting surface (Fig. 10–3).

Complex angular projections with two angle designations are placed between three directional terms that describe the x-ray beam entrance point. An example is an oblique projection of the lateral border of the distal sesamoid bone (navicular) or the third phalanx in an equine. This view would be designated a laterodorsoproximal-mediopalmarodistal oblique view and is made 45 degrees dorsal to the lateromedial line and 50 degrees proximal to the supporting surface. The abbreviation is L45°D50° Pr-MPaDiO (Fig. 10–4).

When radiographs are produced with the patient in other than recumbency for small animals or standing for large animals, a specific designation of the position of the body and orientation of the central x-ray beam is required. For example, a left-to-right lateral projection of a canine thorax made while the animal is standing and with the central beam oriented horizontally would be designated LeRtL (standing/horizontal). A parenthetical open mouth, flexed or hyperextended may also be used to further clarify the examination method.

Since time will be required to become accustomed to this new method of designating radiographic views, the system used in the first edition of this book will be used parenthetically when possibility of confusion exists.

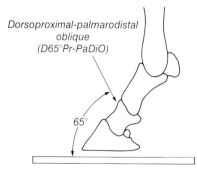

Figure 10–3. Radiographic projection of the equine distal sesamoid bone (navicular) using the direction of the primary x-ray beam from the point of entrance to point of exit. The angular notation is in reference to the supporting surface and indicates the degree of angulation in the proximal direction from the surface. (After Shively et al., 1982.)

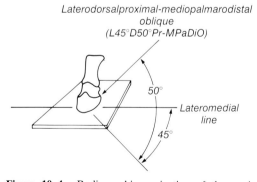

Figure 10–4. Radiographic projection of the equine distal phalanx (PIII) using an oblique primary x-ray beam direction to examine the lateral aspect. The beam direction is described from the point of entrance to the point of exit. The beam is directed 45 degrees from the lateral aspect toward the dorsal aspect and is elevated 50 degrees proximal to the supporting surface. (After Shively et al., 1982.)

Table 10–4. AGE AT APPEARANCE OF OSSIFICATION CENTERS AND OF BONY FUSION IN THE IMMATURE CANINE

Anatomical Site	Age at Appearance of Ossification Center	Age When Fusion Occurs	Anatomical Site	Age at Appearance of Ossification Center	Age When Fusion Occurs
Scapula			Ilium	Birth	4–6 mo
Body	Birth		Ischium	Birth	4–6 mo
Tuber scapulae	7 wk	4–7 mo	Os acetabulum	7 wk	5 mo
			Iliac crest	4 mo	1–2 yr
Humerus			Tuber ischii	3 mo	8–10 mo
Diaphysis	Birth	—	Ischial arch	6 mo	12 mo
Proximal epiphysis	1–2 wk	10–13 mo	Caudal symphysis pubis	7 mo	5 yr
Distal epiphysis		6–8 mo to shaft	Symphysis pubis		5 yr
Medial condyle	2–3 wk	6 wk to lateral condyle	*Femur*		
			Diaphysis	Birth	
Lateral condyle	2–3 wk		Proximal epiphysis (head)	2 wk	7–11 mo
Medial epicondyle	6–8 wk	6 mo to condyles	Trochanter major	8 wk	6–10 mo
			Trochanter minor	8 wk	8–13 mo
Radius			Distal epiphysis		8–11 mo to shaft
Diaphysis	Birth	—	Trochlea	2 wk	3 mo condyles to trochlea
Proximal epiphysis	3–5 wk	6–11 mo			
Distal epiphysis	2–4 wk	8–12 mo	Medial condyle	3 wk	
			Lateral condyle	3 wk	
Ulna					
Diaphysis	Birth		*Patella*	9 wk	
Olecranon	8 wk	6–10 mo			
Distal epiphysis	8 wk	8–12 mo	*Tibia*		
			Diaphysis	Birth	
Carpus			Condyles		6–12 mo to shaft
Ulnar	4 wk		Medial	3 wk	
Radial	3–4 wk				
Central	4–5 wk		Lateral	3 wk	
Intermediate	3–4 wk				
Accessory			Tuberosity	8 wk	6–8 mo to condyles
Body	2 wk				6–12 mo to shaft
Epiphysis	7 wk	4 mo			
First	3 wk		Distal epiphysis	3 wk	8–11 mo
Second	4 wk		Medial malleolus	3 mo	5 mo
Third	4 wk				
Fourth	3 wk		*Fibula*		
Sesamoid bone	4 mo		Diaphysis	Birth	
			Proximal epiphysis	9 wk	8–12 mo
Metacarpus			Distal epiphysis	2–7 wk	7–11 mo
Diaphysis	Birth				
Distal epiphysis (2–5)*	4 wk	6 mo	*Tarsus*		
Proximal epiphysis (1)*	5 wk	6 mo	Talus	Birth–1 wk	
			Calcaneus	Birth–1 wk	
Phalanges			Tuber calcis	6 wk	3–8 mo
First phalanx			Central	3 wk	
Diaphysis (1–5)*	Birth		First	4 wk	
Distal epiphysis (2–5)*	4 wk	6 mo	Second	4 wk	
Distal epiphysis (1)*	6 wk	6 mo	Third	3 wk	
Second phalanx			Fourth	2 wk	
Diaphysis (2–5)*	Birth		Metatarsus and pelvic limb		
Proximal epiphysis (2–5)*	5 wk	6 mo	phalanges are approximately		
Second phalanx absent or			the same as the metacarpus		
fused with first in first			and pectoral limb phalanges.		
digit.					
Third phalanx			*Sesamoids*		
Diaphysis	Birth		Fabellar	3 mo	
Volar sesamoids	2 mo		Popliteal	3 mo	
Dorsal sesamoids	4 mo		Plantar phalangeal	2 mo	
			Dorsal phalangeal	5 mo	
Pelvis					
Pubis	Birth	4–6 mo			

*Digit numbers.

Table 10–5. AGE AT APPEARANCE OF OSSIFICATION CENTERS AND OF BONY FUSION IN THE IMMATURE EQUINE*

Anatomical Site	Age of Appearance of Ossification Center	Age When Fusion Occurs
Scapula		
Proximal end	9–12 mo.	After 3 yrs.
Supraglenoid tubercle and coracoid process	At birth	9–18 mos.
Cranial part of the glenoid cavity	At birth	9–18 mos.
Humerus		
Proximal epiphysis	At birth	26–42 mos.
Greater tubercle	At birth	15–34 mos.
Distal epiphysis	At birth	11–18 mos.
Medial epicondyle	At birth	11–18 mos.
Radius		
Proximal epiphysis	At birth	11–18 mos.
Distal epiphysis	At birth	24–42 mos.
		26–35 in standardbred (Gabel et al., 1977)
Ulna		
Proximal epiphysis (olecranon tuberosity)	At birth	27–42 mos.
Distal epiphysis (styloid process)	At birth	2–9 mos. (some up to 4 yrs.)
Carpals	At birth	C1 absent in about 50% of all horses
Accessory Carpal		
Epiphysis	By 104 days	Variable
Metacarpal III		
Proximal epiphysis	At birth	Before birth
Distal epiphysis	At birth	6–18 mos.
Metacarpals II and IV	By 104 days	
Proximal Phalanx (PI)		
Proximal epiphysis	At birth	6–15 mos.
Distal epiphysis	At birth	Partial at birth—complete at 22 days
Middle Phalanx (PII)		
Proximal epiphysis	At birth	6–12 mos.
Distal epiphysis	At birth	Most fused at birth to 1 wk.
Distal Phalanx	At birth	
Sesamoids (proximal and distal)	At birth	
Femur		
Proximal epiphysis	At birth	36–42 mos.
Greater trochanter	At birth	36–42 mos.
Distal epiphysis	At birth	21–42 mos.
Patella	At birth	
Tibia		
Proximal epiphysis	At birth	12–24 mos.
Tibial tuberosity	At birth	{ 12–24 mos. to proximal epiphysis { 36–42 mos. to metaphysis
Distal epiphysis	At birth	17–24 mos.

Table continued on opposite page

Table 10–5. AGE AT APPEARANCE OF OSSIFICATION CENTERS AND OF BONY FUSION IN THE IMMATURE EQUINE (*Continued*)*

Anatomical Site	Age of Appearance of Ossification Center	Age When Fusion Occurs
Fibula		
Proximal epiphysis	At birth or soon after	42 mos. (variable)
Diaphysis	At birth or soon after	Multiple transverse defects common
Distal epiphysis (lateral malleolus)	At birth	3–24 mos. (most by 1 yr.) to the tibia.
Tarsals	At birth	I and II fuse between 52 and 104 days in about 50% of foals
Calcaneus		
Epiphysis	At birth	22–36 mos.
Bones distal to the tarsus show about the same times of ossification and fusion as those distal to the carpus.		
Skull		
Spheno-occipital suture		2–3 yrs. (Ackerman et al., 1974)

*Compiled from Myers et al., 1975; Getty, 1975; Brown and MacCallum, 1975; Zeskov, 1959; Gabel et al., 1977; Ackerman et al., 1974.

POSITIONING

Positioning small animal patients for radiographic examination demands the judicious use of an anesthetic or sedative and the aid of various positional and restraint devices. Chemical sedation or anesthesia is desirable when positioning patients in pain or those that are apprehensive. Properly relaxed small animal patients may be positioned with the aid of sponge blocks, ropes, tape, compression bands or head positioning devices.

Only a small percentage of small animal patients should be restrained manually. This method of restraint should be used only when chemical restraint is contraindicated. Large animal patients, except those that are anesthetized, usually require the presence of at least two persons to perform radiographic examinations. Strict adherence to radiation safety principles must be observed, especially when manual restraint is necessary (see Chap. 5).

Angular relationships between the primary x-ray beam and the part being examined must be correct for proper projection onto the film. This is particularly true of skull, vertebral and extremity examination. Proper positioning may prevent certain artifacts. For example, when examining the lateral projection of an elbow joint in the immature canine patient, moderate flexion will avoid the superimposition of the medial epicondylar physis of the humerus on the anconeal process, thereby decreasing the possibility of misdiagnosing an ununited anconeal process.

Illustrations of various positional and restraint devices are found in this atlas.

OSSIFICATION CENTERS AND BONY FUSION

Knowledge of the age at which ossification centers appear and the age that these structures fuse to adjacent structures is desirable when interpreting radiographs of the immature patient. Table 10–4 lists a summary of available data for the canine; Table 10–5 provides similar data for the equine. The age at fusion varies with breed; therefore, considerable ranges are listed for some sites.

REFERENCES

Ackerman, N., Coffman, J. R., and Corley, E A.: The spheno-occipital suture of the horse: Its normal radiographic appearance. J. Am. Vet. Radiol. Soc. 15:79–81, 1974.

Brown, M. P., and MacCallum, E. J.: A system of grading ossification in limbs of foals to assist in radiographic interpretation. Am. J. Vet. Res. 36:655–661, 1975.

Chapman, W. L.: Appearance of ossification centers and epiphyseal closures—determined by radiographic techniques. Thesis. Fort Collins, Colorado, Colorado State University, 1963.

Crouch, J. E.: Text-Atlas of Cat Anatomy. Philadelphia, Lea & Febiger, 1969.

Douglas, S. W., and Williamson, H. D.: Principles of Veterinary Radiography. 3rd ed. Baltimore, Williams & Wilkins Co., 1980.

Gabel, A. A., Spencer, C. P., and Pipers, F. S.: A study of correlation of closure of the distal radial physis with performance and injury in the standardbred. J.A.V.M.A. 170:188–194, 1977.

Getty, R.: Sisson and Grossman's The Anatomy of the Domestic Animals, 5th Ed. Philadelphia, W. B. Saunders Co., 1975.

Gillette, E. L., Thrall, D. E., and Lebel, J. L.: Carlson's Veterinary Radiology, 3rd ed. Philadelphia, Lea and Febiger, 1967.

International Committee on Veterinary Anatomical No-menclature. Nomina Anatomica Veterinaria. 2nd ed. Vienna, published by the Committee, 1973.

Meyers, V. S., Bergin, W. C., and Guffy, M. M.: In Getty, R.: Sisson and Grossman's The Anatomy of the Domestic Animals, 5th ed. Philadelphia, W. B. Saunders Co., 1975.

Miller, M. E., Christensen, G. C., and Evans, H. E.: Anatomy of the Dog. Philadelphia, W. B. Saunders Co., 1953.

Schebitz, H., and Wilkens, H.: Atlas of Radiographic Anatomy of Dog and Cat. Berlin, Paul Parey, 1978.

Shively, M. J., Smallwood, J. E., Habel, R. E., and Rendano, V. T.: A Standardized Nomenclature for Radiographic Views Used in Veterinary Medicine. Unpublished report of the Nomenclature Committee, Am. Coll. Vet. Radiol., 1982.

Sisson, S., and Grossman, J. D.: The Anatomy of the Domestic Animals. 5th ed. Philadelphia, W. B. Saunders Co., 1975.

Zeskov, B.: A Study of discontinuity of the fibula in the horse. Am. J. Vet. Res. 20:852, 1959.

11

Thoracic Limb

SCAPULA AND SHOULDER JOINT

Caudocranial (CdCr) View. The patient is placed in dorsal recumbency (supine), and the sternum is rotated (approximately 30 degrees) away from the side being examined in such a manner that the vertical x-ray beam is passed between the scapula and rib cage (Figs. 11–1 and 11–2). The limb is fully extended. For scapular examinations, x-ray beam collimation and film size should be large enough to allow visualization of the entire blade of the scapula and shoulder joint. The central x-ray beam should transect the midscapula. For shoulder joint examination, the x-ray beam should be centered at the joint.

Figure 11–3 illustrates the radiographic anatomy of the mature canine scapula and shoulder joint in the CdCr projection. Excessive abduction of the humerus may result in an artifactual subluxation of the shoulder joint, since a moderate degree of joint laxity is normal. When the scapula, shoulder joint and humerus are positioned in the CdCr projection, this artifact may be avoided by aligning the scapula and humerus.

Mediolateral (ML) View. The patient is placed in lateral recumbency, and the limb to be examined is placed adjacent to the film.

Visualization of the distal aspect of the scapula and shoulder joint is best accomplished by placing the scapula over the caudal cervical region (Fig. 11–4). This is the best position for survey radiographs of the scapular and shoulder region. The limb should be extended and placed at an angle of approximately 45 degrees from the spinal column. This places the shoulder joint over soft tissue, thereby avoiding superimposition over the bony structures of the sternum and ribs. The contralateral limb should be flexed and placed over the cranial aspect of the thorax. The normal radiographic anatomy of the mature canine scapula in this projection is shown in Figure 11–5. The normal radiographic anatomy of the mature canine shoulder joint is shown in Figure 11–6.

If the scapular blade is to be visualized in its entirety, the scapula should be superimposed over the cranial thorax (Fig. 11–7). This places the thin structure of the bone over the radiolucent lung fields and allows better visualization of the borders. The contralateral limb should be extended and placed over the cervical region. The normal radiographic anatomy of the mature canine scapula in this projection is shown in Figure 11–8.

The mediolateral view of the immature canine shoulder shows two physes that are often misdiagnosed as pathological processes (Fig. 11–9). The ossification center of the scapular tuberosity appears between the fifth and the eighth week of age and is seen on the mediolateral view just cranial to the glenoid fossa (Hare, 1959*b*). The ossification center soon becomes wedge-shaped and unites with the body of the scapula between four and six months after birth (Hare, 1959*b*; Chapman, 1963). This normal structure should not be misdiagnosed as a fracture.

The proximal epiphysis of the humerus appears during the first two weeks of life and unites with the diaphysis at 10 to 15 months of age (Hare, 1959*b*; Chapman, 1963). Figure 11–10 illustrates the normal appearance of the physis of the proximal humerus in a six-month-old dog. At this age, the cranial aspect

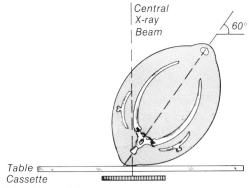

Figure 11–1. Diagrammatic illustration of the relationship of the scapular blade and thoracic wall to the central x-ray beam when producing a caudocranial view of the scapula and shoulder joint. Note that the sagittal plane of the thoracic cavity is placed at an angle of 60 degrees to the x-ray film surface (30° to the central x-ray beam).

of the physis appears widened on the mediolateral view. This normal structure must not be considered an avulsion fracture.

Mature feline shoulder radiographs show well mineralized clavicles (Fig. 11–11). Occasionally, vestiges of these structures are seen in the canine and should be considered normal.

SHOULDER ARTHROGRAPHY

Arthrography is the radiographic demonstration of articular surfaces and joint capsule outlines after introduction of either positive or negative contrast medium into the synovial fluid. Positive contrast medium is superior to negative or double (both positive and negative) medium in canine shoulder joints for the demonstration of articular or capsular defects (Suter and Carb, 1969).

Indications. Shoulder arthrography aids in demonstrating radiolucent articular cartilage defects and joint capsule abnormalities that are not visualized on noncontrast radiographs. The extent of cartilaginous and subchondral bone defects may also be demonstrated with a greater degree of accuracy using arthrography. This information may aid in establishing a diagnosis and in planning a therapeutic regimen.

Method. Anesthesia is induced and an area of approximately 8 cm square is clipped, prepared surgically, and draped. As with all arthrocentesis procedures, asepsis must be maintained. The acromion is palpated with a gloved finger, and a one-inch, 20-gauge needle (with syringe attached) is introduced

Text continued on page 123.

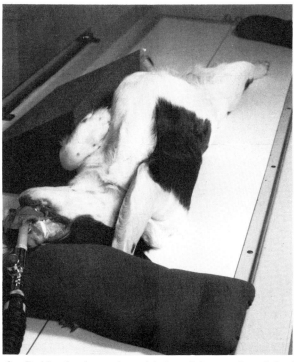

Figure 11–2. Position for the caudocranial view of the scapula and shoulder joint.

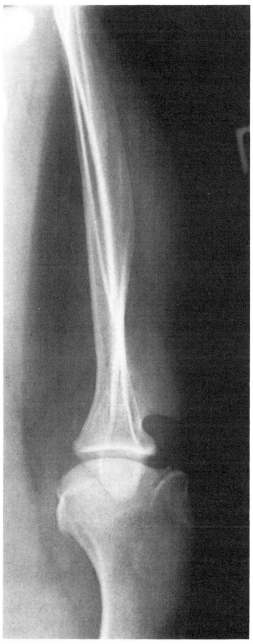
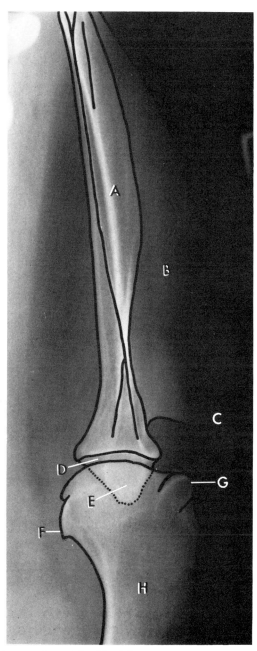

Figure 11–3. Caudocranial view of the canine scapula and shoulder joint.

A. Scapula
B. Spine of scapula
C. Acromion
D. Glenoid cavity

E. Scapular and coracoid
   tuberosities
F. Lesser tubercle
G. Greater tubercle
H. Humerus

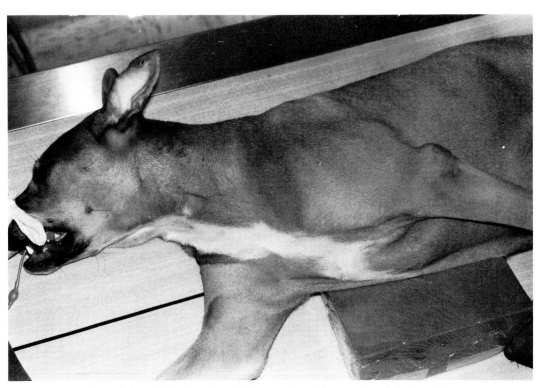

Figure 11–4. Position for the mediolateral view of the scapula and shoulder joint.

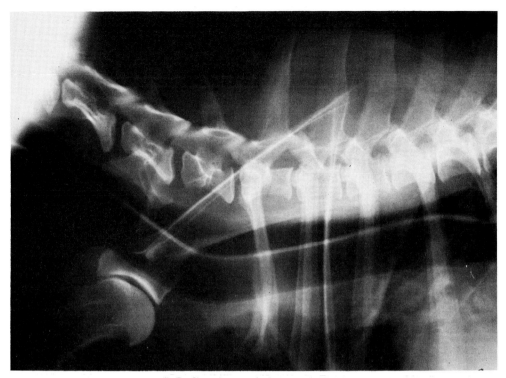

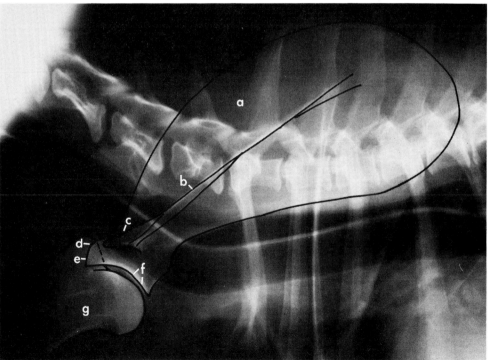

Figure 11–5. Mediolateral view of the canine scapula.

a. Scapula
b. Spine of scapula
c. Acromion
d. Coracoid process
e. Scapular tuberosity
f. Glenoid cavity
g. Humerus

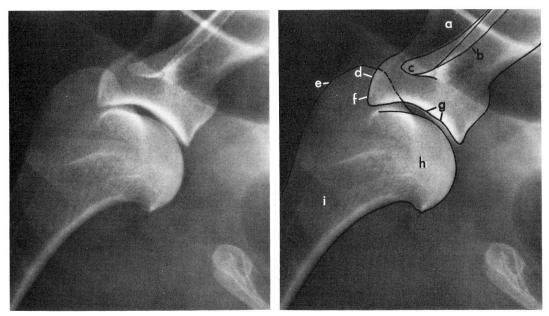

Figure 11–6. Mediolateral view of the canine shoulder joint.
       a. Scapula
       b. Spine of scapula
       c. Acromion
       d. Coracoid process
       e. Greater tubercle
       f. Scapular tuberosity
       g. Glenoid cavity
       h. Humeral head
       i. Humerus

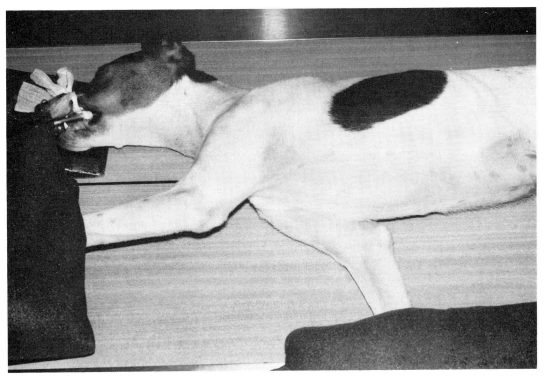

Figure 11–7. Position of the mediolateral view of the scapula projected over the thorax.

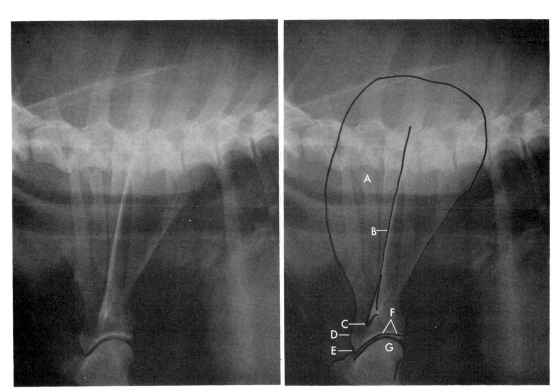

Figure 11–8. Mediolateral view of the canine scapula projected over the thorax.

    A. Scapula
    B. Spine of scapula
    C. Acromion
    D. Coracoid process
    E. Scapular tuberosity
    F. Glenoid cavity
    G. Humerus

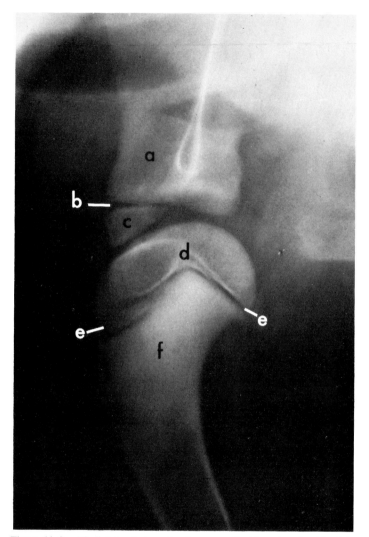

Figure 11–9. Mediolateral view of a three-month-old canine shoulder joint.
a. Scapula
b. Scapular tuberosity physis
c. Scapular tuberosity
d. Epiphysis of proximal humerus (head)
e. Physis proximal humerus
f. Metaphysis of proximal humerus

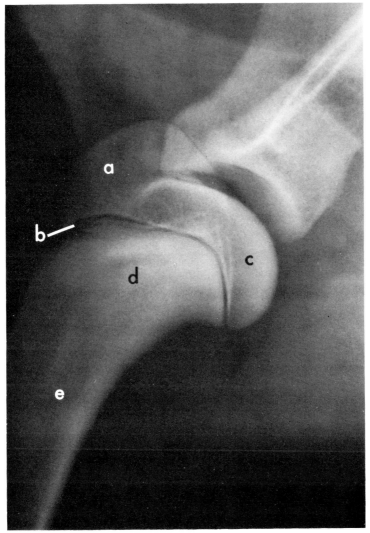

Figure 11–10. Mediolateral view of an immature canine shoulder.
a. Greater tubercle
b. Proximal humeral physis
c. Proximal humeral epiphysis
d. Humeral metaphysis
e. Humeral diaphysis

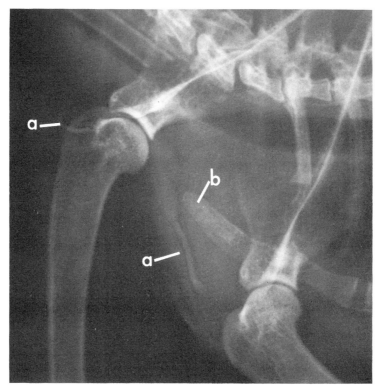

Figure 11–11. Mediolateral view of a mature feline shoulder.
a. Clavicles
b. Manubrium of sternum

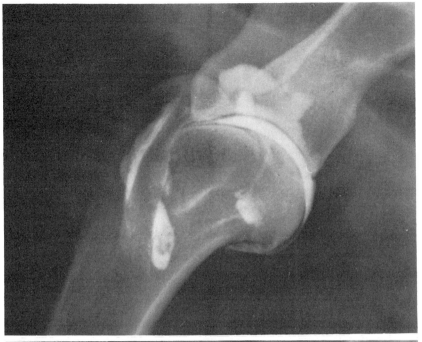

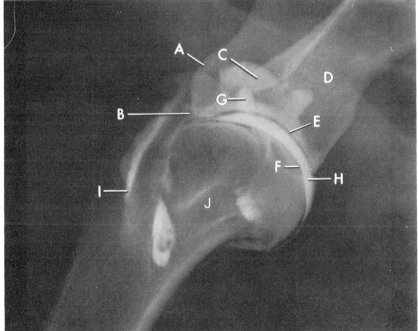

Figure 11–12. Mediolateral view of a canine shoulder arthrogram.

  A. Coracoid process
  B. Scapular tuberosity
  C. Acromion
  D. Scapula
  E. Articular cartilage of glenoid cavity
  F. Articular cartilage of humeral head
  G. Contrast medium in subscapular pouch of joint capsule
  H. Contrast medium in shoulder joint cavity
  I. Contrast medium in tendon sheath of biceps muscle
  J. Humeral head

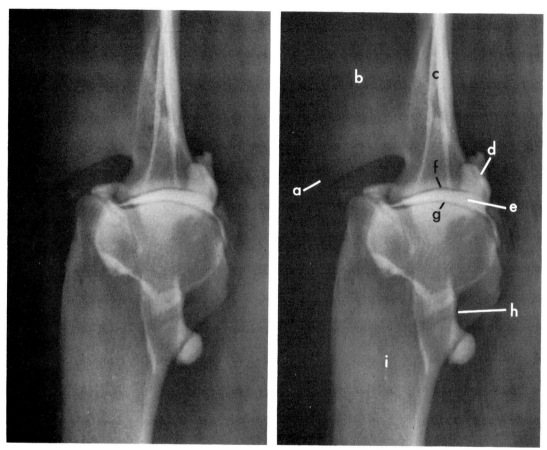

Figure 11–13. Caudocranial view of a canine shoulder arthrogram.
    a. Acromion
    b. Spine of scapula
    c. Scapula
    d. Subscapular pouch
    e. Contrast medium in shoulder joint
    f. Articular cartilage of the glenoid cavity
    g. Articular cartilage of humeral head
    h. Contrast medium in tendon sheath of biceps muscle
    i. Humerus

approximately 1 cm distally. The needle is directed distally and caudally into the shoulder joint. Aspiration of a small amount of synovia confirms the proper location. The syringe is then removed from the needle, and a second syringe containing 4 to 5 ml of sodium diatrizoate solution (Hypaque sodium, 50%, Winthrop Laboratories) is attached. Inject the medium with moderate pressure to avoid reflux of medium around the needle. Withdraw the needle and flex and extend the joint a few times to allow thorough mixing of the medium and synovia. Place the affected shoulder adjacent to the table and produce mediolateral (Fig. 11–12) and caudocranial (Fig. 11–13) views. The radiographs should be produced within one minute after injection, since prolongation of the interval between injection and radiography allows partial absorption of the contrast medium, which reduces the detail at the cartilage-synovia interface.

Considerable variation is found in the normal appearance of the canine shoulder arthrogram. Various degrees of subscapular pouch enlargement and biceps muscle tendon sheath distention may occur without corresponding clinical abnormalities. Large outpouching defects of the area of the infraspinatus and supraspinatus muscles are associated with clinical signs of shoulder lameness and may indicate tear of the joint capsule (Suter and Carb, 1969). Articular surfaces should be well delineated and free from defects. Such defects are commonly seen in cases of osteochondrosis dissecans when detachment of the articular cartilage has occurred.

HUMERUS

Caudocranial (CdCr) View. The patient is placed in dorsal recumbency, and the sternum is rotated slightly away from the limb being examined until a true CdCr projection is obtained (Fig. 11–14). The central x-ray beam is placed at midhumerus. The x-ray beam should be collimated to include both the shoulder and elbow joints. In large dogs, proper exposure of the proximal humerus usually results in overexposure of the distal end. In these cases, two exposures may be necessary. Cats and most dogs may be radiographed adequately with one exposure.

Figure 11–15 illustrates the normal radiographic anatomy of a mature canine humerus in CdCr projection.

Mediolateral (ML) View. The patient is placed in lateral recumbency, with the limb to be examined placed adjacent to the film (Fig. 11–16). The shoulder is extended and the axis of the limb is placed at an angle of approximately 45 degrees from the axis of the spinal column. The sternum is elevated a few centimeters above the table with radiolucent sponges. This prevents overlying radiodensities in the region of the proximal humerus. The x-ray beam collimation and film size should be large enough to include the shoulder and elbow joints.

Figure 11–17 illustrates the normal radiographic anatomy of the mature canine humerus in ML projection.

ELBOW JOINT

Craniocaudal (CrCd) View. The patient is placed in ventral recumbency with the limb extended and pulled forward (Fig. 11–18). The head should be rotated away from the elbow joint. The elbow joint must be in a true CrCd plane, with the olecranon placed at equal distances from the medial and lateral humeral condyles. This is most easily accomplished by elevating the contralateral elbow slightly. If the elbow joint cannot be completely extended, the x-ray beam should be angled approximately 15 degrees in the distal direction from its normal perpendicular orientation (Cranio-15°distal-caudoproximal oblique). This will allow better visualization of the joint surface. Both elbow joints should not be radiographed simultaneously, because malpositioning due to elbow rotation will make radiographic interpretation difficult.

Figure 11–19 illustrates the normal radiographic anatomy of the CrCd view of a mature canine elbow.

The medial aspect of the distal feline humerus contains the supracondyloid foramen, which may be visible on CrCd or oblique views of the elbow region (Fig. 11–20).

Mediolateral (ML) View. The patient is placed in lateral recumbency with the elbow joint to be examined placed adjacent to the film. The elbow joint may be either extended (Fig. 11–21) or flexed (Fig. 11–23). The flexed position is used specifically to examine the anconeal process. The contralateral limb is flexed and placed over the thorax. The sternum may need to be elevated slightly to avoid superimposition of the thoracic bony structures, especially for examination of the flexed position.

Figure 11–22 illustrates the normal radio-
Text continued on page 131.

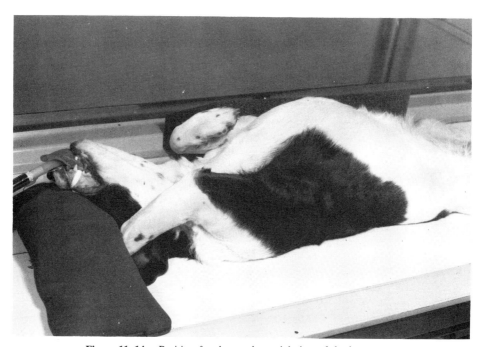

Figure 11–14. Position for the caudocranial view of the humerus.

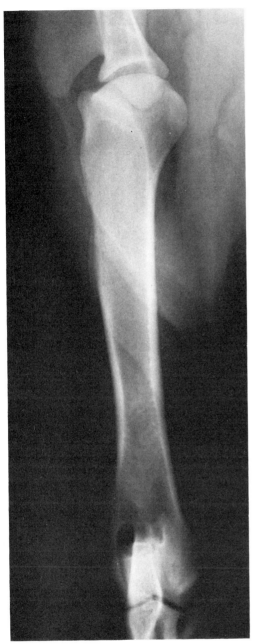
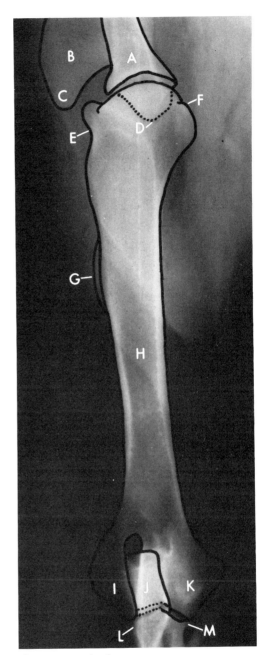

Figure 11–15. Caudocranial view of a mature canine humerus.

A. Scapula
B. Spine of scapula
C. Acromion
D. Scapula and coracoid tuberosities
E. Greater tubercle
F. Lesser tubercle
G. Deltoid tuberosity
H. Humeral diaphysis
I. Lateral condyle
J. Olecranon of ulna
K. Medial condyle
L. Head of radius
M. Medial aspect of ulnar coronoid process

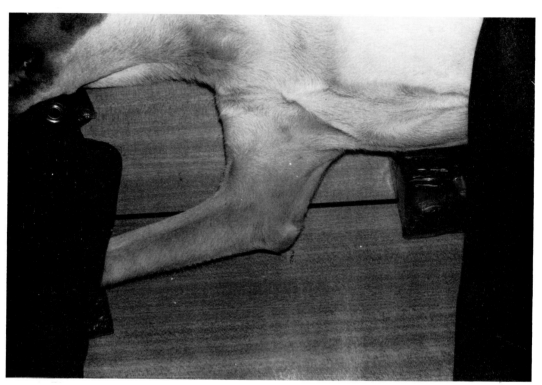

Figure 11–16. Position for the mediolateral view of the humerus.

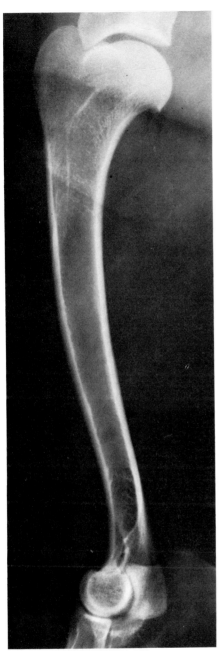
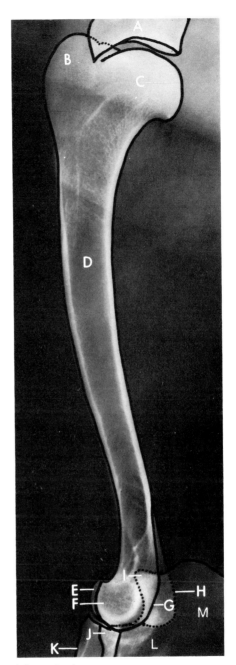

Figure 11–17. Mediolateral view of the canine humerus.

    A. Scapula
    B. Greater tubercle
    C. Humeral head
    D. Humeral diaphysis
    E. Medial condyle
    F. Lateral condyle
    G. Lateral epicondyle
    H. Medial epicondyle
    I. Anconeal process
    J. Coronoid process
    K. Radius
    L. Ulna
    M. Olecranon

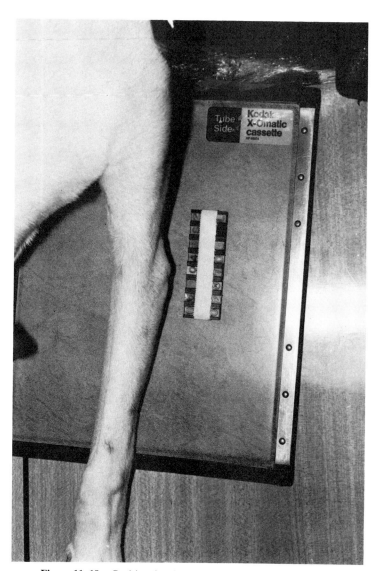

Figure 11–18. Position for the craniocaudal view of the elbow.

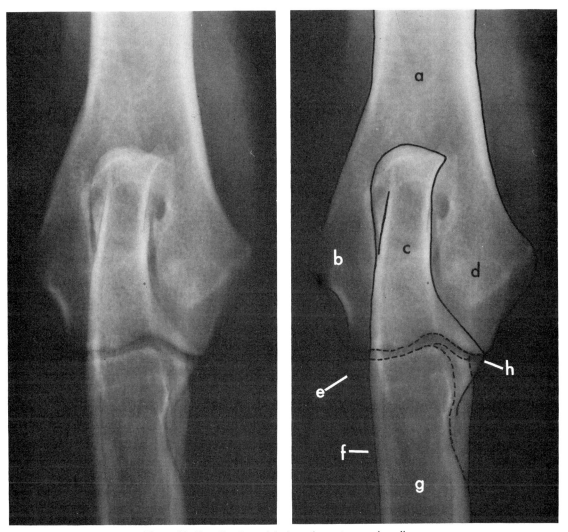

Figure 11–19. Craniocaudal view of a mature canine elbow.

    a. Humerus
    b. Lateral condyle
    c. Olecranon
    d. Medial condyle
    e. Head of radius
    f. Radius
    g. Ulna
    h. Medial aspect of ulnar coronoid process

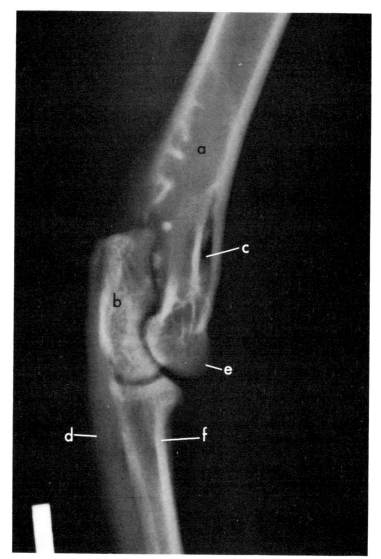

Figure 11–20. Craniolateral-caudomedial oblique view of a feline elbow.
    a. Humerus
    b. Olecranon
    c. Supracondyloid foramen
    d. Ulna
    e. Medial humeral condyle
    f. Radius

graphic anatomy of a mature canine elbow in the extended position. Figure 11–24 illustrates the normal appearance of the anconeal process when the elbow is radiographed in the flexed position.

The center of ossification for the medial humeral epicondyle appears between the sixth and eighth week of life and unites with the medial condyle during the sixth to eighth month of life (Hare, 1959*b*; Chapman, 1963). During this period, a distinct physis is visible radiographically on lateral projection (Fig. 11–25). Note the superimposition of the medial epicondylar physis on the anconeal process. This should not be mistaken for an ununited anconeal process. To avoid this superimposition, the ML projection of the elbow joint in patients less than six months of age should be produced in a flexed position.

RADIUS AND ULNA

Craniocaudal (CrCd) View. The patient is placed in ventral recumbency with the limb to be examined pulled forward and the head rotated toward the contralateral side (Fig. 11–26). If a true CrCd projection of the elbow is obtained, the carpus will be projected in a moderate oblique manner, because there is usually a moderate degree of supination (rotated laterally) of the distal limb. On the other hand, if a true dorsopalmar (DPa) projection of the carpus is obtained, the elbow joint may be shown in a slightly oblique position. Generally, it is preferable to position the elbow joint in a true CrCd projection when examining the radius and ulna. Specific evaluation of the carpal joint should not be attempted on survey radiographs of the radius and ulna.

The x-ray beam should be collimated to include both the elbow and carpal joints. The central x-ray beam is placed at the middiaphyseal region.

Figure 11–27 illustrates the normal radiographic anatomy of the mature canine radius and ulna in CrCd projection. Figure 11–28 illustrates the normal radiographic anatomy of the distal aspect of a mature feline radius and ulna in CrCd projection. Notice the normal appearance of the distal radioulnar articulation (*a*) in the feline.

Mediolateral (ML) View. The patient is placed in lateral recumbency with the limb being radiographed placed adjacent to the film (Fig. 11–29). The contralateral limb is flexed and pulled back over the cranial thorax. The x-ray beam is collimated to include both the elbow and carpal joints. The central x-ray beam is placed at the middiaphyseal region. Slight flexion of the elbow and carpus usually does not interfere with interpretation of the radiograph. Specific evaluation of the elbow or carpal joint should not be attempted on survey radiographs of the radius and ulna.

Figure 11–30 illustrates the normal radiographic anatomy of the mature canine radius and ulna in ML projection.

THORACIC LIMB EXAMINATION FOR SEVERELY INJURED HUMERUS OR RADIUS AND ULNA

The craniocaudal projection of a severely fractured radius and ulna is best performed with the patient in lateral recumbency using a horizontally oriented x-ray beam. This will allow the limb to be placed in a nonstressed, natural position and will prevent additional trauma to the injured site. The patient is placed in opposite lateral recumbency from the injured limb, and the limb is supported by a dry foam block. The cassette is placed on the caudal surface of the limb, and the x-ray beam is directed craniocaudally in a plane parallel to the table top (Fig. 11–31).

A fractured humerus may be examined in caudocranial projection by placing the cassette on the cranial surface and directing the x-ray beam from the caudal direction in the horizontal plane.

CARPUS

Dorsopalmar (DPa) View. The patient is placed in ventral recumbency with the limb to be examined pulled forward (Fig. 11–32). Allow the elbow to abduct slightly so that the natural supination of the distal limb will not cause the carpus to be projected in an oblique manner. The x-ray beam is centered at the carpus.

Figure 11–33 illustrates the normal radiographic anatomy of the mature canine carpus in DPa projection. Figure 11–34 illustrates the normal radiographic anatomy of a four-month-old canine carpus in DPa projection. The normal distal radial epiphysis (*c*) should not be confused with the radial carpal bone

Text continued on page 145.

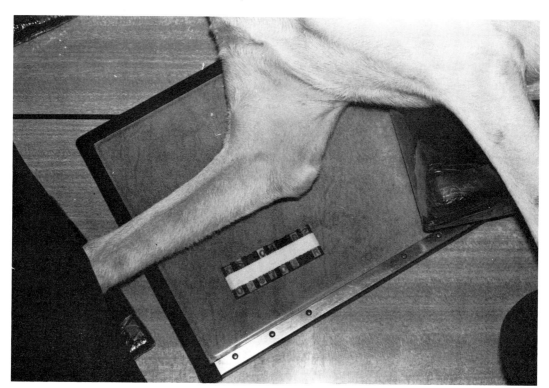

Figure 11–21. Position for the mediolateral view of the elbow.

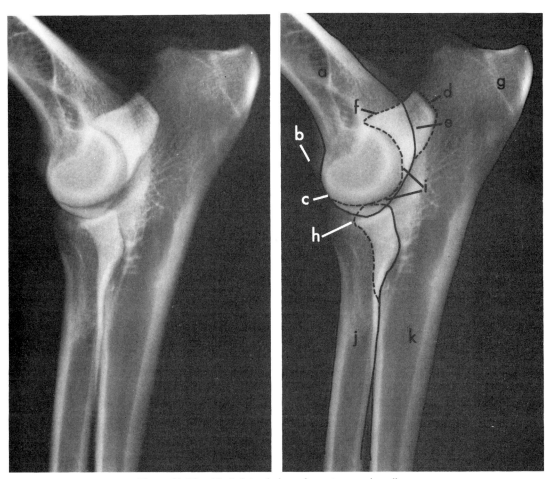

Figure 11–22. Mediolateral view of a mature canine elbow.

    a. Humerus
    b. Medial condyle
    c. Lateral condyle
    d. Medial epicondyle
    e. Lateral epicondyle
    f. Anconeal process
    g. Olecranon
    h. Coronoid process
    i. Trochlear notch
    j. Radius
    k. Ulna

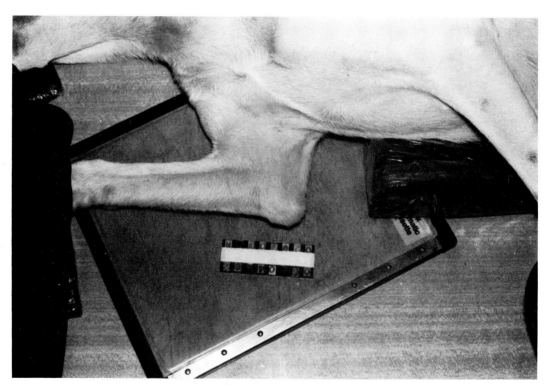

Figure 11–23. Position for flexed mediolateral view of the elbow.

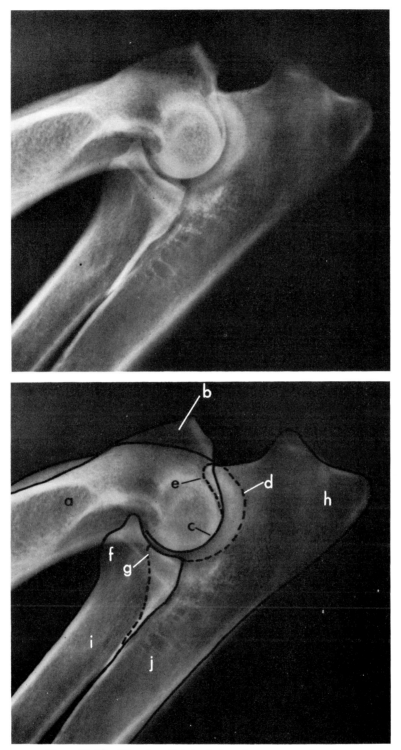

Figure 11–24. Flexed mediolateral view of a mature canine elbow.
  a. Humerus
  b. Medial epicondyle
  c. Medial condyle
  d. Lateral condyle
  e. Anconeal process
  f. Radial tuberosity
  g. Coronoid process
  h. Olecranon
  i. Radius
  j. Ulna

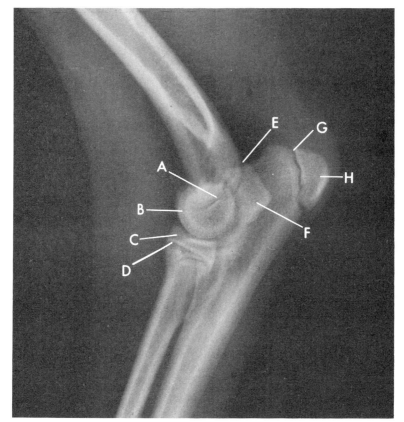

Figure 11–25. Mediolateral view of an immature canine elbow (five-month-old miniature poodle).

A. Physis of humeral condyles
B. Humeral condyles (superimposed)
C. Proximal radial epiphysis
D. Proximal radial physis
E. Medial humeral epicondylar physis
F. Medial humeral epicondylar
G. Olecranon physis
H. Olecranon epiphysis

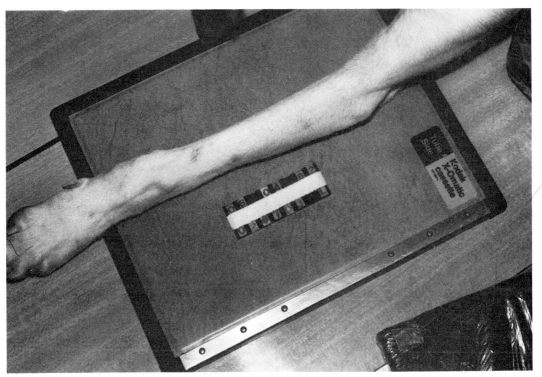

Figure 11–26. Position for the craniocaudal view of the radius and ulna.

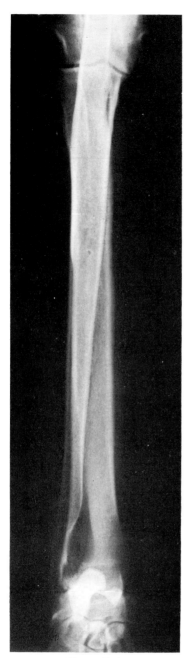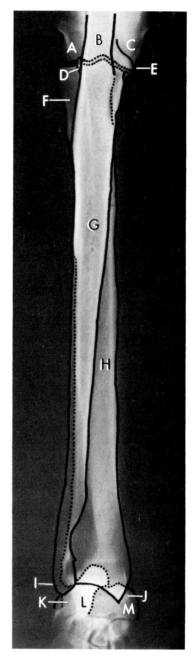

Figure 11–27. Craniocaudal view of the mature canine radius and ulna.
- A. Lateral condyle of humerus
- B. Olecranon
- C. Medial condyle of humerus
- D. Lateral aspect of coronoid process
- E. Medial aspect of coronoid process
- F. Head of radius
- G. Ulna
- H. Radius
- I. Styloid process of ulna
- J. Styloid process of radius
- K. Ulnar carpal bone
- L. Accessory carpal bone
- M. Radial carpal bone

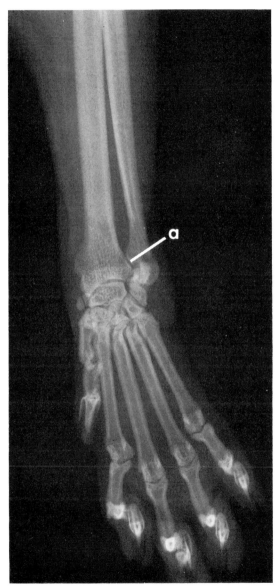

Figure 11–28.   Craniocaudal view of the distal radius and ulna of the feline.
a. Distal radioulnar articulation

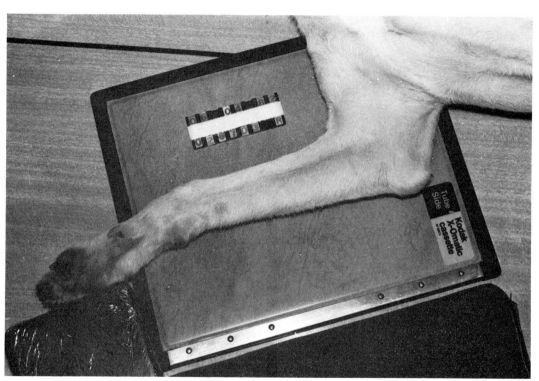

Figure 11–29. Position for mediolateral view of the radius and ulna.

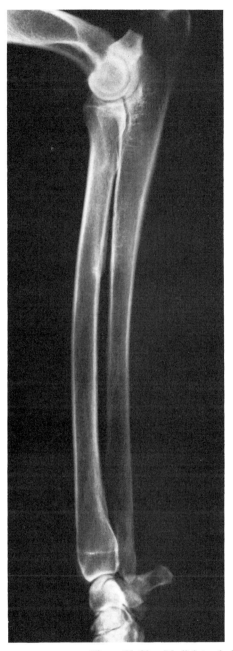
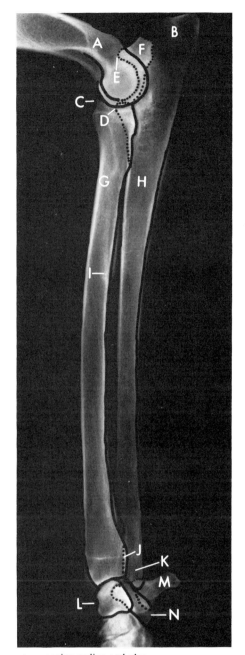

Figure 11–30. Mediolateral view of the mature canine radius and ulna.

A. Humerus
B. Olecranon
C. Radial tuberosity
D. Coronoid process
E. Anconeal process
F. Medial epicondyle
G. Radius
H. Ulna
I. Nutrient foramen of radius
J. Distal radioulnar articulation
K. Styloid process of ulna
L. Radial carpal bone
M. Accessory carpal bone
N. Ulnar carpal bone

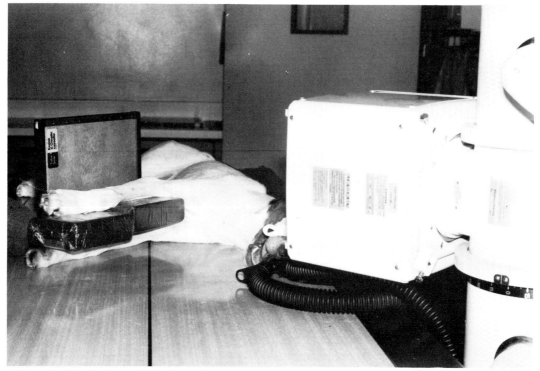

Figure 11–31. Craniocaudal (horizontal) view of the radius and ulna using a horizontally oriented x-ray beam.

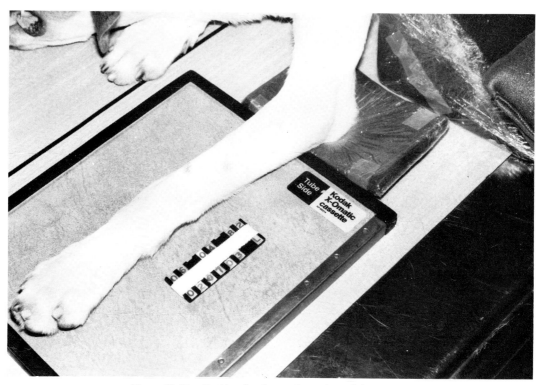

Figure 11–32. Position for dorsopalmar view of the carpus.

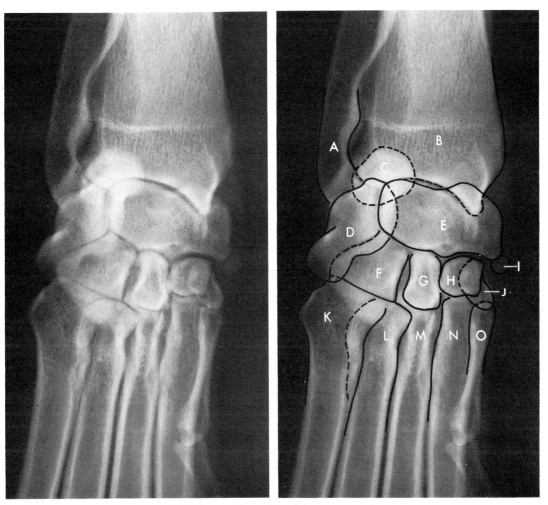

Figure 11–33. Dorsopalmar view of the mature canine carpus.

A. Ulna
B. Radius
C. Accessory carpal bone
D. Ulnar carpal bone
E. Radial carpal bone
F. 4th carpal bone
G. 3rd carpal bone
H. 2nd carpal bone
 I. Sesamoid bone in the tendon of abductor pollicis longus muscle
J. 1st carpal bone
K. 5th metacarpal bone
L. 4th metacarpal bone
M. 3rd metacarpal bone
N. 2nd metacarpal bone
O. 1st metacarpal bone

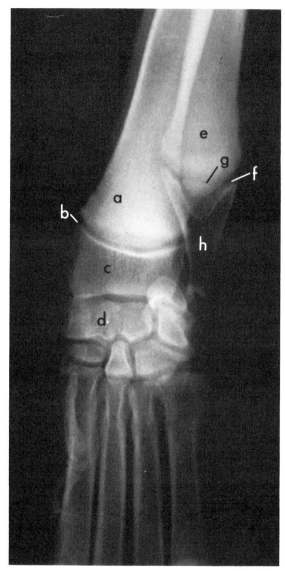

Figure 11–34. Dorsopalmar view of a four-month-old canine carpal region.
  a. Distal radial metaphysis
  b. Distal radial physis
  c. Distal radial epiphysis
  d. Radial carpal bone
  e. Distal ulnar metaphysis
  f. Distal ulnar physis
  g. Lucent line produced by proximal edge of the ulnar epiphysis
  h. Distal ulnar epiphysis

(d) in immature patients. Notice that the distal ulnar physis is cone-shaped and that the proximal edge of the epiphysis produces a radiolucent line (g) across the distal metaphysis (Fig. 11–34).

Mediolateral (ML) View. The patient is placed in lateral recumbency and the limb to be examined is placed adjacent to the film (Fig. 11–35). The contralateral limb is flexed and pulled back over the thorax. The x-ray beam is centered over the carpal joint.

Figure 11–36 illustrates the normal radiographic anatomy of the mature canine carpus in ML projection.

Flexed Mediolateral (ML [flexed]) View. The patient is placed in lateral recumbency and the limb to be examined is placed adjacent to the film (Fig. 11–37). The joint is flexed and the contralateral limb is pulled back over the thorax. The x-ray beam is centered over the carpal joint.

This position is useful at times to delineate the source of chip fractures or to examine the dorsal aspects of the carpal joint surfaces.

Figure 11–38 illustrates the normal radiographic anatomy of the mature canine carpus in the ML (flexed) projection.

Dorsomedial-Palmarolateral Oblique (D45°M-PaLO) View. The patient is placed in ventral recumbency and the limb to be examined is pulled forward. The dorsal surface is then rotated laterally approximately 45 degrees (supinated) (Fig. 11–39). The x-ray beam is then centered on the carpal joint.

The D45°M-PaLO view is used to examine the dorsolateral and palmaromedial aspects of the carpus, and the oblique projection of the first, the second and possibly the third metacarpal bones.

Figure 11–40 illustrates the normal radiographic anatomy of the D45°M-PaLO view of a mature canine carpus.

Palmaromedial-Dorsolateral Oblique (Pa45°M-DLO) View. The patient is placed in lateral recumbency with the limb being examined placed adjacent to the film. The dorsal surface is rotated laterally approximately 45 degrees (supinated) (Fig. 11–41). The x-ray beam is centered at the carpus.

The Pa45°M-DLO view is used to examine the dorsomedial and palmarolateral aspects of the carpal joint and the oblique projection of the distal ulna and the fourth and fifth metacarpal bones.

Figure 11–42 illustrates the normal radiographic anatomy of the Pa45°M-DLO view of the mature canine carpus.

METACARPUS

Dorsopalmar (DPa) View. The patient is placed in ventral recumbency and the limb to be examined is pulled forward (Fig. 11–43). The x-ray beam is centered at the junction of the proximal two thirds to the distal one third of the metacarpal bones. Specific examination of the carpus should not be made using this position, because obliquity of the x-ray beam will not project the carpal articular spaces parallel to the central ray. This view may be used for the dorsopalmar projection of the digits because the natural flexion or extension of the metacarpal-phalangeal and intraphalangeal joints usually prevents adequate evaluation of joint space even with specific placement of the central x-ray beam at the joint space of interest. These spaces are best examined in the lateral projection.

Figure 11–44 illustrates the normal radiographic anatomy of the DPa view of the mature canine metacarpal region.

Mediolateral (ML) View. The patient is placed in lateral recumbency and the limb being examined is placed adjacent to the film (Fig. 11–45). The contralateral limb is pulled back and placed over the thorax. The x-ray beam is centered at the junction of the proximal two thirds to the distal one third of the metacarpal bones. Figure 11–46 illustrates the normal radiographic anatomy of the ML view of the mature canine metacarpal region.

DIGITS

Dorsopalmar (DPa) View. The DPa projection of the digits is similar to the DPa view of the metacarpal region. A radiolucent object such as a wooden spoon may be used to apply pressure to the dorsal surface in order to flatten the digits against the cassette.

Mediolateral (ML) View. The patient is placed in lateral recumbency and the limb to be examined is pulled forward and placed on the film. The specific digit to be examined is pulled dorsally and fixed in this position with tape (Fig. 11–47). The remaining digits may need to be secured with tape in order to maintain traction on the digit being examined. The x-ray beam is centered at the distal end of the first phalanx. If the joint spaces are to be evaluated, the digit must be kept parallel to the film.

Figure 11–48 illustrates the normal radiographic anatomy of the ML view of the mature canine digit.

References follow on page 159

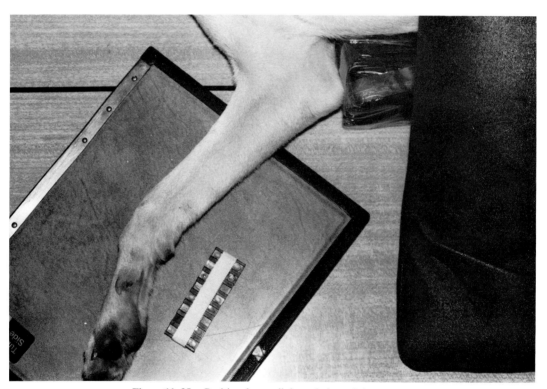

Figure 11–35. Position for mediolateral view of the carpus.

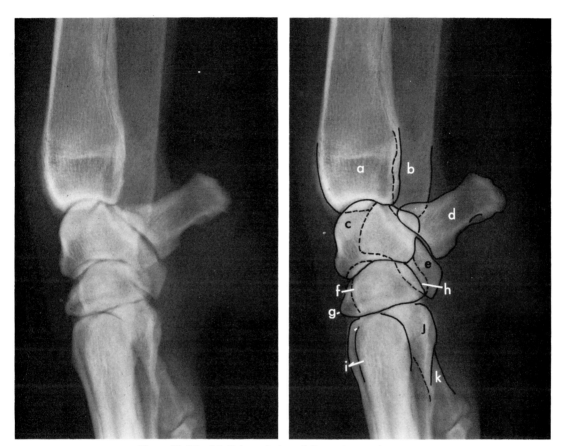

Figure 11–36. Mediolateral view of the mature canine carpus.
  a. Radius
  b. Ulna
  c. Radial carpal bone
  d. Accessory carpal bone
  e. Ulnar carpal bone
  f. 2nd carpal bone
  g. 3rd carpal bone
  h. 4th carpal bone
  i. 2nd, 3rd, and 4th metacarpal bones superimposed
  j. 5th metacarpal bone
  k. 1st metacarpal bone

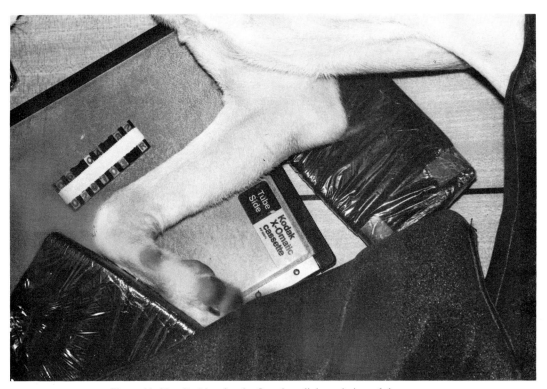

Figure 11–37. Position for the flexed mediolateral view of the carpus.

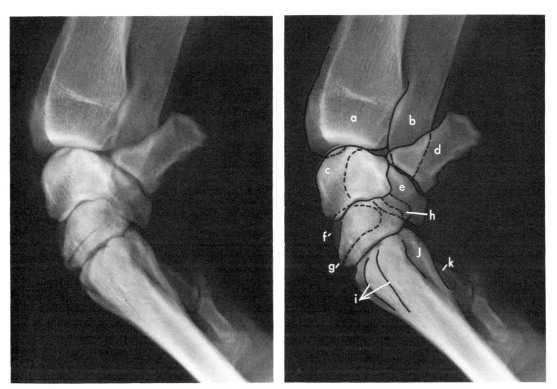

Figure 11–38. Flexed mediolateral view of the mature canine carpus.

a. Radius
b. Ulna
c. Radial carpal bone
d. Accessory carpal bone
e. Ulnar carpal bone
f. 2nd carpal bone
g. 3rd carpal bone
h. 4th carpal bone
i. 2nd, 3rd, and 4th metacarpal bones superimposed
j. 5th metacarpal bone
k. 1st metacarpal bone

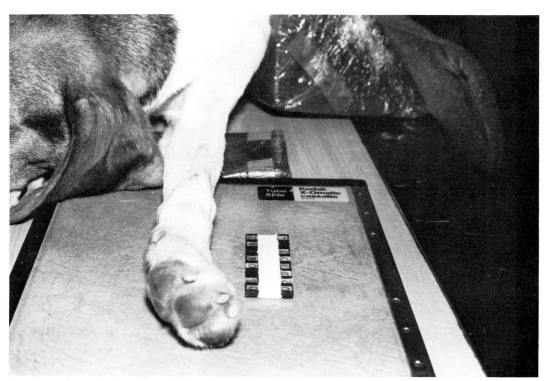

Figure 11–39. Position for dorsomedial-palmarolateral oblique view of the carpus.

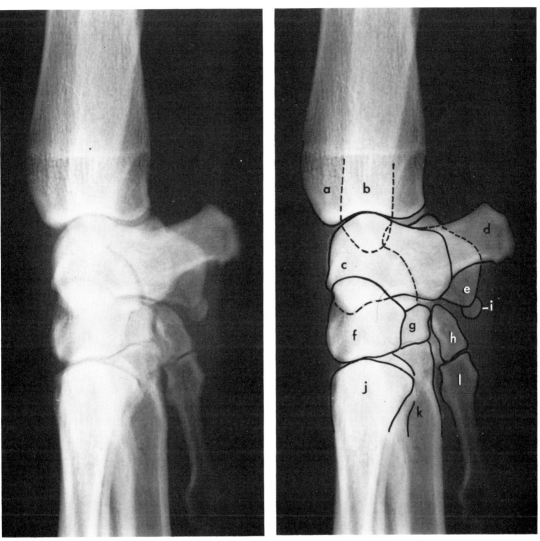

Figure 11–40. Dorsomedial-palmarolateral oblique view of the mature canine carpus.

    a. Radius
    b. Ulna
    c. Radial carpal bone
    d. Accessory carpal bone
    e. Ulnar carpal bone
    f. 4th carpal bone
    g. 3rd carpal bone
    h. 1st carpal bone
    i. Sesamoid bone in the tendon of abductor pollicis longus muscle
    j. 4th and 5th metacarpal bones superimposed
    k. 2nd metacarpal bone
    l. 1st metacarpal bone

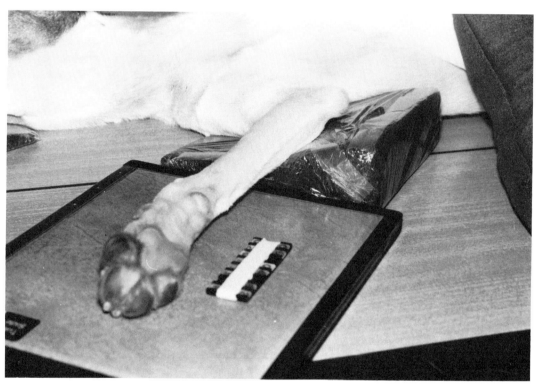

Figure 11–41. Position for palmaromedial-dorsolateral oblique view of the carpus.

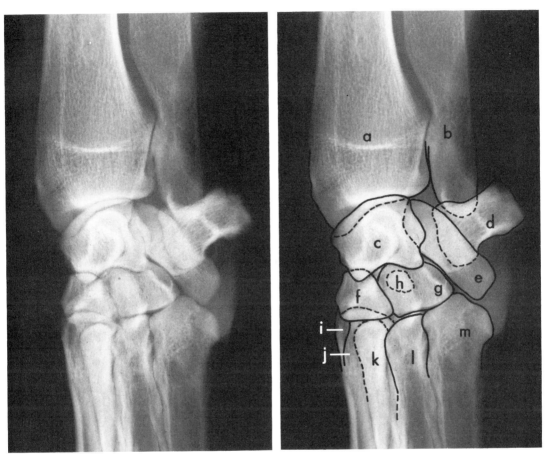

Figure 11–42. Palmaromedial-dorsolateral oblique view of the mature canine carpus.

a. Radius
b. Ulna
c. Radial carpal bone
d. Accessory carpal bone
e. Ulnar carpal bone
f. 2nd carpal bone
g. 4th carpal bone
h. Sesamoid bone in the tendon of abductor pollicis longus muscle
i. 2nd metacarpal bone
j. 3rd metacarpal bone
k. 1st metacarpal bone
l. 4th metacarpal bone
m. 5th metacarpal bone

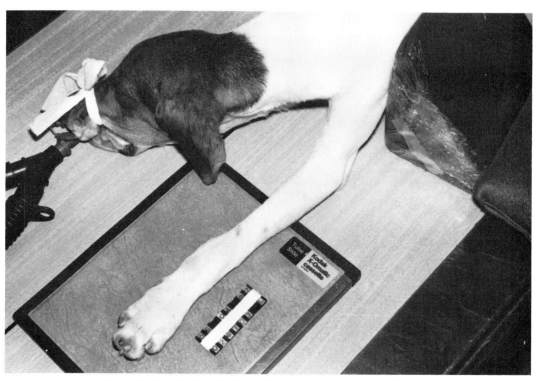

Figure 11–43. Position for dorsopalmar view of the metacarpal region.

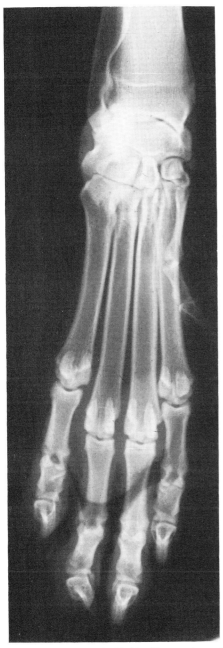
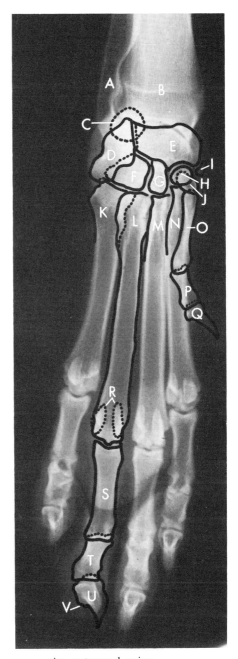

Figure 11–44. Dorsopalmar view of the mature canine metacarpal region.

A. Ulna
B. Radius
C. Accessory carpal bone
D. Ulnar carpal bone
E. Radial carpal bone
F. 4th carpal bone
G. 3rd carpal bone
H. 2nd carpal bone
I. Sesamoid bone in the tendon of abductor pollicis longus muscle
J. 1st carpal bone
K. 5th metacarpal bone

L. 4th metacarpal bone
M. 3rd metacarpal bone
N. 2nd metacarpal bone
O. 1st metacarpal bone
P. 1st and 2nd phalanx (fused), 1st digit
Q. 3rd phalanx, 1st digit
R. Palmar sesamoid bones at metacarpophalangeal articulation of 4th digit
S. 1st phalanx, 4th digit
T. 2nd phalanx, 4th digit
U. 3rd phalanx, 4th digit
V. Ungual crest of 3rd phalanx

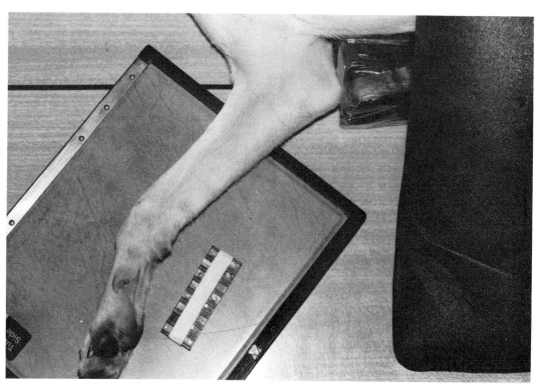

Figure 11–45. Position for the mediolateral view of the metacarpal region.

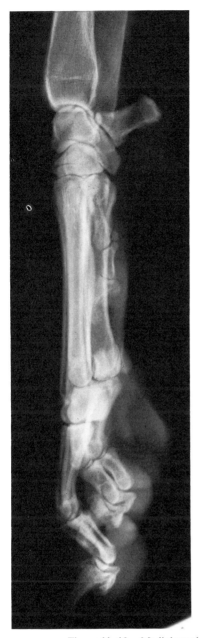

Figure 11–46. Mediolateral view of the mature canine metacarpal region.

A. Radius
B. Ulna
C. Radial carpal bone
D. Accessory carpal bone
E. Ulnar carpal bone
F. 2nd carpal bone
G. 3rd carpal bone
H. 4th carpal bone
I. 1st metacarpal bone
J. Palmar sesamoid bones at metacarpophalangeal
   articulation of 1st digit

K. 1st and 2nd phalanx, 1st digit
L. 3rd phalanx, 1st digit
M. 5th metacarpal bone
N. Dorsal sesamoid bone at metacarpophalangeal
   articulation of 5th digit
O. Palmar sesamoid bone at metacarpophalangeal
   articulation of 5th digit
P. 1st phalanx, 5th digit
Q. 2nd phalanx, 5th digit
R. 3rd phalanx, 5th digit
S. Ungual crest of 3rd phalanx

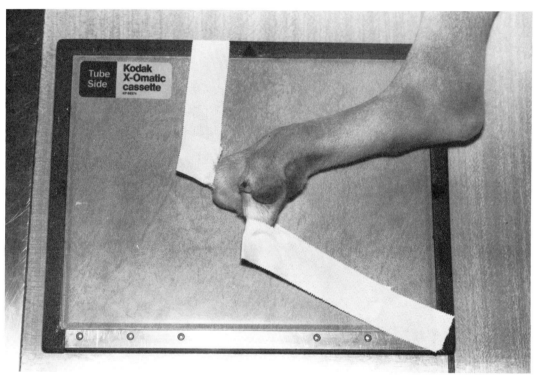

Figure 11–47. Position for the mediolateral view of the digits.

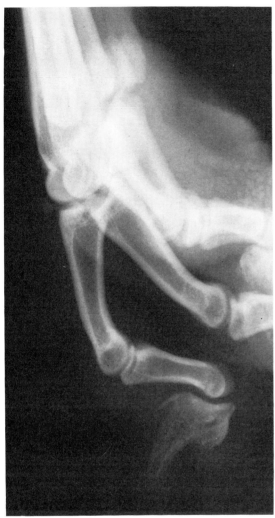 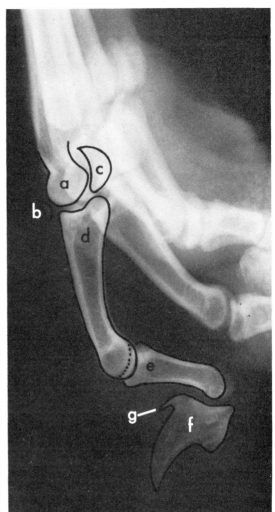

Figure 11–48. Mediolateral view of the mature canine digits.

a. 3rd metacarpal bone
b. Dorsal sesamoid bone
c. Palmar sesamoid bones at metacarpophalangeal articulation of the 3rd digit
d. 1st phalanx of the 3rd digit
e. 2nd phalanx of the 3rd digit
f. 3rd phalanx of the 3rd digit
g. Ungual crest of the 3rd phalanx

REFERENCES

Gillette, E. L., Thrall, D. E., and Lebel, J. L.: Carlson's Veterinary Radiology, 3rd ed. Philadelphia, Lea and Febiger, 1977.

Chapman, W. L.: Appearance of ossification centers and epiphyseal closures—determined by radiographic techniques. Thesis. Fort Collins, Colorado, Colorado State University, 1963.

Crouch, J. E.: Text-Atlas of Cat Anatomy. Philadelphia, Lea & Febiger, 1969.

Douglas, S. W., and Williamson, H. D.: Principles of Veterinary Radiography. 3rd ed. Baltimore, Williams & Wilkins Co., 1980.

Hare, W. C. D.: Radiographic anatomy of the canine pectoral limb. Part I. Fully developed limb. J.A.V.M.A., 135:265, 1959a.

Hare, W. C. D.: Radiographic anatomy of the canine pectoral limb. Part II. Developing limb. J.A.V.M.A., 135:305, 1959b.

Miller, M. E., Christensen, G. C., and Evans, H. E.: Anatomy of the Dog. Philadelphia, W. B. Saunders Co., 1964.

Schebitz, H., and Wilkens, H.: Atlas of Radiographic Anatomy of Dog and Cat. Berlin, Paul Parey, 1978.

Getty, R.: Sisson and Grossman's The Anatomy of the Domestic Animals. 5th ed. Philadelphia, W. B. Saunders Co., 1975.

Suter, P. F., and Carb, A. V.: Shoulder arthrography in dogs—radiographic anatomy and clinical application. J. Sm. An. Pract., 10:407, 1969.

Morgan, J. P., Silverman, S., and Zontine, W. J.: Techniques of Veterinary Radiography. 2nd ed. Davis, CA., Veterinary Radiology Associates, 1977.

12

Pelvic Limb

PELVIS AND HIP JOINT

Ventrodorsal–Extended Hip (VD–extended hip) View. The patient is placed in dorsal recumbency, and the femurs are extended, adducted and placed parallel to a line extended along the vertebral column. The hip joints are fully extended, and cranial aspects of the femurs are rotated medially (Fig. 12–1) so that the patellas are projected over the midportion of the distal femur (Fig. 12–2). The hip joints should be equidistant from the table top. Slight rotation of the pelvis causing elevation or depression of either hip joint will result in an asymmetrical projection of the acetabulums and femoral heads. When properly positioned, the obturator foramens, the hip joints, the hemipelves and the sacroiliac joints appear as mirror images of each other. With imperfect positioning, the side with the smallest obturator foramen will show the shallowest appearing acetabulum (Morgan, 1972a). This side will be the closest to the film (Smith, 1963). Positional correction may be accomplished by elevating the affected side. The side with the largest obturator foramen will show an artifactually deeper acetabulum. For radiographic evaluation of hip joint conformation, pelvic rotation must be prevented.

If inadequate medial rotation of the femurs occurs, the patellas will be projected laterally, and the fovea capitus and lesser trochanter will be more prominent (Smith, 1963). If excessive medial rotation occurs, the patellas will be projected medially, the curvature of the femoral head will appear unbroken, and neither fovea capitus nor lesser trochanter will be well visualized (Morgan, 1972b). These signs vary considerably in different breeds of dogs.

Excessive femoral abduction will force the femoral heads into the acetabulums and change the profile of the femoral necks. This may result in a mistaken diagnosis of a femoral neck valgus deformity (Morgan, 1972a).

Positioning of the dog for a VD–extended hip view of the pelvis is facilitated by the use of general anesthesia or a tranquilizer (Morgan, 1972b). Support devices are also helpful (Olsson, 1962). A foam trough works well for maintaining the patient in dorsal recumbency. Positioning devices may be as simple as a pair of sand bags laid alongside the patient to maintain position while the femurs are extended with ropes or tape. Medial rotation of the patellas and the parallel relationship of the femurs may be maintained with tape placed around the stifle joints. Anesthetized patients in such devices may be maintained in the same position until the first radiograph is developed. Positional adjustments may then be made, using the first film as a reference. Anesthesia-produced relaxation does not allow subluxation of normal hip joints (Dixon, 1972).

The VD–extended hip position is most commonly used to evaluate the canine hip joints for dysplasia (Whittington et al., 1961; Riser, 1962). For the radiographic demonstration of hip joint laxity, an object (wedge) is placed between the femurs while the animal is in the VD–extended hip position (Bardens, 1972). This wedge acts as a fulcrum when medial pressure is applied to the distal aspects of the limbs. Since this technique involves many variables, it should not be used for routine radiographic examination of the hip joints.

Figure 12–2 illustrates the normal radiographic anatomy of a mature canine pelvis in VD–extended hip view.

Ventrodorsal–Flexed Hip (VD–flexed hip) View (Frog-Legged Position). The patient is placed in dorsal recumbency, and the femurs are flexed and abducted so that the stifle joints are lateral to the abdomen (Fig. 12–3). The femurs are placed at an angle of approximately 45 degrees to the vertebral column. It is important that the limbs be positioned identically. Excessive, forceful hip flexion may result in caudal pelvic elevation, which will cause the pelvis to appear shortened (Olsson, 1962; Lawson, 1963; Smith, 1963). This artifact will cause the acetabulums to appear deeper than they are when properly positioned (Morgan, 1972b).

Figure 12–4 illustrates the normal radiographic anatomy of a mature canine pelvis in VD–flexed hip view.

Left-Right, or Right-Left Lateral (LeRtL or RtLeL) View. The patient is placed in lateral recumbency with the dependent limb pulled cranially and labeled with a lead marker (Fig. 12–5). The nondependent limb is elevated with a foam block to a position parallel to the table top. This view is most useful for examining unsuspected pubic or sacral pathology.

Figure 12–6 illustrates the normal radiographic anatomy of a mature canine pelvis in left-right lateral view.

Lateral Oblique (Le20°D-RtVO or Rt20°D-LeVO) View. The patient is placed in lateral recumbency with the dependent limb pulled cranially and labeled (Fig. 12–7). A foam wedge is used to elevate the dorsal aspect of the pelvis approximately 20 degrees from the table in such a manner that there will be no superimposition of the hemipelves and hip joints. In right recumbency, this projection would be termed a left dorsal-right ventral oblique (Le20°D-RtVO) and would result in the dependent right hemipelvis being projected dorsally on the radiograph. This projection may also be produced by placing the patient in true lateral position (without the foam wedge) and adjusting the tube angle so that the x-ray beam is directed 20 degrees toward the dorsal aspect from its normal overhead postion. It is usually simpler to elevate the pelvis, however.

For examination of the left hemipelvis, the patient is placed on the left side and the dorsal aspect of the pelvis is elevated 20 degrees. This will result in a right dorsal–left ventral oblique (Rt20°D-LeVO) view.

Figure 12 8 illustrates the normal radiographic anatomy of a mature canine pelvis in Le20°D-RtVO view.

FEMUR

Craniocaudal (CrCd) View. The patient is placed in dorsal recumbency and the limb to be examined is extended (Fig. 12–9). The x-ray beam is centered at midfemur. The beam collimation and film size should be large enough to include the hip and stifle joints. Slight abduction of the limb will aid in obtaining a proper CrCd alignment.

To prevent underexposure, measurement for exposure calculation should be made at the proximal femur. In some breeds of dogs, this exposure may cause excessive radiographic density of the distal femur and stifle joint, thus requiring two radiographs for adequate examination.

Figure 12–10 illustrates the normal radiographic anatomy of a mature canine femur in the CrCd view.

Mediolateral (ML) View. The patient is placed in lateral recumbency with the limb to be examined placed on the table. The nondependent leg is abducted and rotated out of the line of the x-ray beam (Fig. 12–11). The x-ray beam is centered midfemur. The beam collimation and film size should be large enough to include the hip and stifle joints.

Measurement for exposure calculation should be made at the proximal femur. In some breeds of dogs, this exposure may cause excessive radiographic density of the distal femur, and two radiographs may be required for adequate examination.

Figure 12–12 illustrates the normal radiographic anatomy of a mature canine femur in the ML view.

STIFLE JOINT

Caudocranial (CdCr) View. The patient is placed in ventral recumbency and the limb to be examined is pulled caudally into a position of maximum extension. The contralateral limb is flexed and elevated with a sand bag or foam pad (Fig 12–13). The degree of

Text continued on page 170.

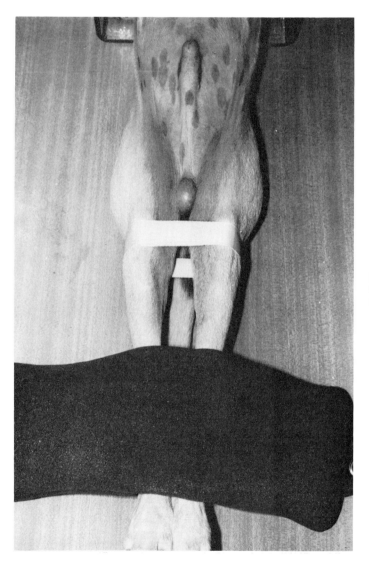

Figure 12–1. Position for ventrodorsal view of the pelvis with femurs extended.

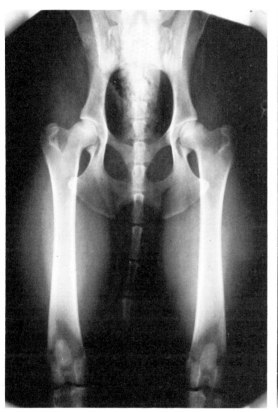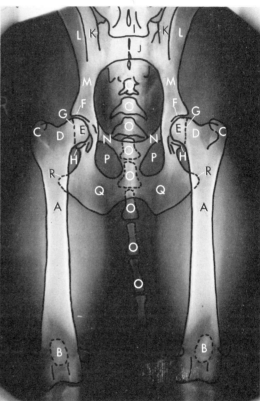

Figure 12–2. Ventrodorsal view of a mature canine pelvis with femurs extended.

A. Femur
B. Patella
C. Greater trochanter
D. Femoral neck
E. Femoral head
F. Cranial acetabular edge
G. Dorsal acetabular edge
H. Caudal acetabular edge
 I. 7th lumbar vertebra

J. Sacrum
K. Sacroiliac joint
L. Wing of the ilium
M. Ilium
N. Pubis
O. Coccygeal vertebrae
P. Obturator foramen
Q. Ischium
R. Ischiatic tuberosity

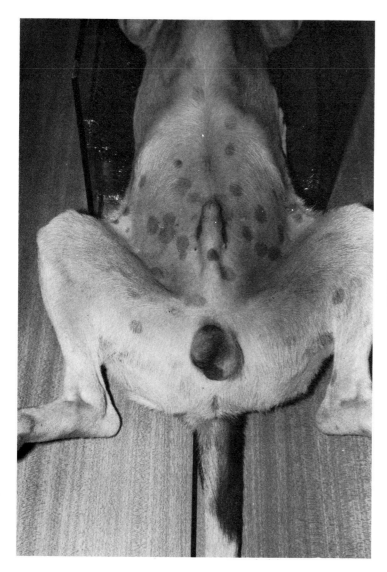

Figure 12–3. Position for ventrodorsal view of the pelvis with femurs flexed.

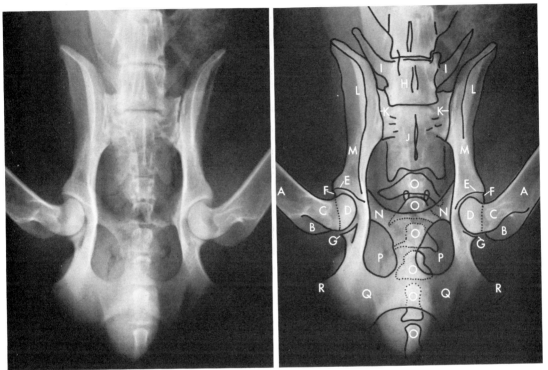

Figure 12–4. Ventrodorsal view of a mature canine pelvis with femurs flexed.

    A. Femur
    B. Greater trochanter
    C. Femoral neck
    D. Femoral head
    E. Cranial acetabular edge
    F. Dorsal acetabular edge
    G. Caudal acetabular edge
    H. 7th lumbar vertebra
    I. Lateral processes of 7th lumbar vertebra
    J. Sacrum
    K. Sacroiliac joint
    L. Wing of the ilium
    M. Ilium
    N. Pubis
    O. Coccygeal vertebrae
    P. Obturator foramen
    Q. Ischium
    R. Ischiatic tubersoity

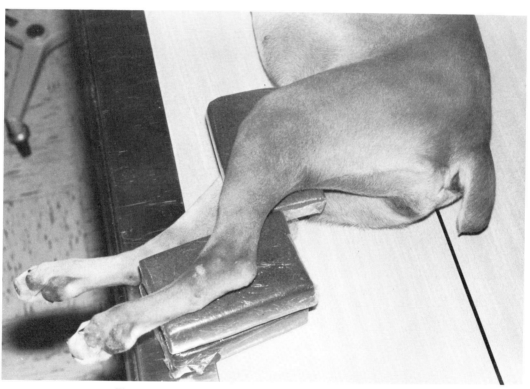

Figure 12–5. Position for the left-right lateral view of the pelvis.

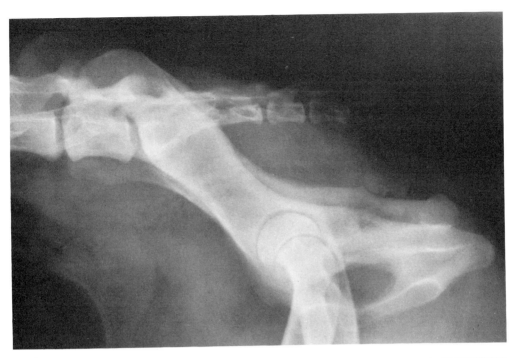

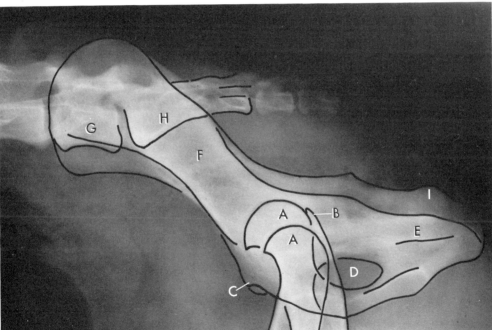

Figure 12–6. Left-right lateral view of a mature canine pelvis.

 A. Femoral heads
 B. Greater trochanter
 C. Pubis
 D. Obturator foramen
 E. Ischium
 F. Ilium
 G. 7th lumbar vertebra
 H. Sacrum
 I. Ischiatic tuberosity

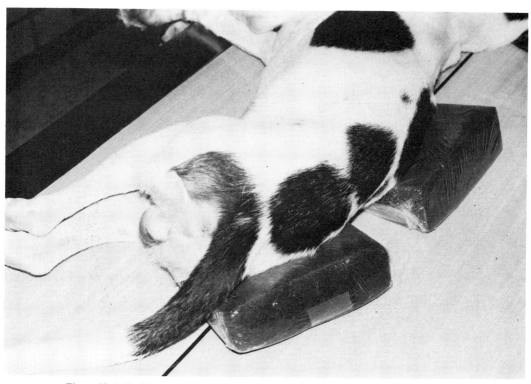

Figure 12–7. Position for the left dorsal–right ventral oblique view of the canine pelvis.

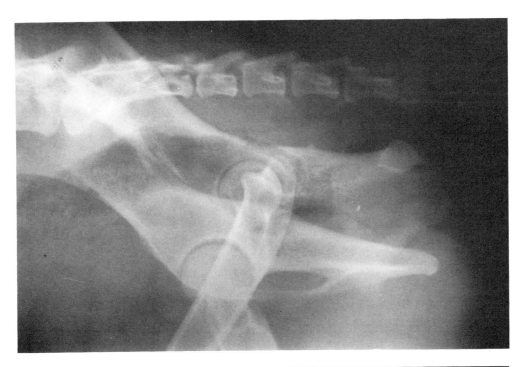

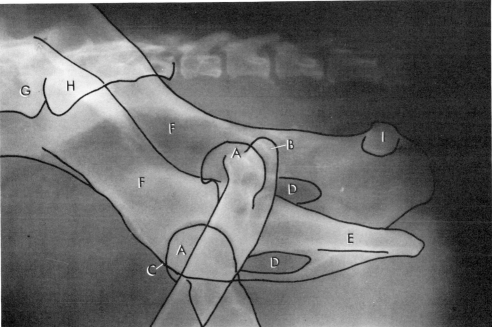

Figure 12–8. Left dorsal–right ventral oblique view of a mature canine pelvis.

A. Femoral heads
B. Greater trochanter
C. Pubis
D. Obturator foramen
E. Ischium
F. Ilium (right side on top)
G. 7th lumbar vertebra
H. Sacrum
I. Ischiatic tuberosity

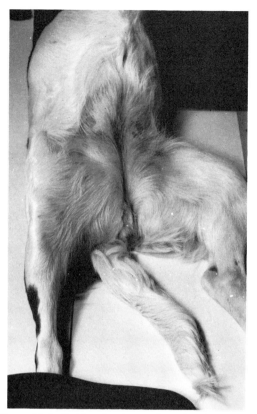

Figure 12–9. Position for the craniocaudal view of the femur.

elevation will control the rotation of the stifle joint being examined. Palpation of the tibial tuberosity assists in determining the proper degree of limb rotation necessary for exact CdCr projection. In large dogs the x-ray beam should be angled approximately 10 degrees in the distal direction from its normal perpendicular orientation to prevent superimposition of the femoral condyles over the proximal tibia. This is termed a caudal 10-degree distal-cranioproximal oblique (Cd10°Di-CaPrO) view. The x-ray beam is centered at the joint space.

Weight-bearing studies using a horizontal x-ray beam centered at the joint space may be useful in evaluating chronic joint disease in small animals (Morgan, 1972a). Because of the difficulty in obtaining an accurate positional relationship between the joint space and the x-ray beam, such studies should be limited to cases that fail to show diagnostic radiographic signs on routine radiographs.

Figure 12–14 illustrates the normal radiographic anatomy of a mature canine stifle point in the CdCr view.

Mediolateral (ML) View. The patient is placed in lateral recumbency and the joint to be examined is placed on the cassette. The contralateral limb is flexed and abducted (Fig. 12–15). The tarsal joint is elevated with a foam pad so that the tibia is parallel to the table surface. The x-ray beam is centered at the joint space.

Figure 12–16 illustrates the normal radiographic anatomy of a mature canine stifle joint in the ML view.

Figure 12–17 illustrates the normal radiographic anatomy of an eight-month-old canine stifle joint region. Note that the distal aspect of the tibial tuberosity physis appears as a widened radiolucent space between the tuberosity epiphysis *(A)* and the proximal tibial metaphysis *(C)*. This normal structure must not be mistaken for an avulsion fracture. The tibial tuberosity epiphysis appears during the third month of life and unites with the proximal tibial epiphysis *(B)* during the eighth or ninth month; together, they unite with the tibial metaphysis during the tenth to twelfth month (Hare, 1960b).

Caudocranial (flexed/horizontal) (CdCr flexed/horizontal) (tangential) View of the Distal Femur. The patient is placed in dorsal recumbency and the joint to be examined is flexed maximally and abducted. The hip is then flexed until the femur is perpendicular to the table surface (Fig. 12–18). The cassette is placed adjacent to the cranial surface of the femoral segment, and the x-ray beam is directed in a plane parallel to the table top (horizontal beam) and centered at the distal end of the femur. This view is useful in examining the depth of the intercondylar groove. This projection was formerly called the tangential view.

Figure 12–19 illustrates the normal radiographic anatomy of a mature canine distal femur in the CdCr (flexed/horizontal) view.

TIBIA AND FIBULA

Caudocranial (CdCr) View. The patient is placed in ventral recumbency and the limb to be examined is pulled caudally into a position of maximum extension. The contralateral limb is flexed and elevated with a sand bag or foam wedge (Fig. 12–20). The degree of elevation will control the rotation of the tibia being examined. Palpation of the tibial crest of the limb assists in determining the

Text continued on page 179.

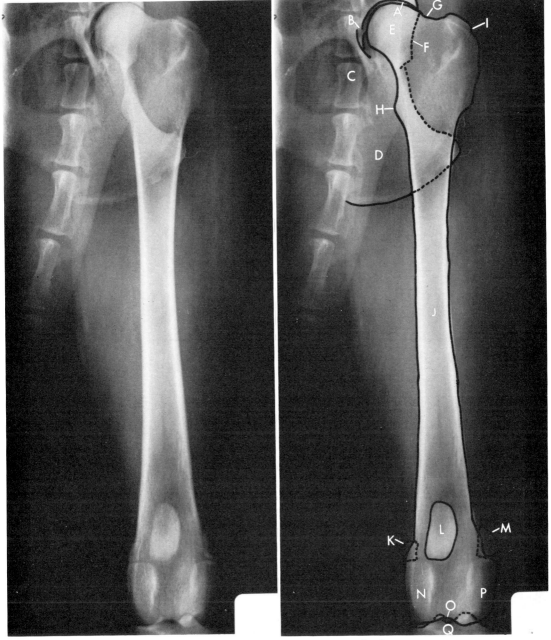

Figure 12–10. Craniocaudal view of a mature canine femur.
  A. Cranial acetabular edge
  B. Acetabular notch
  C. Obturator foramen
  D. Ischium
  E. Femoral head
  F. Dorsal acetabular edge
  G. Femoral neck
  H. Lesser trochanter
  I. Greater trochanter
  J. Femoral diaphysis
  K. Medial fabella in tendon of gastrocnemius muscle
  L. Patella
  M. Lateral fabella in tendon of gastrocnemius muscle
  N. Medial condyle
  O. Intercondyloid fossa
  P. Lateral condyle
  Q. Tibia

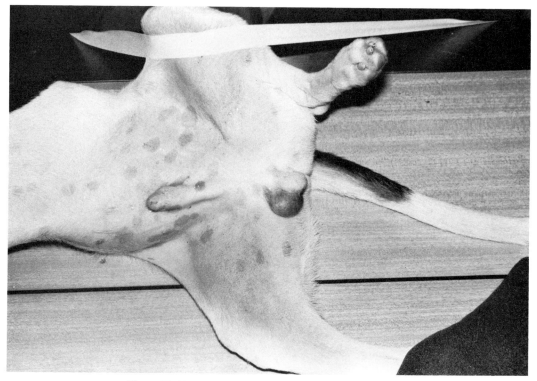

Figure 12–11. Position for the mediolateral view of the femur.

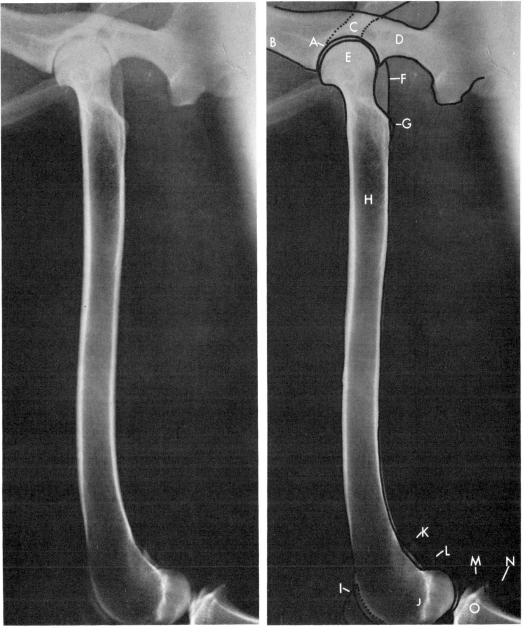

Figure 12–12. Mediolateral view of a mature canine femur.

- A. Acetabulum
- B. Ilium
- C. Pubis
- D. Ischium
- E. Femoral head
- F. Greater trochanter
- G. Lesser trochanter
- H. Femoral diaphysis
- I. Patella
- J. Femoral condylar superimposed
- K. Lateral fabella in tendon of gastrocnemius muscle
- L. Medial fabella in tendon of gastrocnemius muscle
- M. Fabella in tendon of popliteus muscle
- N. Fibula
- O. Tibia

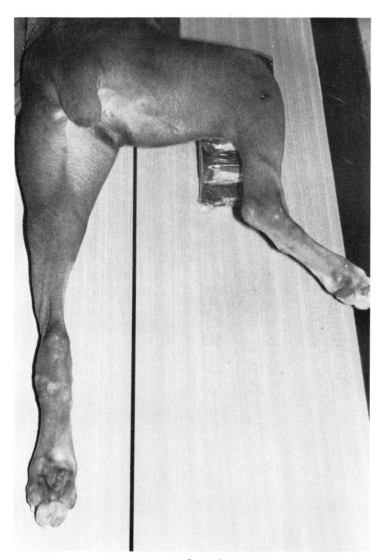

Figure 12–13. Caudocranial view of the stifle joint. Note the contralateral limb is flexed and elevated by foam wedge.

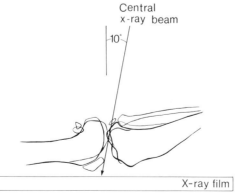

Central
x-ray beam

10°

X-ray film

Preferred x-ray beam angulation for large dogs.

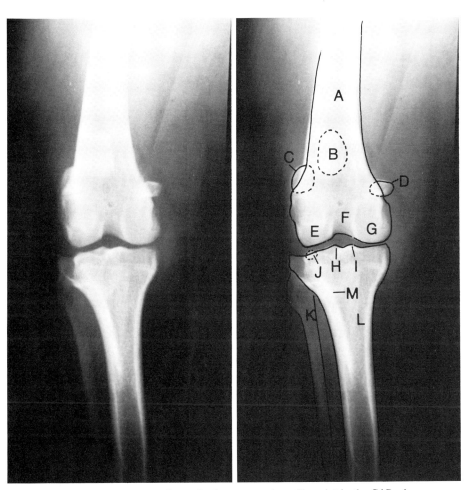

Figure 12–14. Normal radiograph of mature canine stifle point in the CdCr view.

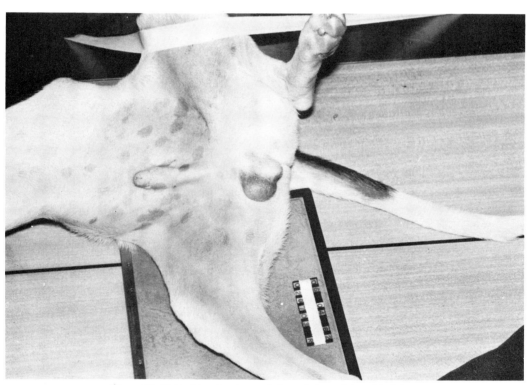

Figure 12–15. Position for the mediolateral view of the stifle joint.

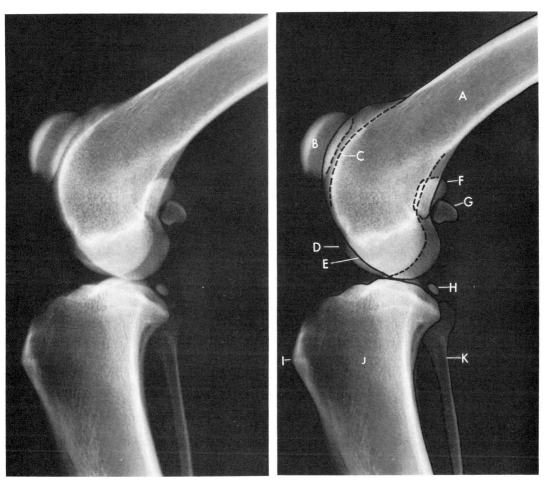

Figure 12–16. Mediolateral view of a mature canine stifle joint.

A. Femur
B. Patella
C. Trochlear groove
D. Lateral condyle
E. Medial condyle
F. Lateral fabella in tendon of gastrocnemius muscle
G. Medial fabella in tendon of gastrocnemius muscle
H. Fabella in tendon of popliteus muscle
I. Tibial tuberosity
J. Tibia
K. Fibula

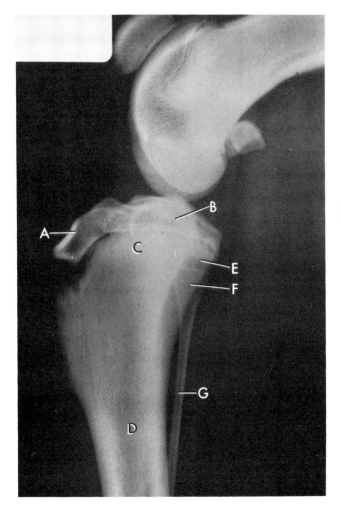

Figure 12–17. Mediolateral view of an immature canine stifle region.
   A. Epiphysis of tibial tuberosity
   B. Epiphysis of proximal tibia
   C. Metaphysis of proximal tibia
   D. Diaphysis of tibia
   E. Epiphysis of proximal fibula
   F. Metaphysis of proximal fibula
   G. Diaphysis of fibula

proper degree of limb rotation necessary for exact CdCr projection.

The x-ray beam should be collimated to include both the stifle and tarsal joints. The central x-ray beam is placed at the middiaphyseal region.

Figure 12–21 illustrates the normal radiographic anatomy of the mature canine tibia and fibula in the CdCr view.

Mediolateral (ML) View. The patient is placed in lateral recumbency and the tibia to be examined is placed on the cassette. The contralateral limb is flexed and abducted (Fig. 12–22).

The x-ray beam is collimated to include both the stifle and tarsal joints. The central x-ray beam is placed at the mid-diaphyseal region.

Figure 12–23 illustrates the normal radiographic anatomy of the mature canine tibia and fibula in the ML view.

PELVIC LIMB EXAMINATION FOR SEVERELY INJURED FEMUR OR TIBIA AND FIBULA

The craniocaudal projection of a severely fractured femur or tibia and fibula is best performed with the patient in lateral recumbency using a horizontally oriented x-ray beam. This will allow the limb to be placed in a nonstressed position and will prevent additional trauma to the injured site. The patient is placed in opposite lateral recumbency from the injured limb. The limb is supported by a dry foam block. The cassette is placed on the caudal surface of the limb and the x-ray beam is directed craniocaudally in a plane parallel to the table top (Fig. 12–24).

TARSUS

Dorsoplantar (DPl) View. The patient is placed in dorsal recumbency, and the limb to be examined is extended behind the patient (Fig. 12–25). The x-ray beam is centered at the proximal intratarsal joint.

Figure 12–26 illustrates the normal radiographic anatomy of the mature canine tarsus in a DPl projection.

Mediolateral (ML) View. The patient is placed in lateral recumbency and the limb to be examined is placed on the cassette. The tibial-tarsal articulation is moderately flexed

(Fig. 12–27). The contralateral limb is retracted caudally. The x-ray beam is centered at the proximal intratarsal joint.

Figure 12–28 illustrates the normal radiographic anatomy of the mature canine tarsus in ML projection.

Dorsolateral-Plantaromedial Oblique (D45°L-PlMO) View. The patient is placed in dorsal recumbency and the limb to be examined is fully extended behind the patient (Fig. 12–29). The dorsal surface of the tarsus is rotated medially (pronated) approximately 45 degrees. The x-ray beam is centered at the proximal intratarsal joint. This view is used to examine the dorsomedial and plantarolateral aspects of the tarsus.

Figure 12–30 illustrates the normal radiographic anatomy of the mature canine tarsus in the D45°L-PlMO view.

Dorsomedial-Plantarolateral Oblique (D45°M-PlLO) View. The patient is placed in dorsal recumbency and the limb to be examined is fully extended behind the patient (Fig. 12–31). The dorsal surface of the tarsus is rotated laterally (supinated) approximately 45 degrees. The x-ray beam is centered at the proximal intratarsal joint. This view is used to examine the dorsolateral and plantaromedial aspects of the tarsus.

Figure 12–32 illustrates the normal radiographic anatomy of the mature canine tarsus in the D45°M-PlLO view.

METATARSUS

Dorsoplantar (DPl) View. The patient is placed in ventral recumbency, and the limb to be examined is flexed at the hip and extended at the stifle and tarsal joints in such a manner that the limb lies alongside the patient (Fig. 12–33). The limb is slightly abducted and the metatarsal region is aligned in a true DPl projection. The x-ray beam is centered at the mid-metatarsal region.

Figure 12–34 illustrates the normal radiographic anatomy of the mature canine metatarsal region in a DPl projection.

Mediolateral (ML) View. The patient is placed in lateral recumbency and the limb to be examined is placed on the cassette. The tarsal joint is moderately flexed (Fig. 12–35). The contralateral limb is retracted caudally. The x-ray beam is centered at the mid-metatarsal region.

Figure 12–36 illustrates the normal radio-

Text continued on page 198.

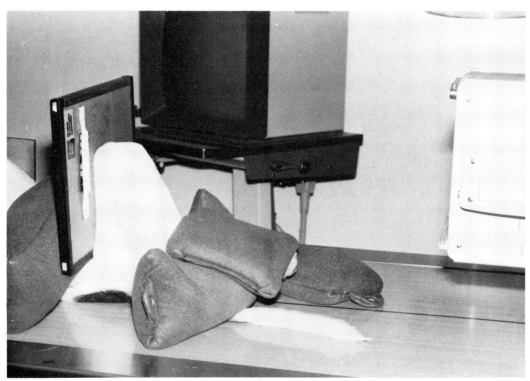

Figure 12–18. Position for the caudocranial (flexed/horizontal) view of the distal femur.

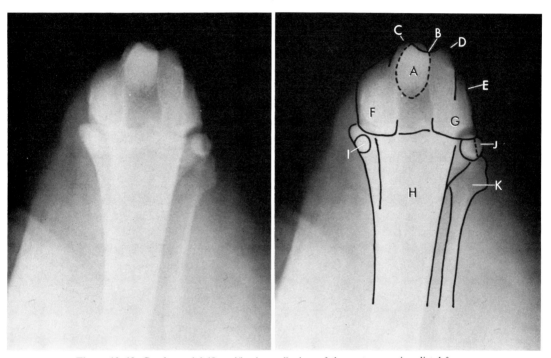

Figure 12–19. Caudocranial (flexed/horizontal) view of the mature canine distal femur.

      A. Patella
      B. Trochlear groove
      C. Medial ridge of trochlear groove
      D. Lateral ridge of trochlear groove
      E. Femur
      F. Medial condyle of femur
      G. Lateral condyle of femur
      H. Tibia
      I. Medial fabella in tendon of gastrocnemius muscle
      J. Lateral fabella in tendon of gastrocnemius muscle
      K. Fibula

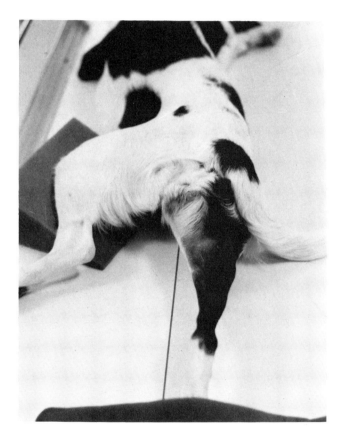

Figure 12–20. Position for the caudocranial view of the tibia and fibula.

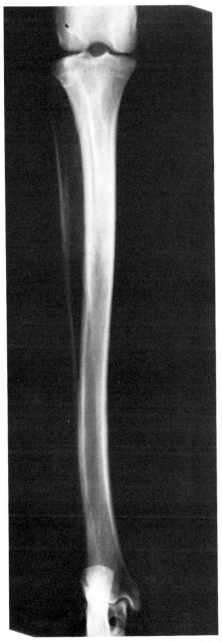

Figure 12–21. Caudocranial view of the mature canine tibia and fibula.

A. Lateral condyle of femur
B. Intercondyloid fossa
C. Medial condyle of femur
D. Lateral intercondyloid tubercle
E. Medial intercondyloid tubercle
F. Fibula
G. Tibial tuberosity

H. Nutrient foramen
 I. Tibia
 J. Lateral malleolus
K. Calcaneal process of fibular tarsal bone
L. Medial malleolus
M. Medial trochlear ridge of tibial tarsal bone

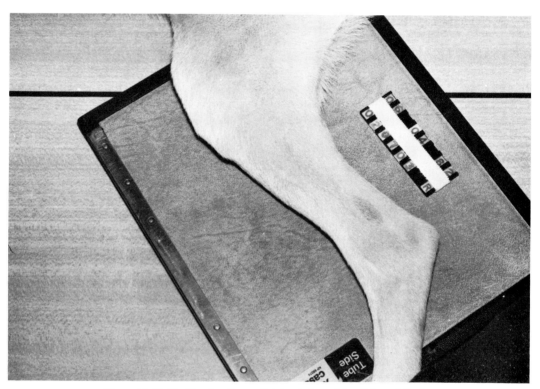

Figure 12–22. Position for the mediolateral view of the tibia and fibula.

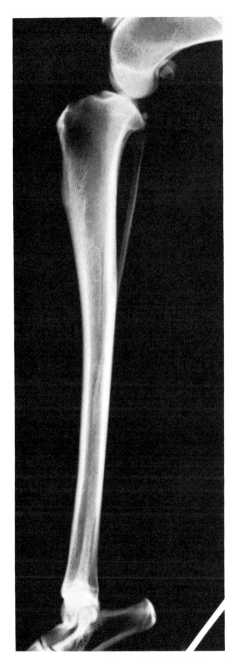
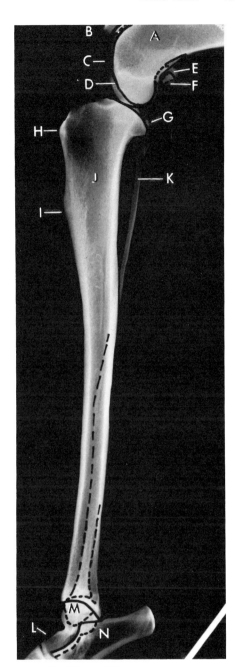

Figure 12–23. Mediolateral view of a mature canine tibia and fibula.

A. Femur
B. Patella
C. Lateral condyle
D. Medial condyle
E. Lateral fabella in tendon of gastrocnemuis muscle
F. Medial fabella in tendon of gastrocnemius muscle
G. Fabella in tendon of popliteus muscle
H. Tibial tuberosity
 I. Tibial crest
J. Tibia
K. Fibula
L. Tibial tarsal bone
M. Distal fibula and trochlea of tibial tarsal bone
N. Fibular tarsal bone

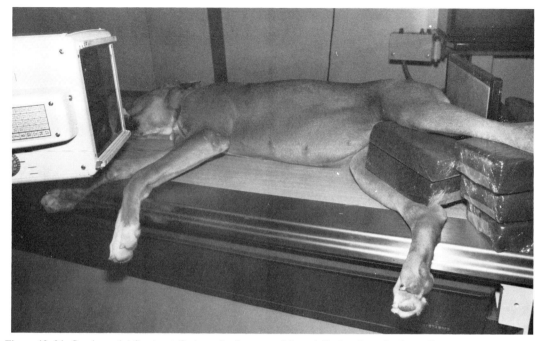

Figure 12–24. Craniocaudal (horizontal) view of a femur or tibia and fibula using a horizontally oriented x-ray beam.

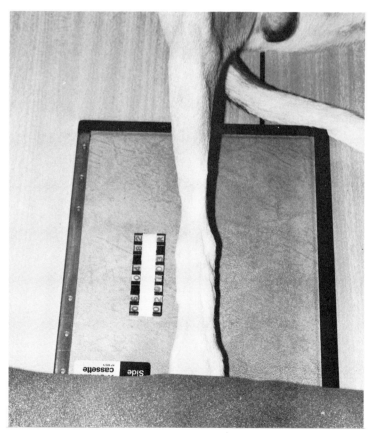

Figure 12–25. Position for the dorsoplantar view of the canine tarsus.

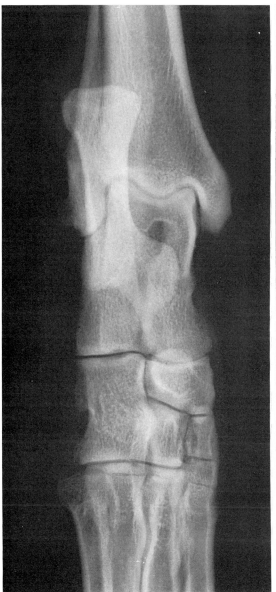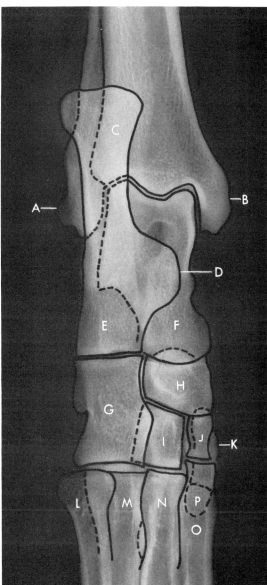

Figure 12–26. Dorsoplantar view of a mature canine tarsus.

A. Lateral malleolus (fibula)
B. Medial malleolus (tibia)
C. Calcaneal process of the calcaneus
D. Sustentaculum tali of the calcaneus
E. Calcaneus
F. Talus
G. 4th tarsal bone
H. Central tarsal bone

I. 3rd tarsal bone
J. 2nd tarsal bone
K. 1st tarsal bone
L. 5th metatarsal bone
M. 4th metatarsal bone
N. 3rd metatarsal bone
O. 2nd metatarsal bone
P. 1st metatarsal bone

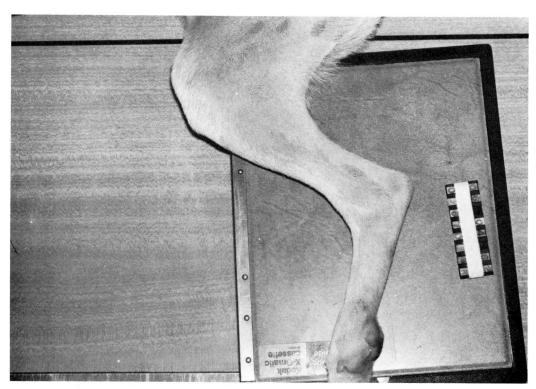

Figure 12–27. Position for the mediolateral view of the tarsus.

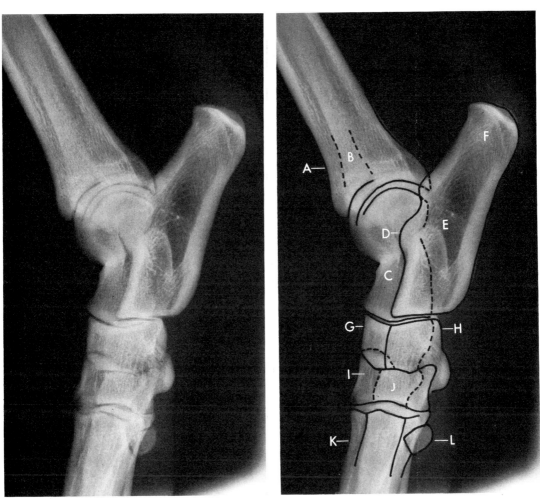

Figure 12–28. Mediolateral view of a mature canine tarsus.
- A. Tibia
- B. Fibula
- C. Talus
- D. Cochlear process of fibular tarsal bone
- E. Calcaneus
- F. Calcaneal process of the calcaneus (tuberosity)
- G. Central tarsal bone
- H. 4th tarsal bone
- I. 3rd tarsal bone
- J. 2nd tarsal bone
- K. 3rd metatarsal bone
- L. 1st metatarsal bone

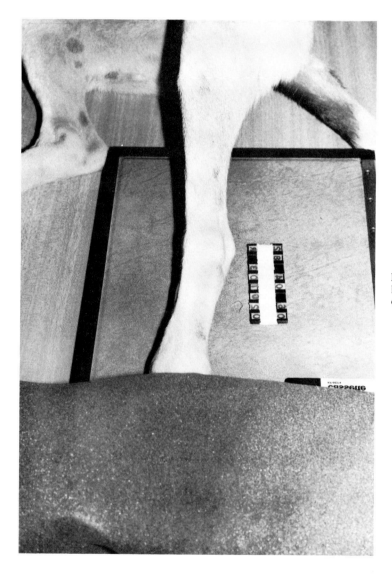

Figure 12–29. Position for Dorso 45° lateral-plantaromedial Oblique view of the tarsus.

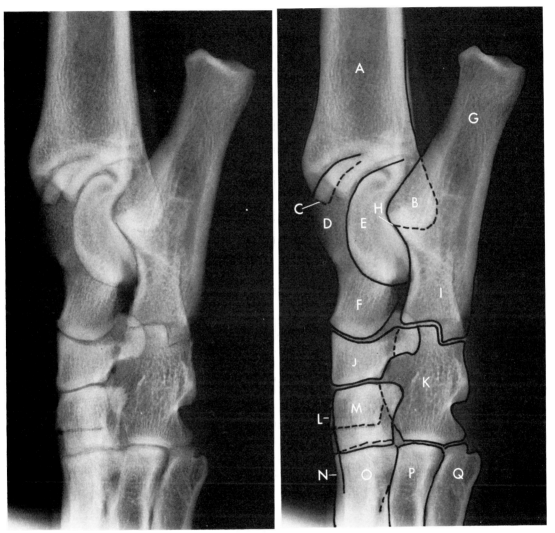

Figure 12–30. Dorso 45 degree lateral-plantaromedial oblique view of a mature canine tarsus.

A. Tibia
B. Lateral malleolus (fibula)
C. Medial malleolus
D. Medial trochlear ridge
E. Lateral trochlear ridge
F. Talus
G. Calcaneal process of the calcaneus
H. Cochlear process of the calcaneus
I. Calcaneus

J. Central tarsal bone
K. 4th tarsal bone
L. 2nd tarsal bone
M. 3rd tarsal bone
N. 2nd metatarsal bone
O. 3rd metatarsal bone
P. 4th metatarsal bone
Q. 5th metatarsal bone

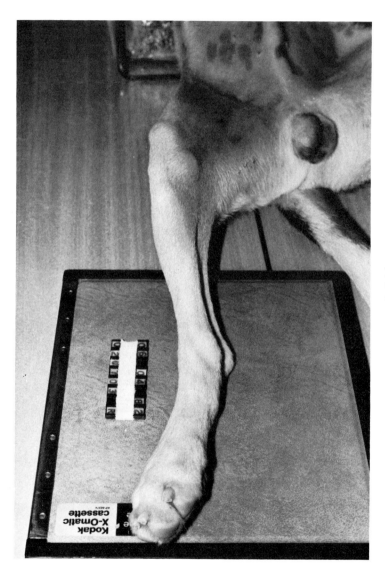

Figure 12–31. Position for dorso 45 degree medial plantarolateral oblique view of the tarsus.

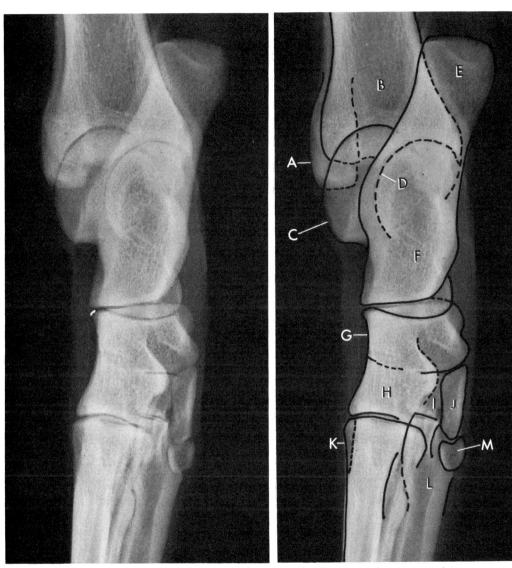

Figure 12–32. Dorso 45 degree medial plantarolateral oblique view of a mature canine tarsus.

A. Lateral malleolus (fibula)
B. Tibia
C. Lateral trochlear ridge of the talus
D. Medial trochlear ridge of the talus
E. Calcaneal process of the calcaneus
F. Calcaneus
G. 4th tarsal bone

H. 3rd tarsal bone superimposed on 4th
I. 2nd tarsal bone
J. 1st tarsal bone
K. 5th metatarsal bone
L. 2nd metatarsal bone
M. 1st metatarsal bone

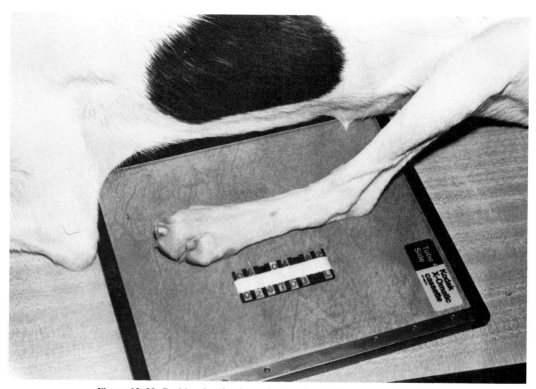

Figure 12–33. Position for the dorsoplantar view of the metatarsal region.

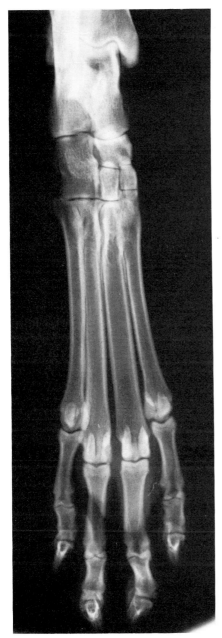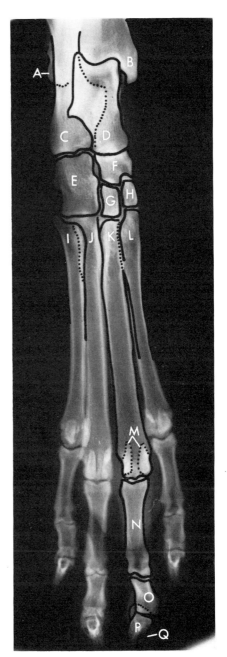

Figure 12–34. Dorsoplantar view of a mature canine metatarsal region.

A. Lateral malleolus (distal fibula)
B. Medial malleolus (distal tibia)
C. Calcaneus
D. Talus
E. 4th tarsal bone
F. Central tarsal bone
G. 3rd tarsal bone
H. 2nd tarsal bone
I. 5th metatarsal bone

J. 4th metatarsal bone
K. 3rd metatarsal bone
L. 2nd metatarsal bone
M. Plantar sesamoid bones at metatarsophalangeal articulation of 3rd digit
N. 1st phalanx, 3rd digit
O. 2nd phalanx, 3rd digit
P. 3rd phalanx, 3rd digit
Q. Ungual crest, 3rd phalanx

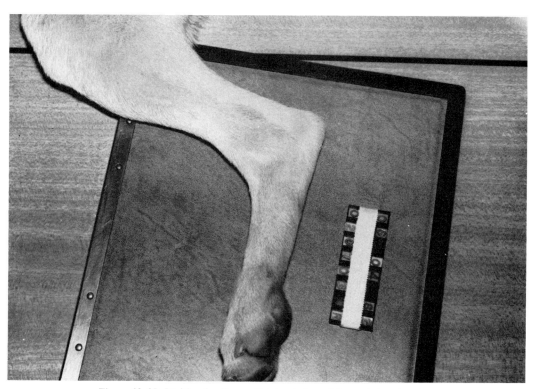

Figure 12–35. Position for the mediolateral view of the metatarsal region.

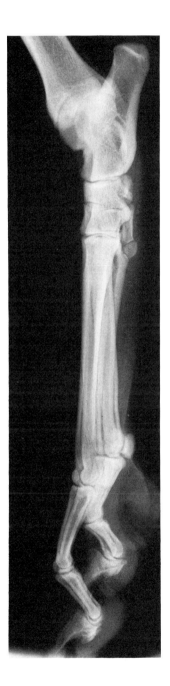 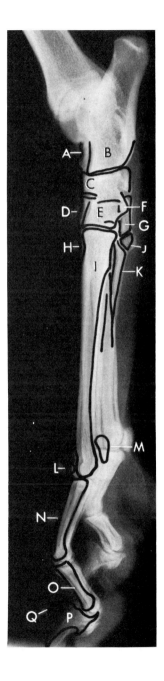

Figure 12–36. Mediolateral view of a mature canine metatarsal region.

A. Talus
B. Calcaneus
C. Central tarsal bone
D. 3rd tarsal bone
E. 2nd tarsal bone
F. 4th tarsal bone
G. 1st tarsal bone
H. 4th metatarsal bone
I. 3rd metatarsal bone
J. 1st metatarsal bone
K. 2nd metatarsal bone
L. Dorsal sesamoid bone
M. Plantar sesamoid bones at the metatarsophalangeal articulation of the 3rd digit
N. 1st phalanx, 3rd digit
O. 2nd phalanx, 3rd digit
P. 1st phalanx, 3rd digit
Q. Ungual crest, 3rd phalanx

graphic anatomy of the mature canine metatarsal region in ML projection.

REFERENCES

Bardens, J. W.: Palpation for the detection of dysplasia and wedge technique for pelvic radiography. Proceedings of the 39th Annual Meeting, American Animal Hospital Association, Las Vegas, Nevada, 1972, p. 468.

Getty, R.: Sisson and Grossman's: The Anatomy of the Domestic Animals. 5th ed. Philadelphia, W. B. Saunders Co., 1975.

Gillette, E. L., Thrall, D. E., and Lebel, J. L.: Carlson's Veterinary Radiology, 3rd ed. Philadelphia, Lea & Febiger, 1977.

Dixon, R. T.: The effect of limb positioning on the radiographic diagnosis of canine hip dysplasia. Vet. Rec., *91*:644, 1972.

Douglas, S. W., and Williamson, H. D.: Principles of Veterinary Radiography. 3rd ed. Baltimore, Williams & Wilkins Co., 1980.

Hare, W. C. D.: Radiographic anatomy of the canine pelvic limb. Part I. Fully developed limb. J.A.V.M.A., *136*:542, 1960*a*.

Hare, W. C. D.: Radiographic anatomy of the canine pelvic limb. Part II. Developing limb. J.A.V.M.A., *136*:603, 1960b.

Lawson, D. D.: The radiographic diagnosis of hip dysplasia in the dog. Vet. Rec., *75*:445, 1963.

Miller, M. E., Christensen, G. C., and Evans, H. E.: Anatomy of the Dog. Philadelphia, W. B. Saunders Co., 1964.

Morgan, J. P.: Radiography in Veterinary Orthopedics. Philadelphia, Lea & Febiger, 1972*a*.

Morgan, J. P.: Radiographic diagnosis of hip dysplasia in skeletally mature dogs. *In* Canine Hip Dysplasia Symposium and Workshop, St. Louis, Missouri, October, 1972*b*.

Olsson, S. E.: Roentgen examination of the hip joints of German shepherd dogs. Advanc. Sm. An. Pract., *3*:117, 1962.

Riser, W. H.: Producing diagnostic pelvic radiographs for canine hip dysplasia. J.A.V.M.A., *141*:600, 1962.

Schebitz, H., and Wilkens, H.: Atlas of Radiographic Anatomy of Dog and Cat. Berlin, Paul Parey, 1978.

Smith, R. N.: The normal radiological anatomy of the hip joint of the dog. J. Sm. An. Pract., *4*:1, 1963.

Whittington, K., Banks, W. C., Carlson, W. D., Hoerlein, B. F., Husted, P. W., Leonard, E. F., McClave, P. L., Rhodes, W. H., Riser, W. H., and Schnelle, G. B.: Report of the panel on canine hip dysplasia. J.A.V.M.A., *139*:791, 1961.

13

Vertebral Column

CERVICAL VERTEBRAE

Right-Left or Left-Right Lateral (LeRtL or RtLeL) View. Proper radiographic examination of the vertebral column can only be performed on patients that are relaxed, having been given either general anesthesia or sedation. This is particularly true for the lateral view of the cervical region.

The patient is placed in lateral recumbency and the forelimbs are retracted over the cranial thorax (Fig. 13–1). The vertebrae are elevated from the x-ray table with dry foam blocks so that the cervical and the thoracic vertebrae are on the same level.

The occipital-atlantal joint is moderately flexed (at approximately 45 degrees to the vertebral column) and the rostral aspect of the head is elevated to eliminate skull obliquity.

The x-ray beam is centered mid-cervically in small dogs. The x-ray beam should be collimated to include the caudal skull and the first few thoracic vertebrae and to exclude most cervical soft tissue. In large dogs (over 40 lb), it is generally preferable to produce two radiographs, one with the central x-ray beam at the C2–C3 interspace and another at the C5–C6 interspace. This technique will prevent obliquity of the intervertebral spaces at the edges of the x-ray beam and will also allow an increased exposure necessary to properly examine the relatively thick caudal cervical region without overexposing the cranial cervical region.

Figure 13–2 illustrates the normal radiographic anatomy of mature canine cervical vertebrae in left-right lateral view.

Occipital-Atlantal Articulation Left-Right or Right-Left Lateral Flexed (LeRtL or RtLeL [flexed]) View. The occipital-atlantal articulation may be flexed approximately 90 degrees to the vertebral column for studies of suspected odontoid process (dens) luxation. Positioning is the same as for the lateral cervical view except for the flexion (Fig. 13–3). The x-ray beam is centered at the joint. Extreme caution should be used during flexion since increased spinal cord injury may occur if severe ligamentous disruption is present.

Figure 13–4 illustrates the normal radiographic anatomy of a mature canine in flexed occipital-atlantal left-right lateral view.

Atlantal-Axial Articulation Left Ventral–Right Dorsal Oblique (Le20°V–RtDO) View. The patient is placed in lateral recumbency and the ventral aspect of the head and sternum are elevated 20 degrees (Fig. 13–5). The x-ray beam is centered at the atlantal-axial articulation. This examination is useful for evaluating suspected odontoid process (dens) pathology other than luxation. The oblique projection artifactually elevates the process from the floor of the atlas and rotates the usually superimposed wings of the atlas from the plane of the process.

Figure 13–6 illustrates the normal radiographic anatomy of a mature canine atlantal-axial region in Le20°V–RtDO view.

Ventrodorsal (VD) View. The patient is placed in dorsal recumbency with the forelimbs secured lateral to the thoracic walls (Fig. 13–7). The central x-ray beam is placed at the mid-cervical region. Measurement to determine the proper exposure should be made in the mid-cervical region in small patients in order to adequately expose both the cranial and caudal aspects of the cervical vertebrae. It may be necessary to produce

Text continued on page 218.

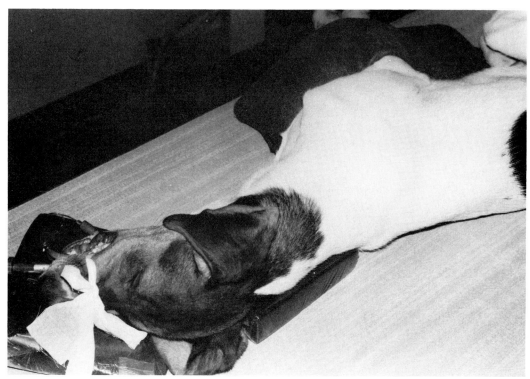

Figure 13–1. Position for left-right lateral view of the cervical vertebrae. Note the foam blocks elevating the midcervical region and rostral skull.

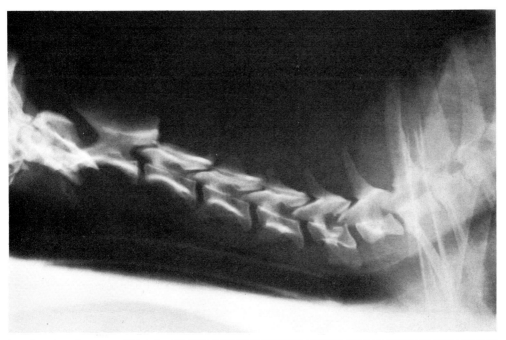

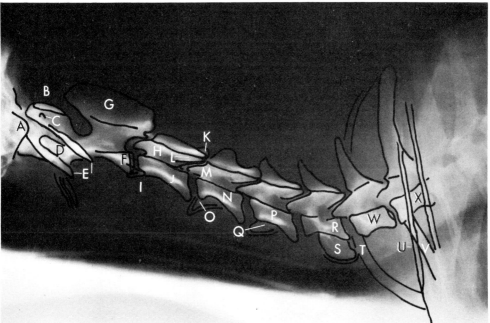

Figure 13–2. Left-right lateral view of the canine cervical vertebrae.

A. Occipital condyle
B. Dorsal arch of the atlas (C2)
C. Transverse foramen
D. Dens
E. Wings of the atlas
F. Body of the axis (C2)
G. Spinous process of the axis
H. Neural canal
I. Transverse process of the axis
J. Body of C2
K. Tubercle of the caudal articular process of C3
L. Caudal articular process of C3

M. Cranial articular process of C4
N. Body of C4
O. Transverse processes of C4
P. Body of C5
Q. Transverse processes of C5
R. Body of C6
S. Transverse processes of C6
T. Blade of the scapula
U. Spine of the scapula
V. 1st rib
W. Body of C7
X. Body of T1

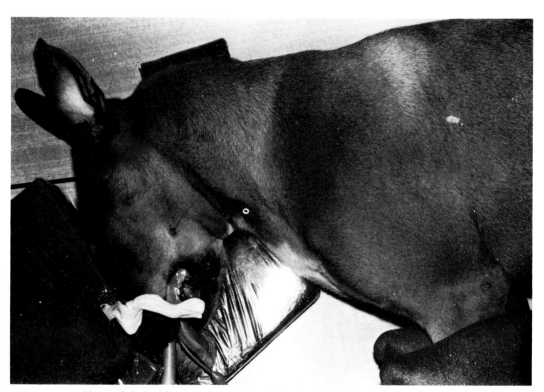

Figure 13–3. Position for left-right lateral flexed occipital-atlantal articulation view.

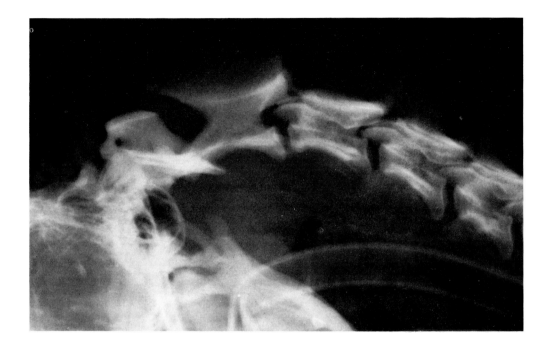

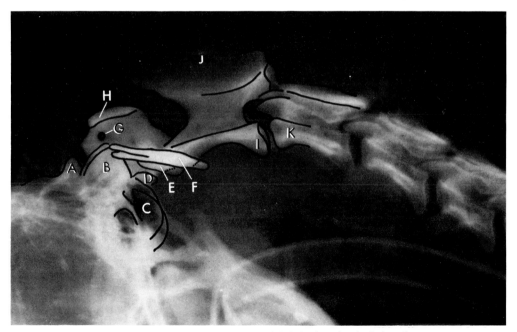

Figure 13–4. Left-right lateral flexed occipital-atlantal articulation view.

A. Nuchal tubercle
B. Occipital condyles
C. Tympanic bullae
D. Ventral arch (floor) of the atlas (C1)
E. Dens
F. Lateral processes of the atlas (C1)

G. Transverse foramen
H. Dorsal arch of atlas (C1)
I. Body of axis (C2)
J. Spinous process of axis (C2)
K. Body of C3

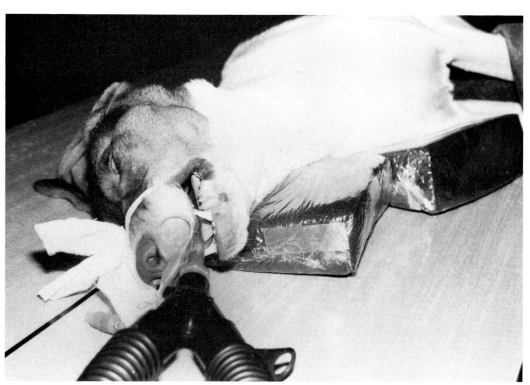

Figure 13–5. Position for atlantal-axial articulation, left 20-degree ventral—right dorsal oblique view.

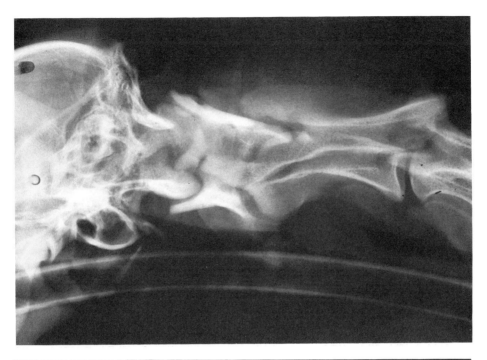

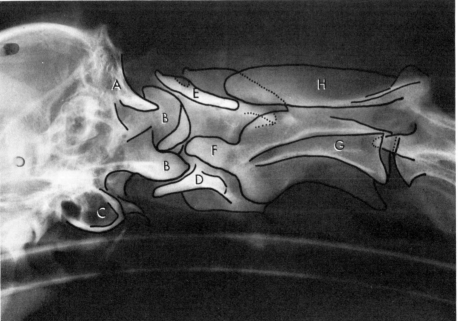

Figure 13–6. Atlantal-axial articulation of the canine, left 20 degree ventral—right dorsal oblique view.

A. Squamous part of the occipital bone
B. Occipital condyles
C. Tympanic bulla
D. Ventral arch (floor) of the atlas (C1)
E. Dorsal arch of the atlas (C1)
F. Dens
G. Body of the axis (C2)
H. Spinous process of the axis (C2)

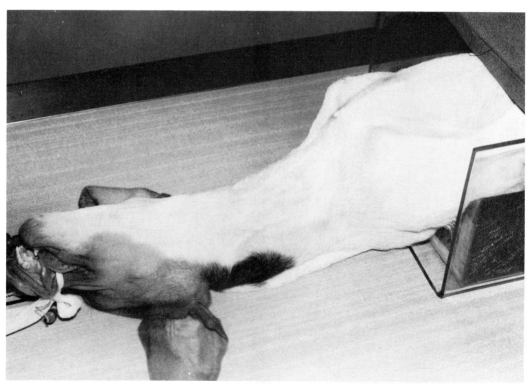

Figure 13–7. Position for ventrodorsal view of the cervical vertebrae.

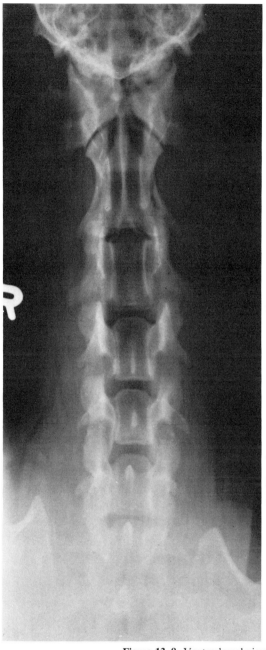
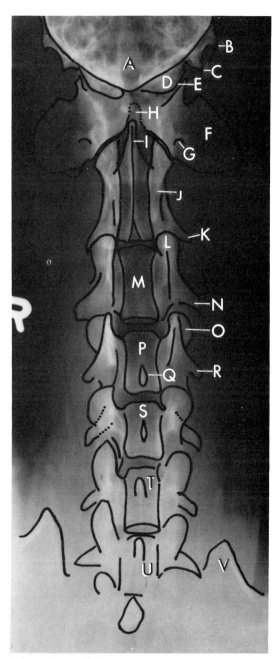

Figure 13–8. Ventrodorsal view of the canine cervical vertebrae.

A. Skull
B. Mastoid process
C. Jugular process
D. Occipital condyle
E. Occipital-atlantal articulation
F. Wings of the atlas (C1)
G. Transverse foramen
H. Dens
I. Spinous process of the axis (C2)
J. Axis (C2)
K. Transverse process of the axis

L. Cranial articular process of C3
M. C3
N. Transverse process of C3
O. Caudal articular process of the C3–C4 articulation
P. C4
Q. Spinous process of C4
R. Transverse process of C4
S. C5
T. C6
U. C7
V. Scapula

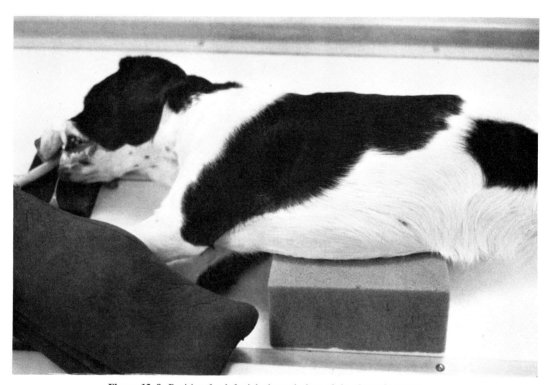

Figure 13–9. Position for left-right lateral view of the thoracic vertebrae.

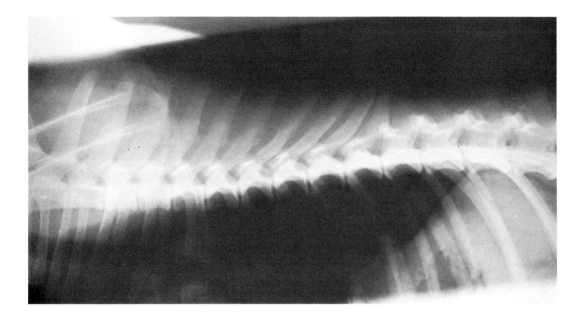

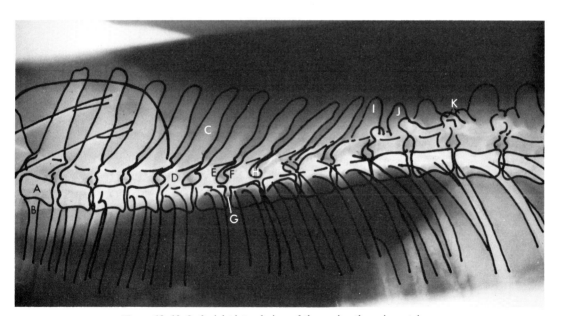

Figure 13–10. Left-right lateral view of the canine thoracic vertebrae.

A. Body of T1
B. 1st ribs
C. Spinous process of T5
D. Neural canal
E. Caudal articular process of T6
F. Cranial articular process of T7

G. Intervertebral disc space between T6–T7
H. Intervertebral foramen between T7–T8
I. Spinous process of T10
J. Spinous process of T11
K. Articular processes

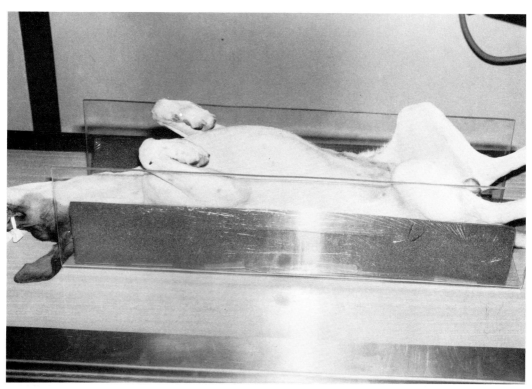

Figure 13–11. Positioning for ventrodorsal view of the thoracic vertebrae.

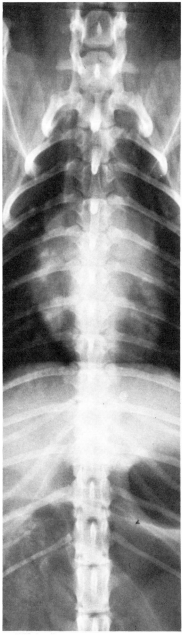

Figure 13–12. VD view of the canine thoracic vertebrae.

A. C7
B. T1
C. Spinous process of T1
D. Head of 2nd rib
E. Tubercle of 2nd rib
F. 2nd rib
G. Intervertebral disc space between T3–T4
H. Heart
I. T13
J. L1
K. Cranial articular process of T12

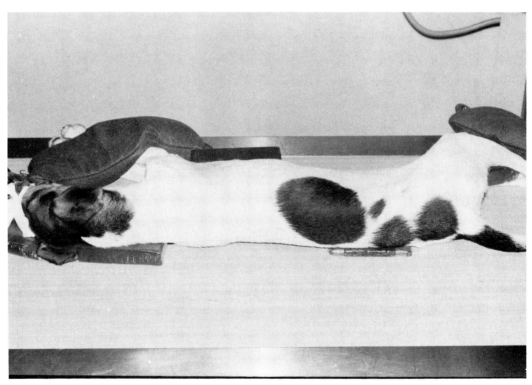

Figure 13–13. Positioning for right-left lateral view of the lumbar vertebrae.

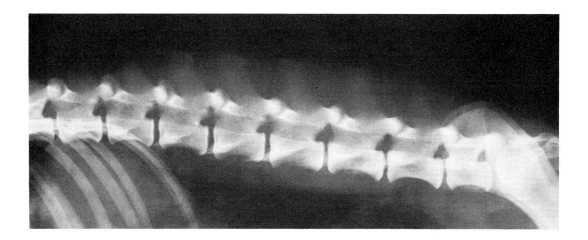

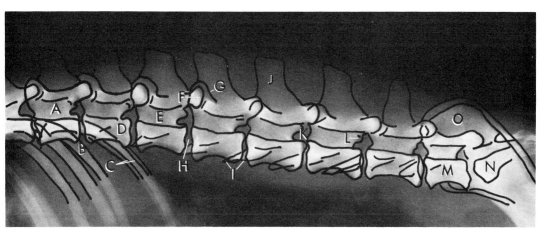

Figure 13–14. Left-right lateral view of the canine lumbar vertebrae.

A. T13
B. 12th rib
C. 13th rib
D. L1
E. Neural canal
F. Caudal articular process of L2
G. Cranial articular process of L3
H. Intervertebral disc space between L2–L3

I. Transverse processes of L4
J. Spinous process of L4
K. Intervertebral foramen between L4–L5
L. Accessory process
M. L7
N. Sacrum
O. Wings of the ilia

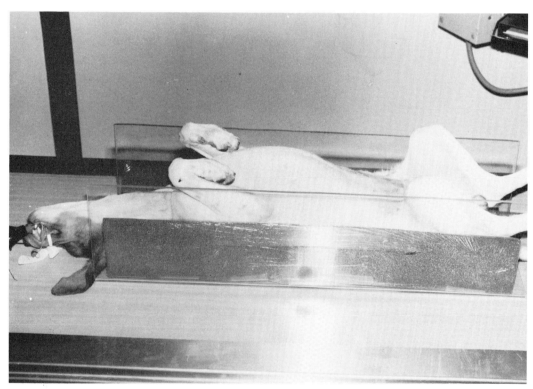

Figure 13–15. Positioning for ventrodorsal view of the lumbar vertebrae.

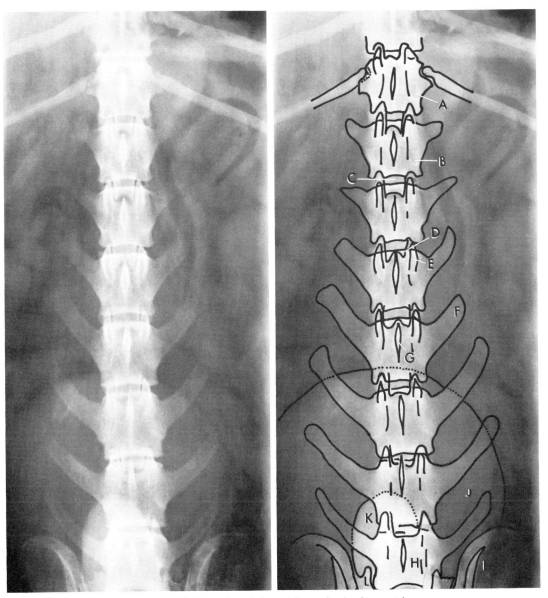

Figure 13–16. Ventrodorsal view of the canine lumbar vertebrae.

A. T13
B. L1
C. Intervertebral disc space between L1–L2
D. Caudal articular process of L2
E. Cranial articular process of L3
F. Transverse process of L4

G. Spinous process of L4
H. L7
I. Wing of the ilium
J. Urinary bladder
K. Prepuce
L. Sacrum

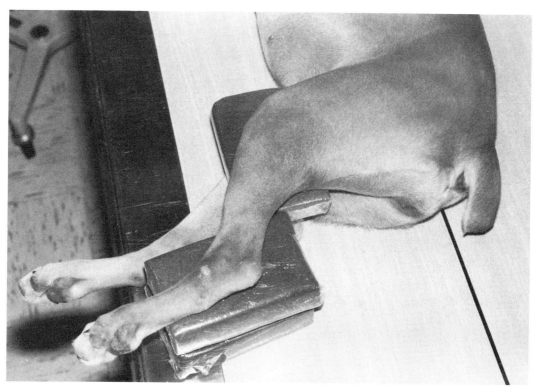

Figure 13–17. Positioning for left-right lateral view of the sacrum.

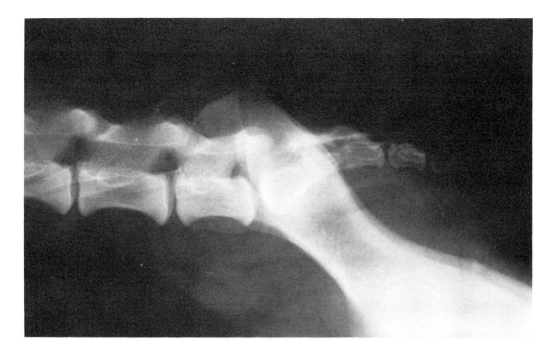

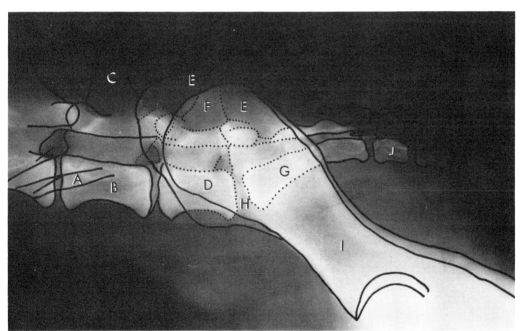

Figure 13–18. Left-right lateral view of the canine sacrum.

A. Transverse processes of L6
B. L6
C. Spinous process of L6
D. L7
E. Wings of the ilia

F. Spinous process of L7
G. Sacrum
H. Lumbosacral joint
I. Ilia superimposed
J. 1st coccygeal vertebra

two exposures in large dogs to prevent over-exposure of the cranial vertebrae and/or underexposure of the caudal vertebrae. A lead marker should be used to identify the left and right sides. Opaque tracheal tubes should be removed prior to exposure in order to avoid confusing overlying images. The x-ray beam is collimated to exclude excessive soft tissue.

Figure 13–8 illustrates the normal radiographic anatomy of mature canine cervical vertebrae in VD view.

THORACIC VERTEBRAE

Left-Right or Right-Left Lateral (LeRtL or RtLeL) View. The patient is placed in lateral recumbency and the forelimbs are extended to lie cranial to the thorax (Fig. 13–9). The sternum is elevated above the table to the level of the thoracic vertebrae in order to avoid obliquity. At times, moderate obliquity may be necessary for proper visualization of the intervertebral foramen if rib overlay becomes a problem. However, the initial examination should be performed without obliquity.

The x-ray beam is centered at the region of suspected pathology. If a survey examination is preferred, the x-ray beam is centered at the T6–T7 interspace. The x-ray beam is collimated to exclude excessive soft tissue.

Figure 13–10 illustrates the normal radiographic anatomy of mature canine thoracic vertebrae in LeRtL view.

Ventrodorsal (VD) View. The patient is placed in dorsal recumbency and the forelimbs are extended and placed beside the cervical region (Fig. 13–11). Moderate thoracic obliquity (approximately 5 degrees) may be necessary to avoid sternebral overlay, especially in large dogs.

The x-ray beam is centered at the T6–T7 interspace and collimated to exclude soft tissue.

Vertebral radiographs in the VD projection are produced without a parallel relationship between the x-ray film and the axis of the vertebral bodies because of the varying heights of the dorsal spinous processes in the thorax. This produces artifactual narrowing of some intervertebral spaces.

Figure 13–12 illustrates the normal radiographic anatomy of mature canine thoracic vertebrae in VD view.

LUMBAR VERTEBRAE

Left-Right or Right-Left Lateral (LeRtL or RtLeL) View. The patient is placed in lateral recumbency with the sternum elevated above the table to a height equal to that of the thoracic vertebrae (Fig. 13–13). In patients with a wide rib spring and a relatively narrow abdominal region, the lumbar vertebrae are elevated with a dry foam block to the level of the thoracic vertebrae. The nondependent rear limb should be elevated to avoid obliquity of the caudal lumbar vertebrae. Measurement for determining exposure should be made at the thickest part (usually the cranial aspect) to avoid underexposure.

The x-ray beam is centered at the level of suspected pathology. For survey radiographs, the x-ray beam is centered at the thoracolumbar junction, and a second radiograph is produced with the x-ray beam centered at the L3–L4 interspace.

Figure 13–14 illustrates the normal radiographic anatomy of mature canine lumbar vertebrae in LeRtL view.

Ventrodorsal (VD) View. The patient is placed in dorsal recumbency and the x-ray beam is centered at the level of suspected pathology or at the L3–L4 interspace for survey radiographs (Fig. 13–15). Measurement for determining exposure should be made at the thickest part (usually the cranial aspect) to avoid underexposure. The x-ray beam is collimated to exclude excessive soft tissue.

Figure 13–16 illustrates the normal radiographic anatomy of mature canine lumbar vertebrae in VD view.

SACRUM

Left-Right or Right-Left Lateral (LeRtL or RtLeL) View. The patient is placed in lateral recumbency with the nondependent rear limb elevated to avoid obliquity (Fig. 13–17). The x-ray beam is centered at mid-sacrum. Exposure factors indicated on the technique chart must be approximately doubled in dogs weighing over 40 lb in order to compensate for the increased tissue density provided by the superimposed ilial wings.

Figure 13–18 illustrates the normal radiographic anatomy of mature canine sacrum in LeRtL view.

Ventrodorsal (VD) View. The patient is placed in dorsal recumbency and the rear limbs are placed in semiflexion (Fig. 13–19). The x-ray beam is centered at mid-sacrum.

Figure 13–20 illustrates the normal radiographic anatomy of mature canine sacrum in VD view.

COCCYGEAL VERTEBRAE

Left-Right or Right-Left Lateral (LeRtL or RtLeL) View. The patient is placed in lateral recumbency and the tail is extended (Fig. 13–21). A cassette is placed beneath the tail and elevated above the table with a foam block to the level of the lumbar and sacral vertebrae. The x-ray beam is centered at the region of pathology.

Figure 13–22 illustrates the normal radiographic anatomy of mature canine coccygeal vertebrae in lateral view.

Ventrodorsal (VD) View. The patient is placed in dorsal recumbency and the tail is extended (Fig. 13–23). The x-ray beam is centered at the region of pathology.

Figure 13–24 illustrates the normal radiographic anatomy of mature canine coccygeal vertebrae in VD view.

MYELOGRAPHY

Myelography is a radiographic examination performed after the introduction of a contrast medium into the spinal subarachnoid space for the purpose of evaluating intramedullary, extramedullary-intradural, or extradural disease (Suter et al., 1971).

Indications

Myelography is of value in evaluating clinical transverse myelopathies but not disseminated myelopathies or meningopathies (Bailey and Holliday, 1975). These patients usually have herniated intervertebral disks (Morgan et al., 1972; Ticer and Brown, 1974; Morgan, 1972) and may have neoplasms, abscesses, hematomas, congenital malformations or some effect of trauma (Bailey and Holliday, 1975; Morgan, 1972).

Myelography should be performed only on patients that have inconclusive findings on the noncontrast radiographic examination (Hoerlein, 1965; Olsson, 1966; Bailey and Holliday, 1975). When the neurologic examination suggests a diagnosis of a disease amenable to surgical treatment, myelography may be used to confirm the diagnosis and delineate the location of the lesion. In these cases, the relative risk involved in the myelographic procedure is acceptable when the information obtained is taken into account (Bullock and Zook, 1967; Morgan et al., 1972; Bailey and Holliday, 1975; Wortman, 1974). A study comparing noncontrast radiographs with myelograms performed for the diagnosis and localization of disk disease concluded that myelograms yielded information unobtainable from the noncontrast studies in almost 70 per cent of cases (Wortman, 1974). This information included diagnoses when the noncontrast radiographs were either nondiagnostic or only suggestive. Spinal cord edema, hematomyelia (before clinically evident), and laterality of the lesion were also demonstrated myelographically. It is therefore evident that the benefits of myelography outweigh the risks in the canine patient with transverse myelopathy requiring decompressive surgery.

Contraindications

Myelography is not indicated in cases in which a definitive diagnosis can be made on the noncontrast radiographic examination. If disseminated myelopathy or meningopathy is suspected, myelography is not indicated (Ticer and Brown, 1974; Bailey and Holliday, 1975). Cerebrospinal fluid (CSF) analysis must be performed prior to myelography if these disseminated disorders are suggested clinically (Ticer and Brown, 1974; Bailey and Holliday, 1975). Evidence of infection in the cerebrospinal fluid makes myelography a contraindicated procedure. Myelography is also contraindicated unless the neurologic deficit appears reversible and unless decompressive surgery is planned should the myelographic findings suggest it (Bailey and Holliday, 1975).

Technique

Patient Preparation. The patient is anesthetized and a survey radiographic examina-
Text continued on page 226.

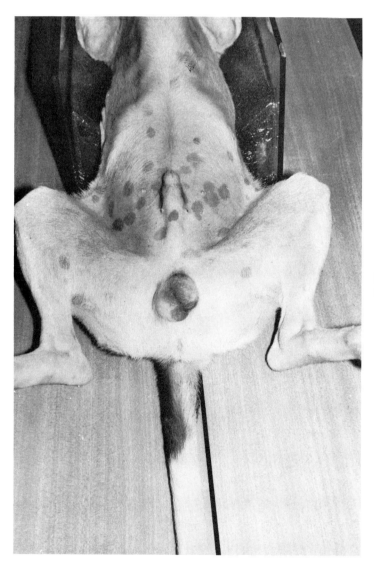

Figure 13–19. Positioning for ventro-dorsal view of the sacrum.

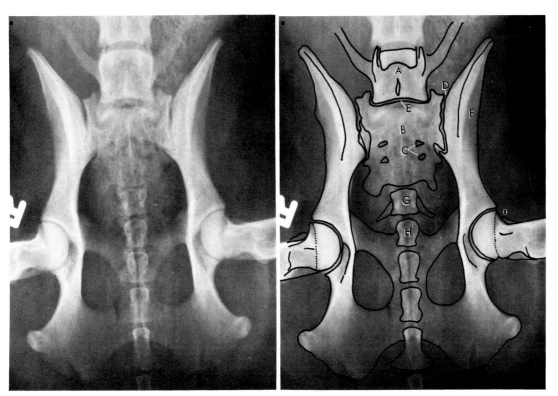

Figure 13–20. Ventrodorsal view of a mature canine sacrum.

    A. L7
    B. Sacrum
    C. Sacral foramina
    D. Sacroiliac joint
    E. Lumbosacral joint
    F. Wing of the ilium
    G. 1st coccygeal vertebra
    H. 2nd coccygeal vertebra

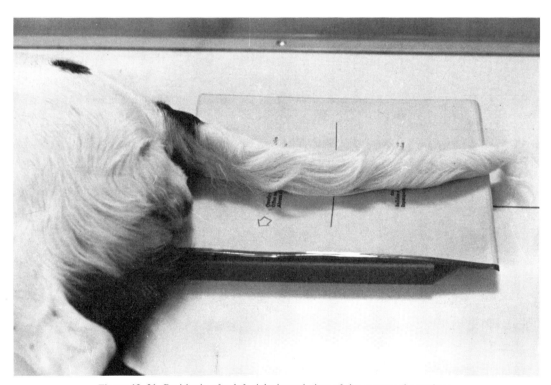

Figure 13–21. Positioning for left-right lateral view of the coccygeal vertebrae.

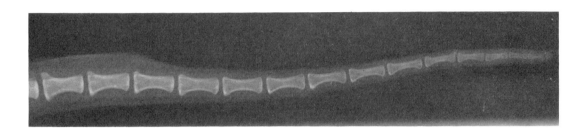

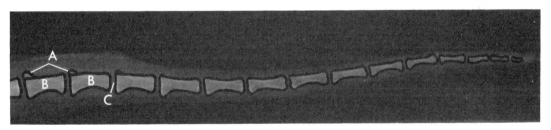

Figure 13–22. Left-right lateral view of the canine coccygeal vertebrae.
    A. Cranial articular processes
    B. Coccygeal vertebral bodies
    C. Intervertebral space

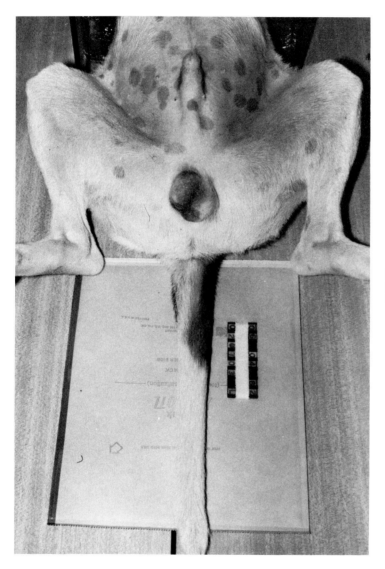

Figure 13–23. Positioning for ventrodorsal view of the coccygeal vertebrae.

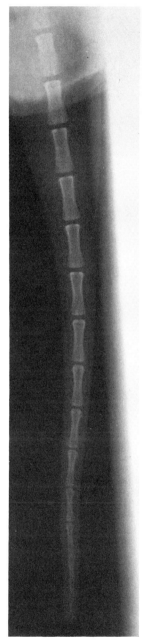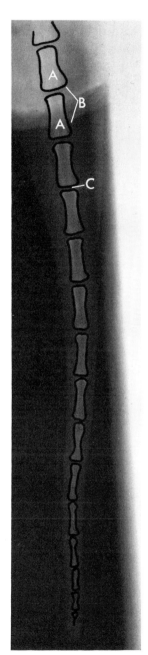

Figure 13–24. Ventrodorsal view of the canine coccygeal vertebrae.
    A. Coccygeal vertebral bodies
    B. Transverse processes
    C. Intervertebral space

tion is performed. If the differential diagnosis includes disseminated myelopathies or meningopathies, a cerebrospinal fluid analysis should be performed to rule out the presence of infectious myelitis, since the injection of a positive contrast medium into the subarachnoid space may disseminate the infection and the medium may further damage the spinal cord (Bailey and Holliday, 1975). The caudal lumbar or occipitocervical region is clipped, scrubbed, and draped.

Materials. All myelographic contrast media have technical drawbacks and postmyelographic complications. Recently metrizamide, a nonionic, water soluble, iodine-containing medium has been used extensively for myelography in dogs and horses (Stowater and Kneller, 1979; Funkquist, 1975; Lord and Olsson, 1976; Nyland et al., 1980; Beech, 1979). When used in concentrations of 170 mg I/ml, its osmolality (0.300 mol. kg^{-1}) is nearly the same as that of CSF. It has good miscibility and flow characteristics, and good to excellent radiographic visualization detail (Bartels et al., 1977). When treated preanesthetically with diazepam (Valium, Hoffman-LaRoche), dogs anesthetized with thiobarbiturate (Surital, Parke Davis) and maintained on a halothane (Fluothane, Ayerst), nitrous oxide, and oxygen showed no changes in the clinical neurologic examination or on EEG or EMG (Spencer et al., 1982). Seizures were not observed. Histologically, there was a patchy hemorrhagic leptomeningitis observed 24 hours after injection and there was a transient mononuclear response in the CSF (Spencer et al., 1982). Seizure activity has been reported in dogs not pretreated with diazepam (Bartels et al., 1977; Stowater and Kneller, 1979) when injections were made cisternally but not when the medium was administered by lumbar puncture at a dose of 0.3 ml/kg body weight (Stowater and Kneller, 1979).

Metrizamide is available in analytical grade powder form* and is reconstituted with sterile water to a concentration of 170 mg I/ml. Preweighed quantities of 1.87 g and 3.75 g may be stored in stoppered vials for ready use by adding 4.5 ml and 8.9 ml of sterile water, respectively. The medium is unstable in solution for long periods and must be prepared prior to each use. Since the solution is not heat tolerant, it may not be autoclaved.

It is therefore necessary to pass the final solution through a millipore filter† into the administration syringe. Metrizamide is also available in preweighed, single dose vials that, when reconstituted, have a volume of 20 ml and 50 ml of sterile solution.‡ These volumes are excessive for small animal myelography and therefore result in waste of the unused portion. The expense of this material is considerably greater than that of the analytical grade powder.

A 3 inch, 20 or 22 gauge, short beveled needle with stylet ("Pitkin" needle, catalogue #1161, Becton-Dickinson) is used to make the injection. The short beveled needle decreases epidural spill of contrast medium (Ticer and Brown, 1974). A suitable-sized syringe is needed to inject the contrast medium.

A volume of 0.3 ml/kg body weight is used for both cisternal and lumbar sites, and usually results in filling the subarachnoid space cranially to about the midthoracic region from lumbar puncture and caudally to about T1–T2 with cisternal injections (Stowater and Kneller, 1979). A volume of 0.4 ml/kg body weight may be injected from the lumbar site to fill the cervical region. If the subarachnoid space is unobstructed, the medium can be caused to flow either caudally or cranially by positioning on a slope.

Lumbar Puncture. The patient is placed in lateral or ventral recumbency, depending on personal preference, and the spinal needle is inserted through the dorsal intervertebral space between L5 and L6. This procedure is facilitated by passing the needle lateral to the dorsal spinous process of L6 and directing the needle point medioventrally to enter the spinal canal. This increases the needle angulation and simplifies spinal canal entry (Ticer and Brown, 1974). Moderate flexion of the patient's trunk will aid in opening the dorsal intervertebral space, making spinal canal entry easier. The beveled edge of the spinal needle is directed cranially.

An attempt should be made to enter the dorsal subarachnoid space. The needle is advanced slowly until a slight contraction of the rear limb musculature is detected. The stylet is then removed and the needle hub is observed for signs of cerebrospinal fluid. The needle may be slightly advanced or retracted

---

*Accurate Chemical and Scientific Corp., 28 Tec St., Hicksville, N.Y. 11801

†Millex Disposable Filter Unit, 0.22 μ, Millipore Corp., Ashby Rd., Bedford, Mass. 01730

‡Amipaque, Winthrop Laboratories, New York, N.Y. 10016

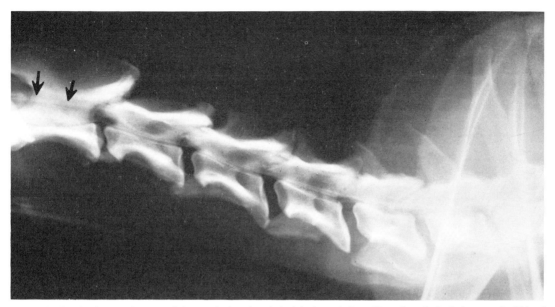

Figure 13–25. Canine myelogram of the cervical region, left-right lateral view. Note the relatively increased width of the subarachnoid space in the dorsal aspect of the C_2 cord (arrows).

until CSF flow is obtained. Compression of the jugular veins may cause a rise in CSF pressure and thus aid in producing flow. The calculated dose of contrast medium is then injected slowly (over a period of one or two minutes) to prevent epidural spill.

If the dorsal subarachnoid space cannot be entered, the needle is advanced to the ventral floor of the spinal canal. The stylet is then removed and the needle hub is checked for cerebrospinal fluid. In chondrodystrophoid breeds, the lumen of the needle is usually located in the subarachnoid space when the needle tip is on the ventral floor of the spinal canal. In other breeds, the needle may need to be retracted slightly from the ventral canal floor before CSF flow is obtained.

If CSF flow is not readily obtainable, excessive needle manipulation is not indicated. In the absence of CSF flow, to confirm the location of the needle lumen, a small dose (0.25 ml) of contrast medium may be in-

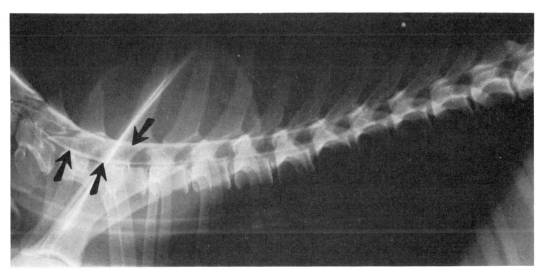

Figure 13–26. Canine myelogram of the thoracic region, left-right lateral view. Note the relatively increased width of the subarachnoid space in the caudal cervical and cranial thoracic region (arrows).

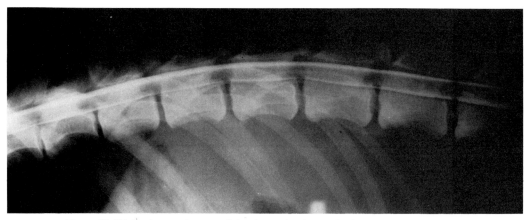

Figure 13–27. Canine myelogram of the thoracolumbar region in left-right lateral view.

jected unless either CSF flow or conformation of needle location is obtained, since epidural injections are generally not of diagnostic quality and intraparenchymal injections are disastrous. After proper needle placement is attained, the calculated dose of contrast medium is injected slowly. The needle is then removed.

Positioning the patient with the caudal trunk elevated slightly may aid in the cranial flow of the medium when the cranial thoracic or caudal cervical region needs to be visualized.

Metrizamide will remain visible and produce good diagnostic detail for a period of one and a half hours or longer (Lord and Olsson, 1976). Repeat radiographs may be produced after additional postural repositioning of the medium, if necessary.

Care should be taken not to allow flexion of the trunk during lateral recumbent radiography, since this may cause an artifactual narrowing of the ventral subarachnoid space at the thoracolumbar region (Ticer and Brown, 1974).

Cisterna Magna Puncture. When clinical signs indicate cervical spinal cord involvement, the contrast medium may be administered into the CSF at the cisterna magna. The puncture is made through the flexed atlanto-occipital joint with the patient in either ventral or lateral recumbency. The needle bevel is directed caudally and the medium is injected slowly. A moderate elevation of the head will cause the majority of the medium to flow caudally. After completion of the injection the needle is removed and the head is maintained in an elevated position. Elevation should be maintained between exposures.

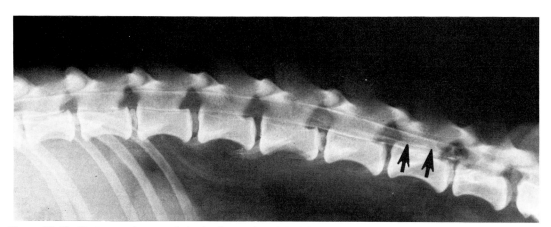

Figure 13–28. Canine myelogram of the lumbar region, left-right lateral view. Note the radiopaque longitudinal striations of the cauda equina (arrows).

isfactorily controlled by small intravenous doses of diazepam (Valium, Hoffman-La-Roche) given as indicated.

Interpretation. The myelographic outline should approximate the normal subarachnoid space (Figs. 13–25 to 13–31). The width of the radiopaque column should be of uniform magnitude over most of its course. A slight narrowing of the ventral subarachnoid space may occur over the intervertebral spaces, especially in chrondrodystrophoid breeds. The lateral view of the cranial cervical (Fig. 13–25) and caudal cervical and cranial thoracic (Fig. 13–26) regions usually shows an increased width of the subarachnoid space. The radiopaque medium delineates the longitudinal striations of the cauda equina (Fig.

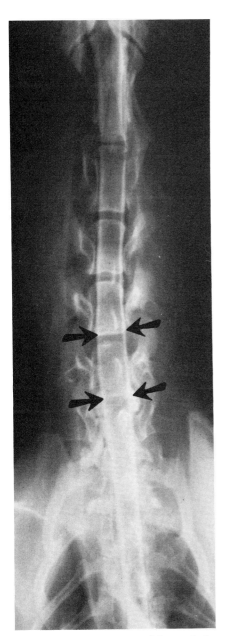

Figure 13–29. Canine myelogram of the cervical region, ventrodorsal view. Note the relatively increased diameter of the spinal cord in the caudal cervical region (arrows).

Radiographs are then produced in left-right or right-left lateral recumbency and in ventrodorsal position.

Aftercare. Recovery from anesthesia is usually uncomplicated; however, postmyelographic convulsions may be a problem in some patients. Elevation of the head may decrease this problem. Seizures may be sat-

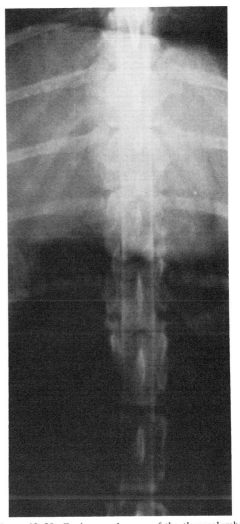

Figure 13–30. Canine myelogram of the thoracolumbar region in ventrodorsal view.

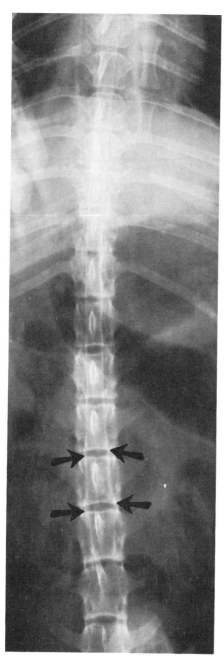

Figure 13–31. Canine myelogram of the lumbar region, ventrodorsal view. Note the relatively increased diameter of the spinal cord in the region of L4–L5 (arrows).

the diameter of the spinal cord is disproportionately smaller than the spinal canal in large breeds of dogs.

REFERENCES

Bailey, C. S., and Holliday, T. A.: Diseases of the Spinal Cord. *In* Ettinger, S. J. (Ed.): Textbook of Veterinary Internal Medicine: Diseases of the Dog and Cat. Philadelphia, W. B. Saunders Co., 1975.

Bartels, J. E., Braund, K. G., and Redding, R. W.: An Experimental Evaluation of a non-ionic agent Amipaque (metrizamide) as a neuroradiologic medium in the dog. J. Am. Vet. Radiol. Soc., *18*(4):117–123, 1977.

Beech, J: Metrizamide myelography in the horse. J. Am. Vet. Radiol. Soc., *20*:22–32, 1979.

Bullock, L. P., and Zook, B. C.: Myelography in dogs using water-soluble contrast mediums. J.A.V.M.A., *151*:321, 1967.

Funquist, B.: Myelographic localization of spinal cord compression in dogs: A comparison between cisternal and lumbar injections of metrizamide, "Amipaque," in diagnosing and locating spinal compression. Acta Vet. Scand., *15*:269, 1975.

Hoerlein, B. F.: Canine Neurology: Diagnosis and Treatment. 2nd ed. Philadelphia, W. B. Saunders Co., 1965.

Lord, P. F., and Olsson, S. E.: Myelograph with metrizamide in the dog: A clinical study on the use for the demonstration of spinal cord lesions other than those caused by intervertebral disc protrusions. J. Am. Vet. Radiol. Soc., *17*:42–50, 1976.

Morgan, J. P., Suter, P. F., and Holliday, T. A.: Myelography with water-soluble contrast medium: Radiographic interpretation of disc herniation in dogs. Acta Radiol. Suppl., *319*:217, 1972.

Nyland, T. G., Blythe, L. L., Pool, R. R., Helphrey, M. G., and O'Brien, T. R.: Metrizamide myelography in the horse: Clinical, radiographic, and pathologic changes. Am. J. Vet. Res., *41*(2):204–211, 1980.

Olsson, S. E.: *In* Pettit, G. D. (Ed.): Intervertebral Disc Protrusion in the Dog. New York, Appleton-Century-Crofts, 1966.

Spencer, C. P., Chrisman, C. L., Mayhew, I. G., and Kaude, J. V.: The neurotoxicological effects of a non-ionic contrast agent (Iopamidol) on the leptomeninges of the dog. Am. J. Vet. Res., 1982 (in press).

Stowater, J. L., and Kneller, S. K.: Clinical evaluation of metrizamide as a myelographic agent in the dog. J.A.V.M.A., *175*(2):191–195, 1979.

Suter, P. F., Morgan, J. P., Holliday, T. A., and O'Brien, T. R.: Myelography in the dog: Diagnosis of tumors of the spinal cord and vertebrae. J. Amer. Vet. Radiol. Soc., *12*:29, 1971.

Ticer, J. W., and Brown, S. G.: Water-soluble myelography in canine intervertebral disc protrusion. J. Amer. Vet. Radiol. Soc., *15*:3, 1974.

Wortman, J. A.: Radiographic diagnosis of intervertebral disc disease in the dog: A comparison of noncontrast and myelographic studies. Scientific Presentations and Seminar Synopses of the 41st Meeting, American Animal Hospital Association, 1974, p. 689.

13–28). The spinal cord usually shows an increased diameter in caudal cervical regions (Fig. 13–29) and the area of the fourth and fifth lumbar vertebrae (Fig. 13–31), especially when viewed in VD projection. Generally,

14

Head and Cervical Region

SKULL

Anatomic variations among species and breeds of animals often necessitate comparison of skull radiographs for disturbances in the bilateral symmetry. Radiographic examination of the skull, therefore, requires accurate positioning. This can be accomplished in most patients only with the aid of chemical restraint, preferably general anesthesia.

Pathologic processes, such as those resulting from trauma, may contraindicate anesthesia, but in most cases restraint assistance may be obtained by some form of sedation.

Exposure factors for skull radiography are generally determined by measuring the widest part of the cranium, since underexposure of this area usually results in a nondiagnostic radiograph. Regional measurements are made when anatomic features such as the nasal, maxillary or mandibular structures are specifically examined.

Some patients, such as brachycephalic canines, have increased bone content per unit thickness compared with the average density composition of other anatomic regions and therefore require increased exposure. Generally, the addition of 10 to 15 per cent kv or doubling the mas will produce satisfactory radiographic density for these patients.

Table 14–1 lists suggested views for examining specific regions of the skull.

Left-Right or Right-Left Lateral (LeRtL or RtLeL) View. The patient is placed in lateral recumbency and the rostral aspect of the skull is elevated with a dry foam block to create a parallel relationship between the sagittal plane of the skull and the film, and to prevent obliquity (Fig. 14–1).

If the base of the skull is of primary interest, the mandibles may be opened to avoid overlay of the mandibular coronoid processes.

Figure 14–2 illustrates the normal radiographic anatomy of an oligocephalic canine skull in LeRtL view.

Left Ventral-Right Dorsal Oblique (Le20°V-RtDO) or Right Ventral-Left Dorsal Oblique (Rt20°V-LeDO) View. Oblique views are utilized to examine the dorsal or ventral aspects of the skull in lateral projection without the interference created by the overlying contralateral side.

By elevating the ventral aspect of the skull so that the sagittal plane is rotated approximately 20 degrees to the film, adequate visualization of the dependent tympanic bulla and temporomandibular joint regions may be obtained (Fig. 14–3). The contralateral frontal sinus is also projected in a manner that will allow visualization.

Figure 14–4 illustrates the normal radiographic anatomy of the canine os bulla and temporomandibular joint regions in Le20°V-RtDO view.

Left Dorsal-Right Ventral Oblique (Le20°D-RtVO) or Right Dorsal-Left Ventral Oblique (Rt20°D-LeVO) View. If examination of the frontal sinus region is the primary objective, the dorsal aspect of the

Table 14–1. SUGGESTED VIEWS FOR DEMONSTRATION OF VARIOUS REGIONS OF THE SKULL

Regions	View
Routine survey	Le-Rt; VD; RCd and R20°D-CdV0
Base of skull	Le-Rt (open mouth); VD and R30°V-CdDO (open mouth/beam bisecting mandibulo-maxillary angle)
Frontal sinus and ethmoid regions and nasal passage	Le20°D-RtVO or Rt20°D-LeVO; RCd and V20°R-DCdO (open mouth)
Middle and inner ear	Le20°V-RtDO and Rt20°V-LeDO; VD and R30°V-CdD (open mouth/beam bisecting mandibulo-maxillary angle)
Mandibles	Le20°V-RtDO or Rt20°V-LeDO; VD
Temporomandibular joints	Le20°V-RtDO or Rt20°V-LeDO; Le20°R-RtCdO or Rt20°R-LeCdO; VD and R30°V-CdDO (open mouth/beam bisecting mandibulo-maxillary angle)
Zygomatic and orbital	Le20°D-RtVO or Rt20°D-LeDO; VD; V20°R-DCdO (open mouth) and RCd
Maxillary premolars and molars	Le45°V-RtDO (open mouth) or Rt45°V-LeDO (open mouth); V20°R-DCdO (open mouth)
Mandibular premolars and molars	Le45°D-RtVO (open mouth) or Rt45°D-LeVO (open mouth); VD (intraoral film)
Maxillary incisors	Le-RtL and D20°R-VCdO (intraoral film)
Mandibular incisors	Le-RtL and V20°R-DCdO (intraoral film)

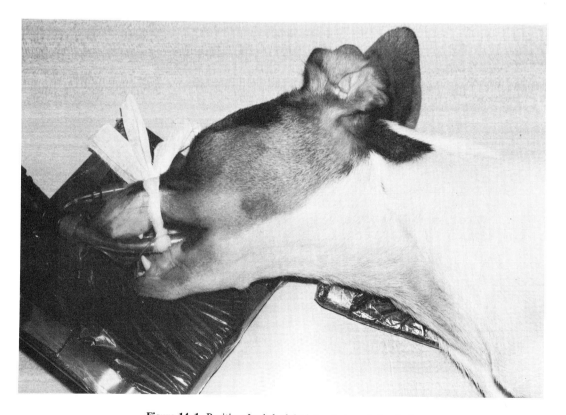

Figure 14–1. Position for left-right lateral view of the skull.

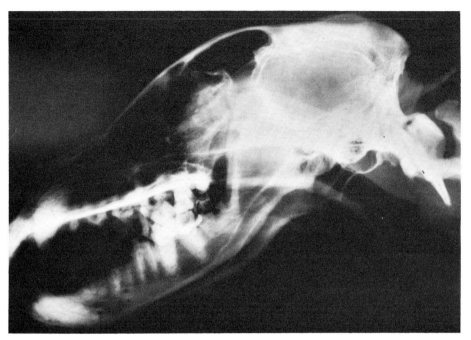

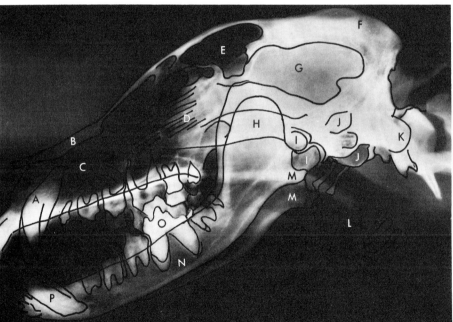

Figure 14–2. Left-right lateral view of the canine skull. In some small canine breeds the frontal sinuses are diminished in size or absent.

A. Maxillary canine teeth superimposed
B. Nasal bone
C. Nasal passage
D. Ethmoid turbinates
E. Frontal sinuses
F. Sagittal crest
G. Cranium
H. Coronoid processes of the mandibles superimposed

I. Mandibular condyles
J. Tympanic bullae
K. Occipital condyles
L. Hyoid bones
M. Angular process of the mandible
N. Mandible
O. 1st molar
P. Mandibular canine teeth superimposed

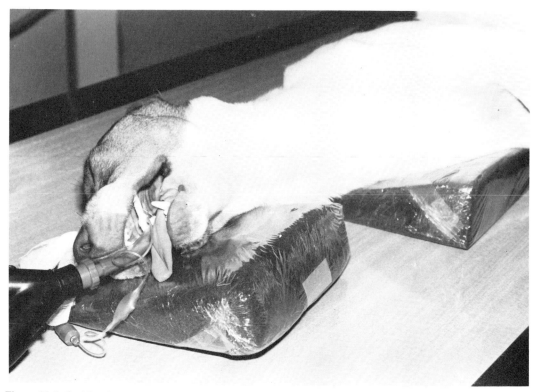

Figure 14–3. Position for the left 20 degree ventral—right dorsal oblique view of the canine skull for demonstration of the right tympanic bulla, temporomandibular joint, and mandible.

skull should be elevated 20 degrees (Fig. 14–5). This will profile the dependent frontal sinus region.

Figure 14–6 illustrates the normal radiographic anatomy of the canine frontal sinus region in Le20°D-RtVO view.

Left Rostral-Right Caudal Oblique (Le20°R-RtCdO) or Right Rostral-Left Caudal Oblique (Rt20°R-LeCdO) View of the Temporomandibular Joint. The patient is placed in lateral recumbency, the rostral aspect of the skull is elevated so that the sagittal plane of the skull is rotated rostrocaudally approximately 20 degrees to the film and the mouth is opened with a dry foam block (Fig. 14–7). The joint to be examined should be placed down.

The central x-ray beam is directed at the joint being examined. This position aligns the long axis of the mandibular condyle perpendicular to the film and allows better evaluation of the intra-articular space in the canine (Douglas and Williamson, 1980).

Figure 14–8 illustrates the normal radiographic anatomy of the right canine temporomandibular joint in Le20°R-RtCdO view.

Left Ventral-Right Dorsal Oblique (Le45°V-RtDO) or Right Ventral-Left Dorsal Oblique (Rt45°V-LeDO) Open Mouth View of the Maxillary Dental Arcades. The patient is placed in lateral recumbency and the mouth is opened maximally, with a dry foam block used as a gag. The dental arcade to be examined is placed down. Views of the maxillary arcade are produced by elevating the ventral aspect of the skull so that the sagittal plane is rotated approximately 45 degrees to the film (Fig. 14–9). The use of nonscreen film or detail screens provides increased detail for dental radiography.

Figure 14–10 illustrates the normal radiographic anatomy of the canine maxillary dental arcade in Le45°V-RtDO (open mouth) view.

Left Dorsal-Right Ventral Oblique (Le45°D-RVO) or Right Dorsal-Left Ventral Oblique (Rt45°D-LeVO) Open Mouth View of the Mandibular Dental Arcade. The mandibular dental arcade is examined by elevating the dorsal aspect of the skull approximately 45 degrees. The mouth is opened with a dry foam block (Fig. 14–11).

Text continued on page 242

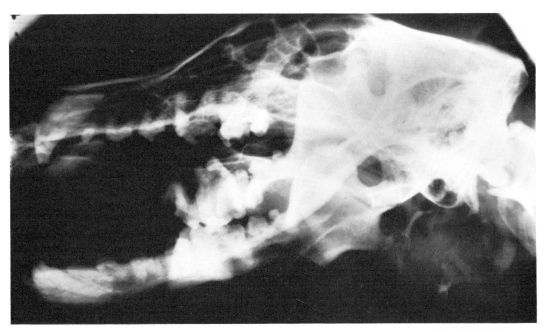

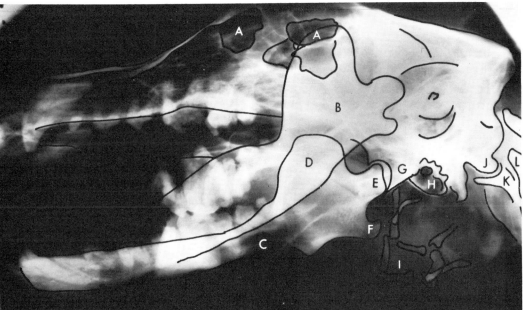

Figure 14–4. Left 20 degree ventral—right dorsal oblique view of the canine skull for demonstration of the right tympanic bulla, temporomandibular joint, and mandibular ramus.

A. Frontal sinuses
B. Upper mandible
C. Lower mandible
D. Coronoid process of lower mandible
E. Mandibular condyle
F. Angular process of the mandible
G. Retroglenoid process
H. Tympanic bulla
I. Hyoid bones
J. Occipital condyle
K. Atlas (C2)
L. Dens

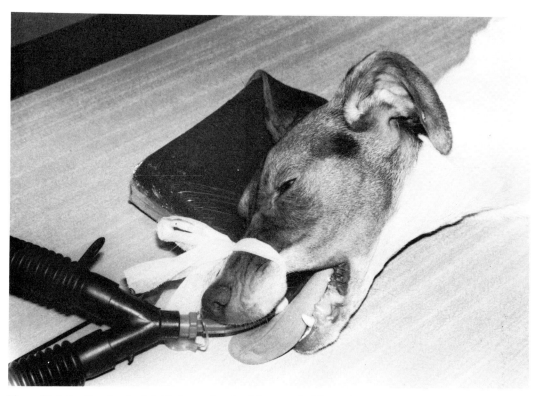

Figure 14–5. Position for the left 20 degree dorsal—right ventral oblique view of the canine skull for demonstration of the right frontal sinus region.

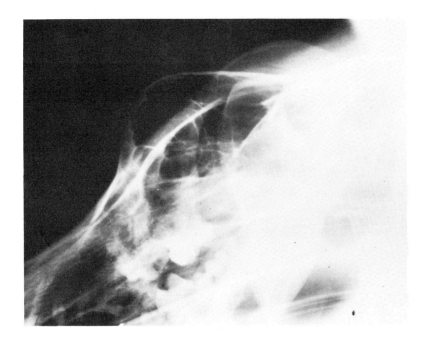

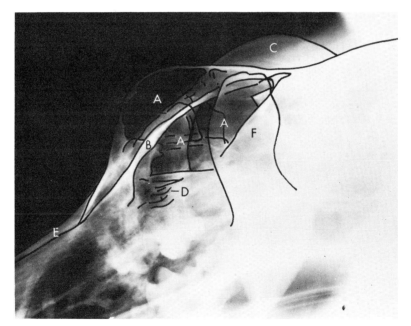

Figure 14–6. Left 20 degree dorsal—right ventral oblique view of the canine skull for demonstration of the right frontal sinus region.

A. Frontal sinus
B. Frontal bone
C. Zygomatic arch
D. Ethmoid region
E. Nasal bone
F. Coronoid process of the mandible

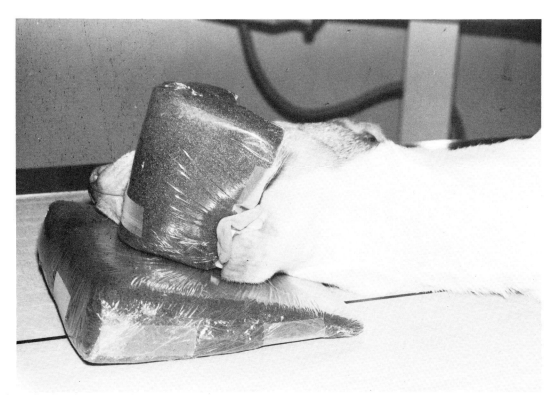

Figure 14–7. Position for the left 20 degree rostral—right caudal oblique (20 degree sagittal/oblique) view of the right temporomandibular joint.

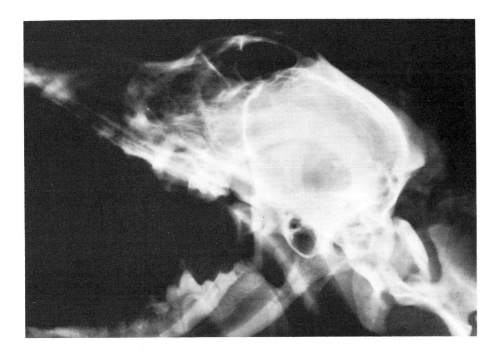

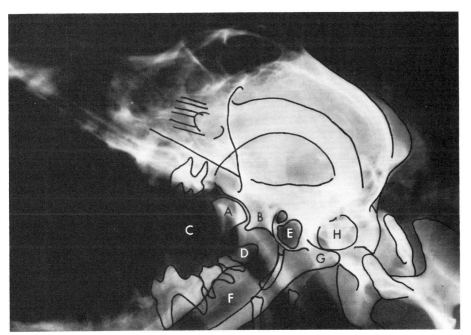

Figure 14–8. Left 20 degree rostral—right caudal oblique view of the canine right temporomandibular joint.
A. Mandibular condyle (condyloid process)
B. Retroglenoid process
C. Coronoid process
D. Angular process
E. Tympanic bulla
F. Contralateral mandible
G. Contralateral angular process
H. Contralateral tympanic bulla

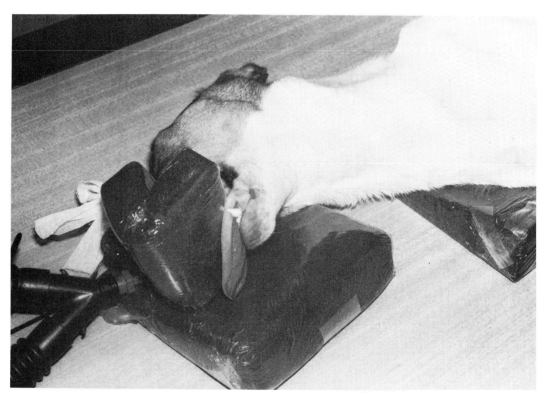

Figure 14–9. Position for left 45 degree ventral—right dorsal oblique open mouth view of the right maxillary dental arcade.

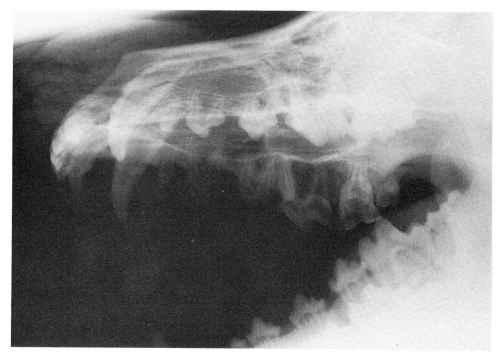

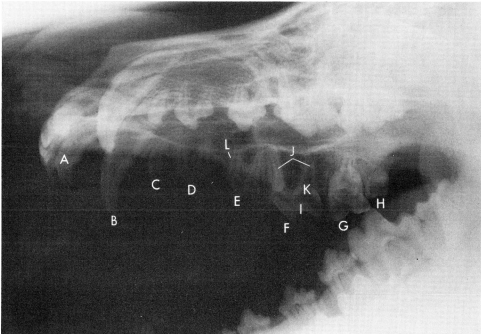

Figure 14–10. Left 45 degree ventral—right dorsal oblique open mouth view of the canine right maxillary dental arcade.

A. Incisor teeth
B. Canine tooth
C. 1st premolar tooth
D. 2nd premolar tooth
E. 3rd premolar tooth
F. 4th premolar tooth (carnasial tooth)

G. 1st molar tooth
H. 2nd molar tooth
I. Crown
J. Roots
K. Pulp cavity
L. Lamina dura

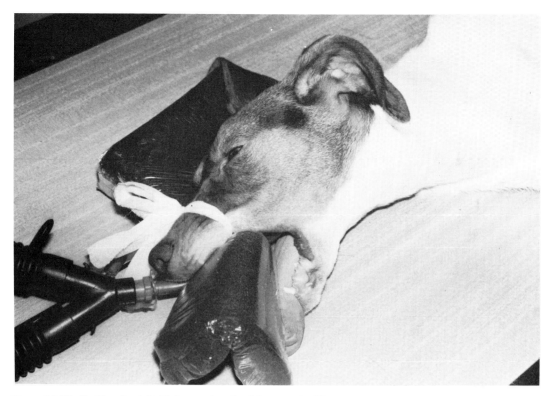

Figure 14–11. Position for left 45 degree dorsal—right ventral oblique open mouth view of the right mandibular dental arcade.

Figure 14–12 illustrates the normal radiographic anatomy of the canine mandibular arcade in Le45°D-RtVO (open mouth) view.

VD View. The patient is placed in dorsal recumbency and the occipital-atlantal articulation is extended so that the hard palate is parallel to the film (Fig. 14–13). The tracheal tube, if radiopaque, should be removed just prior to exposure.

Figure 14–14 illustrates the normal radiographic anatomy of the canine skull in VD view.

Ventral Rostral-Dorsocaudal Oblique (V20°R-DCdO) Open Mouth View of the Nasal and Ethmoid Regions. The patient is placed in dorsal recumbency, and the mouth is opened maximally by tape or a positioning device (Fig. 14–15). The hard palate is positioned parallel to the film. The central x-ray beam is angled from the rostral aspect into the mouth 20 degrees and is centered at the level of the upper third premolar.

This position allows visualization of the entire nasal passage and frontal sinuses without overlying mandibular shadows.

Figure 14–16 illustrates the normal radiographic anatomy of the canine nasal cavity in V20°R-DCdO (open mouth) view.

Dorsorostral-Ventrocaudal Oblique (D20°R-VCdO) (Intraoral Film) View of the Maxillary Incisor Teeth. The patient is placed in ventral recumbency and a cassette is placed intraorally (Fig. 14–17). The x-ray beam is angled from the rostral aspect approximately 20 degrees so that it is more perpendicular to the longitudinal axis of the incisor teeth roots.

Figure 14–18 illustrates the normal radiographic anatomy of the canine maxillary incisor teeth in D20°R-VCdO (intraoral film) view.

Ventrorostral-Dorsocaudal Oblique (V20°R-DCdO) (Intraoral Film) View of the Mandibular Incisor Teeth. The patient is placed in dorsal recumbency and a cassette is placed intraorally (Fig. 14–19). The x-ray beam is angled from the rostral aspect approximately 20 degrees so that it is more perpendicular to the longitudinal axis of the incisor teeth.

Figure 14–20 illustrates the normal radiographic anatomy of the canine mandibular

Text continued on page 252

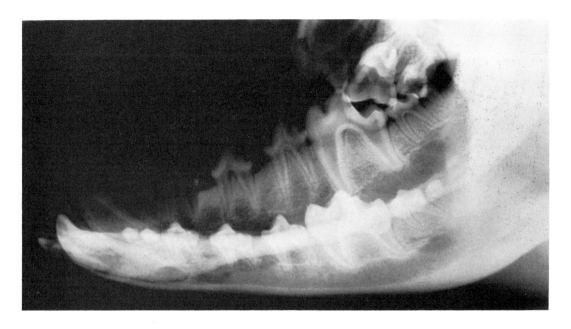

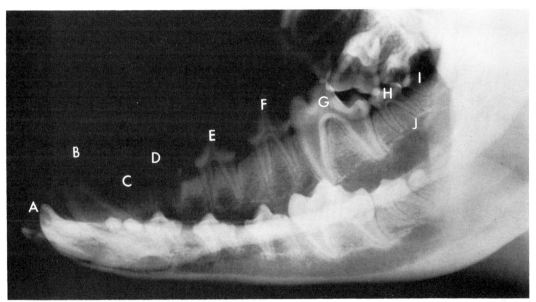

Figure 14–12. Left 45 degree dorsal—right ventral oblique open mouth view of the canine right mandibular dental arcade.

A. Incisor teeth
B. Canine tooth
C. 1st premolar tooth
D. 2d premolar tooth
E. 3rd premolar tooth
F. 4th premolar tooth
G. 1st molar (carnasial tooth)
H. 2nd molar tooth
I. 3rd molar tooth
J. Lamina dura

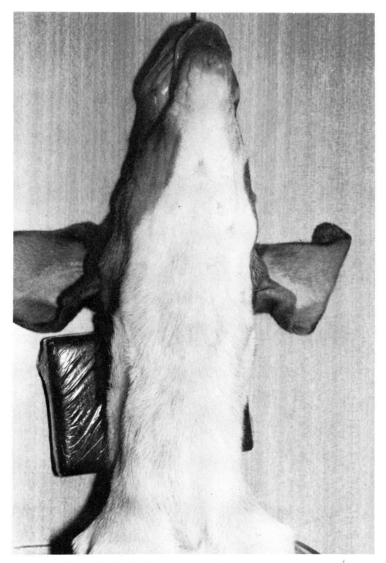

Figure 14–13. Position for ventrodorsal view of the skull.

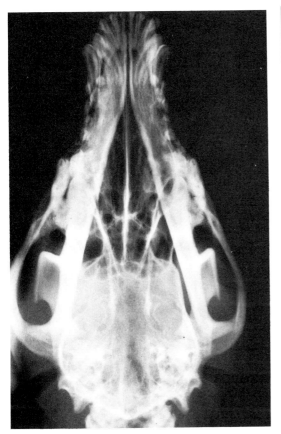
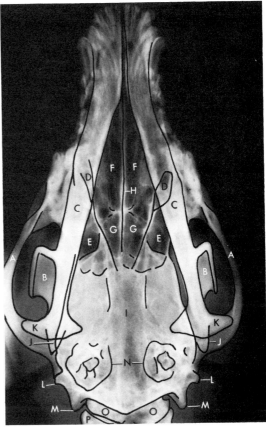

Figure 14–14. Ventrodorsal view of the canine skull.

A. Zygomatic arch
B. Coronoid process of the mandible
C. Mandible
D. Maxillary sinus
E. Frontal sinus
F. Nasal passage
G. Ethmoid turbinates
H. Nasal septum (palatine suture)
I. Cranium
J. Angular process of the mandible
K. Mandibular condyle (condyloid process)
L. Mastoid process
M. Jugular process
N. Tympanic bullae
O. Occipital condyles
P. Atlas (C1)

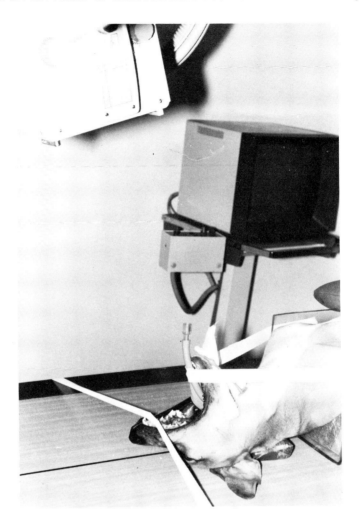

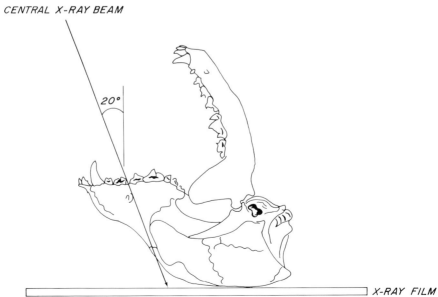

Figure 14–15. Position for ventral 20 degree rostral—dorsocaudal oblique open mouth view of the nasal and ethmoid regions.

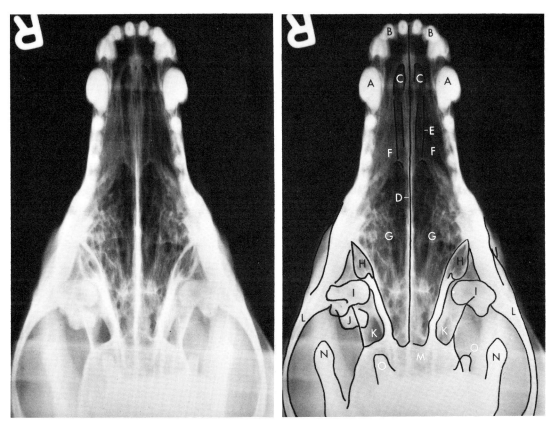

Figure 14–16. Ventral 20 degree rostral—dorsocaudal oblique open mouth view of the canine nasal and ethmoid regions.

A. Maxillary canine teeth
B. Maxillary incisor teeth
C. Palatine fissure
D. Nasal septum (palatine suture)
E. Base of vomer bone
F. Maxilloturbinates
G. Ethmoturbinates
H. Maxillary sinus
I. 1st molar
J. 2nd molar
K. Frontal sinus
L. Zygomatic arch
M. Cranium
N. Coronoid process of mandible
O. Mandibular canine teeth

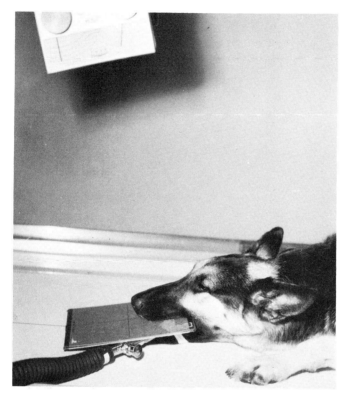

Figure 14–17. Position for dorsal 20 degree rostral—ventrocaudal oblique (intraoral film) view of the maxillary incisor teeth.

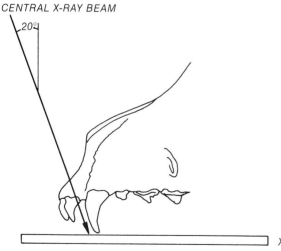

CENTRAL X-RAY BEAM

20°

X-RAY FILM

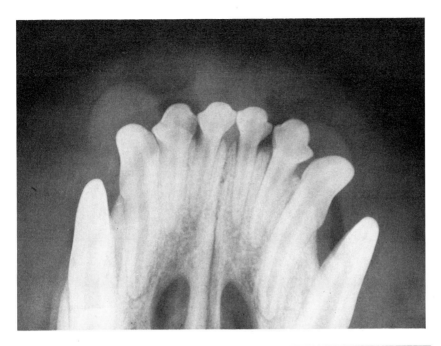

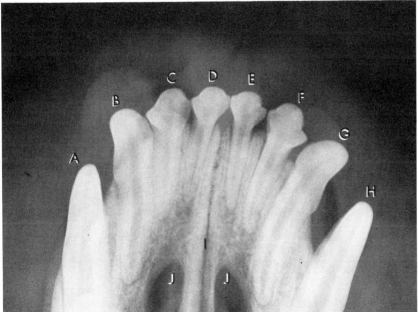

Figure 14–18. Dorsal 20 degree rostral—ventrocaudal oblique (intraoral film) view of the canine maxillary incisor teeth.

A. Canine tooth, left side
B. 3rd incisor tooth, left side
C. 2nd incisor tooth, left side
D. 1st incisor tooth, left side
E. 1st incisor tooth, right side
F. 2nd incisor tooth, right side
G. 3rd incisor tooth, right side
H. Canine tooth, right side
I. Palatine suture
J. Palatine fissure

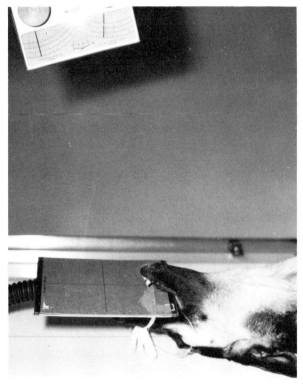

Figure 14–19. Position for ventral 20 degree rostral—dorsocaudal oblique (intraoral film) view of the mandibular incisor teeth.

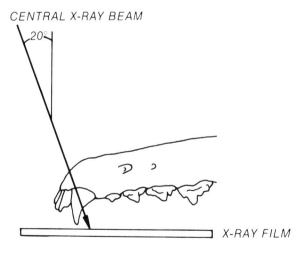

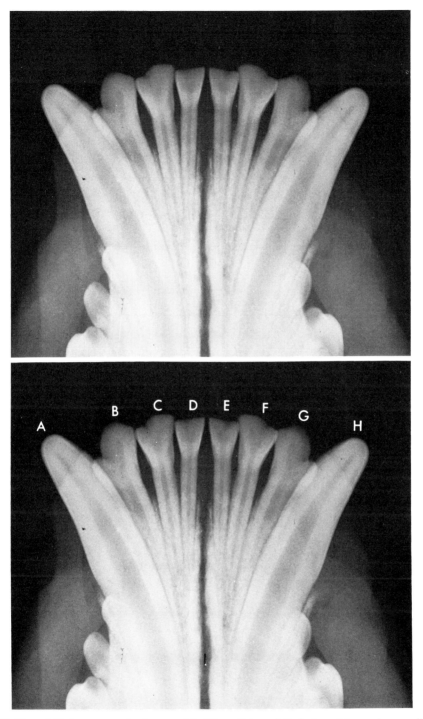

Figure 14–20. Ventral 20 degree rostral—dorsocaudal oblique (intraoral film) view of the canine mandibular teeth.

A. Canine tooth, right side
B. 3rd incisor tooth, right side
C. 2nd incisor tooth, right side
D. 1st incisor tooth, right side
E. 1st incisor tooth, left side
F. 2nd incisor tooth, left side
G. 3rd incisor tooth, left side
H. Canine tooth, left side
I. Mandibular symphysis

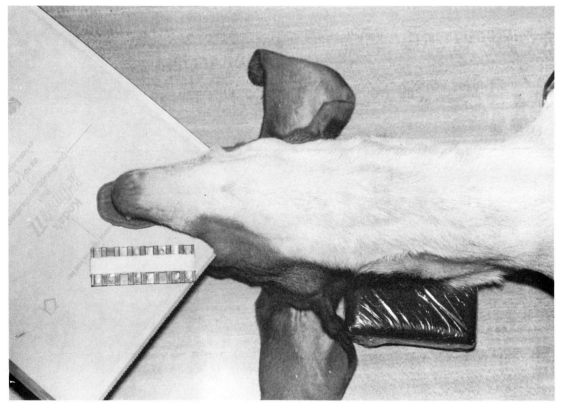

Figure 14–21. Position for ventrodorsal (intraoral film) view of the mandible.

incisor teeth in V20°R-DCdO (intraoral film) view.

Ventrodorsal (VD) (Intraoral Film) View of the Mandible. The patient is placed in dorsal recumbency and a cassette is placed intraorally to the commissure of the mouth. The central x-ray beam is centered at the midmandible (Fig. 14–21).

Figure 14–22 illustrates the normal radiographic anatomy of the canine mandible in VD (intraoral film) view.

Rostrocaudal (RCd) View of the Frontal Sinuses. The patient is placed in dorsal recumbency and the occipital-atlantal articulation is flexed approximately 90 degrees to the vertebral column so that the hard palate is perpendicular to the film and parallel to the central x-ray beam (Fig. 14–23). Measurement to determine exposure is made from the occipital protuberance to approximately one half the distance from the intrapupillary line to the tip of the nose.

This examination is indicated when a frontal view of frontal sinuses is desired.

Figure 14–24 illustrates the normal radiographic anatomy of the canine skull in RCd view.

Rostral 20° Dorsal-Caudoventral Oblique (R20°D-CdVO) View of the Cranium. The patient is placed in dorsal recumbency and the occipital-atlantal articulation is flexed so that the hard palate is approximately 70 degrees from the vertebral column and the frontal sinuses are superimposed over the ventral skull in a manner that profiles the middle and caudal cranium (Fig. 14–25).

Measurement to determine exposure is made from the occipital protuberance to the intrapupillary line.

This examination is indicated when a frontal view of the cranium is desired without superimposition of the frontal sinuses and nasal passages.

Figure 14–26 illustrates the normal radiographic anatomy of the canine cranium in R20°D-CdVO view.

Rostroventral-Caudodorsal Oblique (R30°V-CdDO) (open mouth) View. The patient is placed in dorsal recumbency and the occipital-atlantal articulation is flexed approximately 60 degrees. The mouth is opened in such a manner that the central x-ray beam (which is 90 degrees to the film) bisects the angle of the opened temporomandibular articulation (Fig. 14–27). The hard palate and the mandible are angled approximately 30 degrees to the central x-ray beam in opposite directions. Measurement to determine exposure is made from the occipital protuberance to the commissure of the mouth.

This examination is indicated when a frontal view of the middle (os bullae) or inner ear regions and the temporomandibular joints is needed.

Figure 14–28 illustrates the normal radiographic anatomy of the canine skull in R30°V-CdDO (open mouth) view.

Text continued on page 260

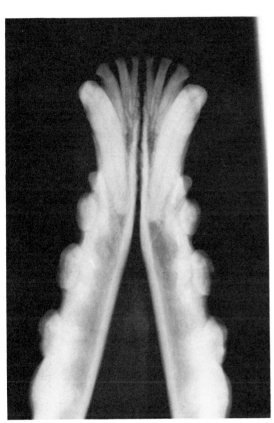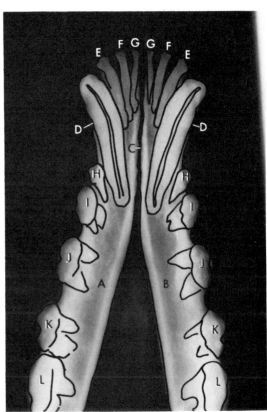

Figure 14–22. Ventrodorsal (intraoral film) view of the canine mandible.

    A. Right mandible
    B. Left mandible
    C. Mandibular symphysis
    D. Canine teeth
    E. 3rd incisor teeth
    F. 2nd incisor teeth
    G. 1st incisor teeth
    H. 1st premolar teeth
    I. 2nd premolar teeth
    J. 3rd premolar teeth
    K. 4th premolar teeth
    L. 1st molar

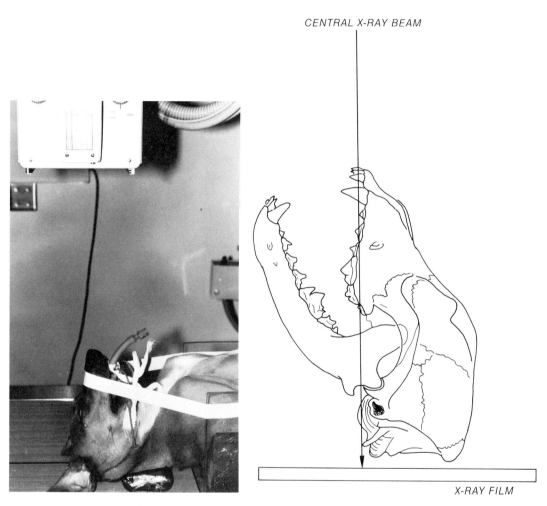

Figure 14–23. Position for the rostrocaudal view of the skull.

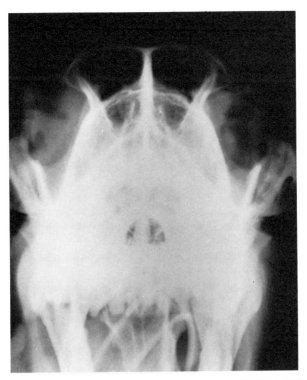

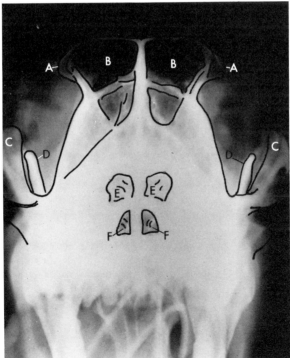

Figure 14–24. Rostrocaudal view of the canine skull. In some small canine breeds the frontal sinuses are diminished in size or absent.

A. Zygomatic processes of the frontal bones
B. Frontal sinuses
C. Zygomatic arch
D. Coronoid process of the mandible
E. Nasal passages
F. Nasopharynx

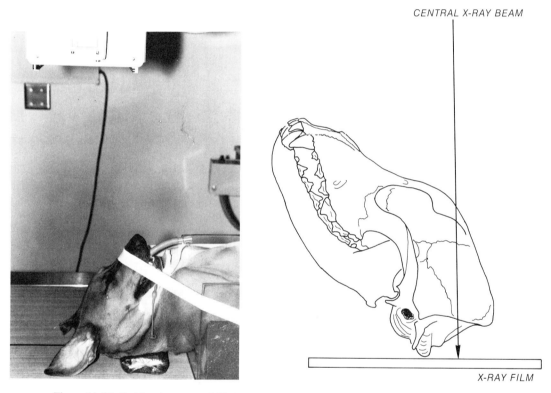

Figure 14–25. Position for a rostral 20 degree dorsal—caudoventral oblique view of the cranium.

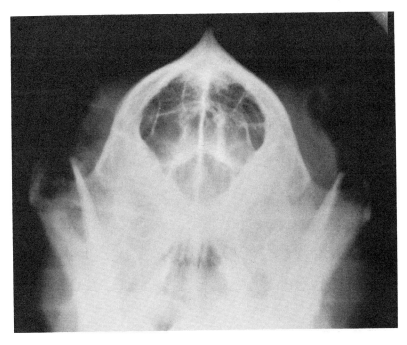

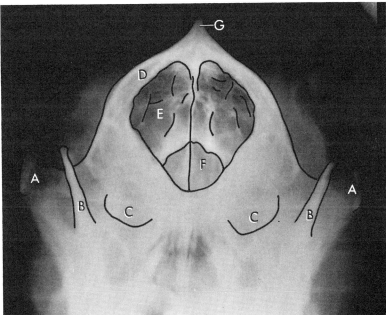

Figure 14–26. Rostral 20 degree dorsal—caudoventral oblique view of the canine cranium.

A. Zygomatic arch
B. Coronoid process of the mandible
C. Tympanic bulla
D. Calvarium
E. Cranial cavity
F. Foramen magnum
G. Sagittal crest

CENTRAL X-RAY BEAM

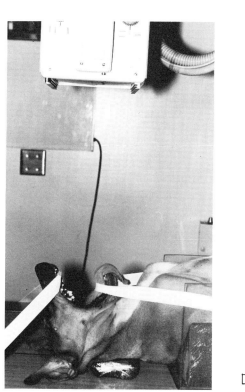

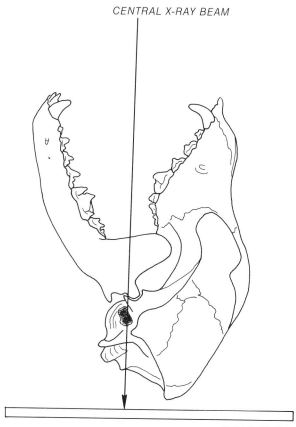

X-RAY FILM

Figure 14–27. Position for the rostral 30 degree ventral—caudodorsal (open mouth) view of the skull.

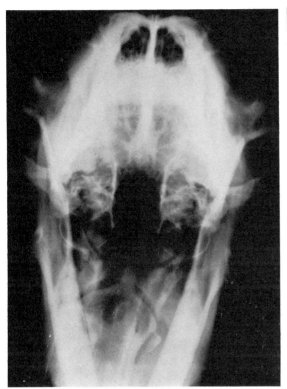 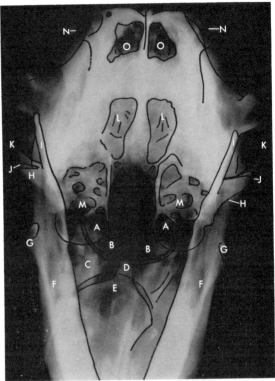

Figure 14–28. Rostral 30 degree ventral—caudodorsal (open mouth) view of the canine skull.

A. Tympanic bullae
B. Occipital condyles
C. Atlas (C1)
D. Des
E. Axis (C2)
F. Mandibular ramus
G. Angular process of the mandible
H. Mandibular condyle
I. Coronoid process of the mandible
J. Temporomandibular joint
K. Zygomatic arch
L. Nasal passages
M. Inner ear region of petrous temporal bone
N. Zygomatic process of the frontal bone
O. Frontal sinuses

CERVICAL REGION

Left-Right or Right-Left Lateral (LeRtL or RtLeL) View. The patient is placed in lateral recumbency and the forelimbs are retracted over the cranial thorax (Fig. 14–29). The cervical vertebrae are elevated from the x-ray table with a dry foam block so that the cervical and thoracic vertebrae are on the same level. The occipital-atlantal articulation is moderately flexed (45 degrees to the vertebral column).

The x-ray beam is centered mid-cervically. The beam is collimated to include the caudal aspect of the skull and the thoracic inlet.

Figure 14–30 illustrates the normal radiographic anatomy of the canine cervical region in LeRtL view.

A marked variation in the position of the laryngeal structures may occur and is related to function (O'Brien et al., 1969). Mineralization of the larynx may occur in all dogs, particularly large breeds, in which the cricoid cartilage may mineralize at an early age. Table 14–2 lists the relationship between age and mineralization of laryngeal cartilages in dogs.

The basihyoid bone normally appears mineralized in the lateral view in all dogs. Tracheal rings may also appear mineralized, especially in large dogs.

VD View. The patient is placed in dorsal recumbency with the forelimbs secured laterally to the thoracic walls (Fig. 14–31).

The x-ray beam is centered mid-cervically and is collimated to include the caudal aspect of the skull and the thoracic inlet.

Figure 14–32 illustrates the normal radiographic anatomy of the canine cervical region in VD view.

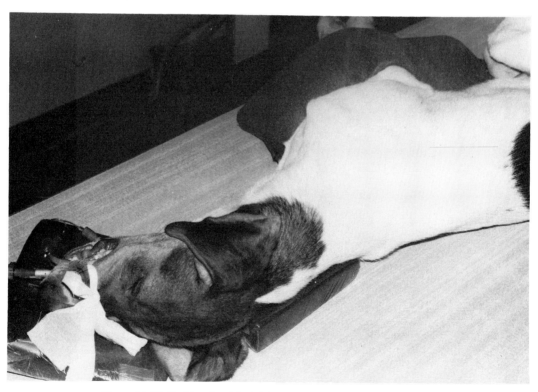

Figure 14–29. Position for right-left lateral view of the cervical region.

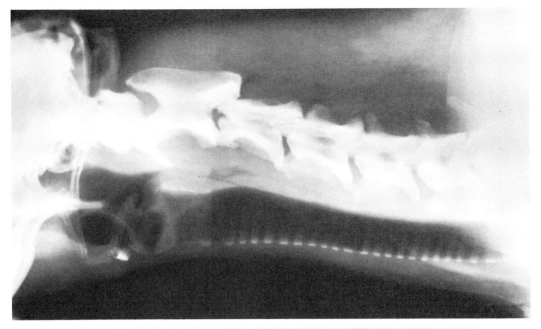

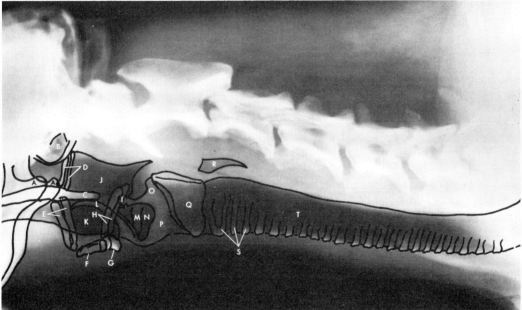

Figure 14–30. Left-right lateral view of the canine cervical region.

A. Angular processes of the mandible
B. Tympanic bullae
C. Soft palate
D. Stylohyoid bones
E. Epihyoid bones
F. Keratohyoid bones
G. Basihyoid bone
H. Thyrohyoid bones
I. Cranial cornu of the thyroid cartilage
J. Nasopharynx

K. Oropharynx
L. Epiglottis
M. Vocal cord
N. Lateral ventricular saccules
O. Corniculate process of arytenoid cartilage
P. Thyroid cartilage
Q. Cricoid cartilage
R. Air in esophagus
S. Tracheal cartilaginous rings
T. Tracheal lumen

Table 14–2. THE RELATIONSHIPS BETWEEN AGE AND MINERALIZATION OF LARYNGEAL CARTILAGES IN DOGS (FROM GASKELL, 1974)

Age	No. of Dogs Examined	Percentage of Dogs Showing Radiographic Evidence of Mineralization			
		Cricoid	Thyroid	Arytenoid	Epiglottis
0–6 mo	18	0	0	0	0
6 mo–1 yr	23	78	65	0	30
1–4 yr	39	97	64	15	28
5–8 yr	46	93	68	30	48
8 + yr	14	100	71	64	57

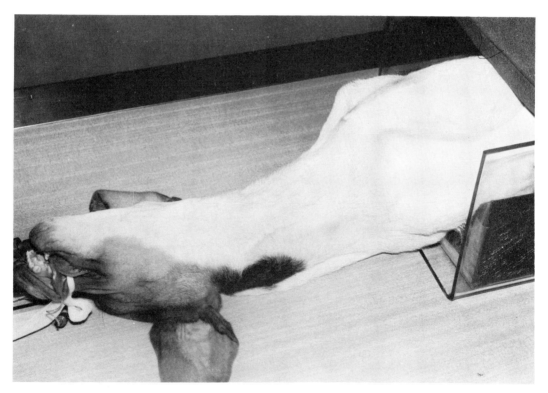

Figure 14–31. Position for ventrodorsal view of the cervical region.

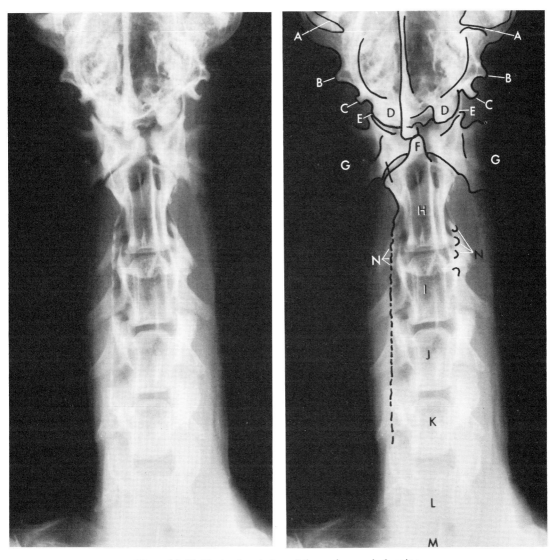

Figure 14–32. Ventrodorsal view of the canine cervical region.
A. Temporomandibular joints
B. Mastoid processes
C. Jugular processes
D. Occipital condyles
E. Atlanto-occipital joint
F. Dens
G. Wings of the atlas (C1)
H. Axis (C2)
I. C3
J. C4
K. C5
L. C6
M. C7
N. Tracheal rings

Orbital Angiography

Orbital angiography may be accomplished by simple retrograde injection of contrast medium through the infraorbital artery.

INDICATIONS

Orbital angiography may assist in diagnosing neoplasms (Gelatt et al., 1970) and vascular abnormalities (Rubin and Patterson, 1965). Visualization of deviation of the large orbital vessels and increased vascularity (tumor blush) caused by certain neoplasms can aid in surgical planning (Gelatt et al., 1970). Exact radiographic location of the eye within the orbit is made possible by angiographic outline of the choroid.

CONTRAINDICATIONS

No specific contraindications for orbital angiography in the dog have been reported; however, orbital pain, ocular hemorrhage, and transient to permanent blindness have been reported in man (Lombardi, 1967).

TECHNIQUE

Patient Preparation

Patient preparation consists of routine preanesthetic procedures. General anesthesia is required.

Materials

A 21-gauge vein infusion set (Butterfly 21 Infusion Set, Abbott Laboratories) and a 5- or 10-ml syringe are used to make the injection of contrast medium. Heparinized physiologic saline solution is needed to flush the infusion set. A 50 to 60 per cent iodine-based, water-soluble contrast medium is used (Hypaque 50%, Winthrop Laboratories; Renografin-60, Squibb & Sons). Surgical instrumentation for simple arteriotomy is used to isolate the artery.

Dosage

Five to 10 ml of contrast medium is used for each injection.

Procedure

The patient is anesthetized and the region of the infraorbital foramen is prepared for surgery. The skin is incised over the foramen, and the superficial facial muscles are bluntly separated to expose the infraorbital artery, nerve and vein. The infraorbital artery is usually located medial or ventral to the nerve but may occasionally be found in the infraorbital nerve bundle (Gelatt et al., 1970). A segment of the artery approximately 1 cm long is isolated and elevated with two lengths of nonabsorbable suture material. The artery is then cannulated in a proximal direction with a 21-gauge vein infusion set, and the needle is tied into place with the previously placed ligature. Heparinized physiologic saline solution is used to flush the needle and tubing periodically to maintain patency.

After the patient has been placed with the side to be examined next to the film, 5 to 10 ml of contrast medium is injected with moderate pressure to produce retrograde flow into the infraorbital artery. A lateral radiograph is produced near the end of the injection period. The injection and radiographic procedure are repeated in the V20°R-DCdO (open mouth) projection (see p. 246). Radiographic exposure technique should be increased from 5 to 7 kv above the normal factors.

The cannula is then removed and moderate digital pressure is applied to the artery for a

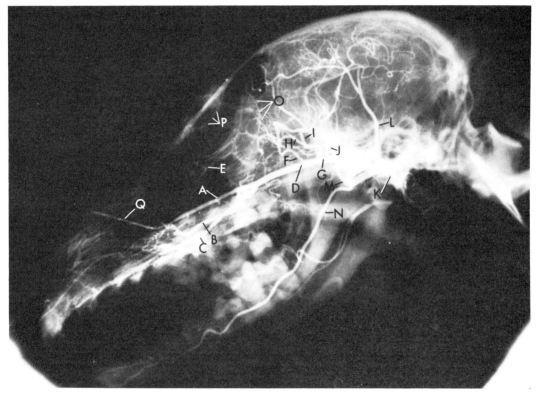

Figure 14–33. Orbital angiogram, canine left-right lateral view. Radiograph was produced after a retrograde injection of contrast medium into the infraorbital artery.

    A. Infraorbital artery
    B. Sphenopalatine artery
    C. Major palatine artery
    D. Maxillary artery
    E. Malar artery
    F. Anterior deep temporal artery
    G. Orbital artery
    H. Ventral muscular branch
    I. External ethmoid artery
    J. External ophthalmic artery
    K. External carotid artery
    L. Superficial temporal artery
    M. Posterior deep temporal artery
    N. Mandibular alveolar artery
    O. Choroid
    P. Ciliary body
    Q. Cannula

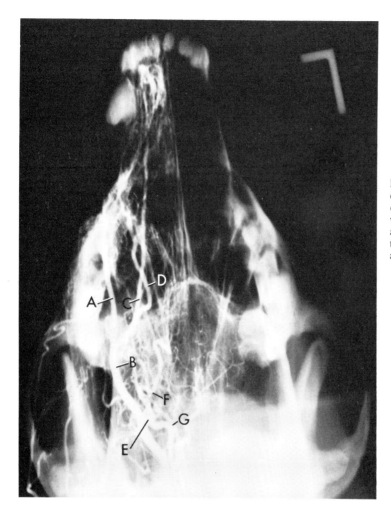

Figure 14–34. Orbital angiogram, canine, ventral 20 degree rostral—dorsocaudal oblique open mouth view. Radiograph was produced after a retrograde injection of contrast medium into the infraorbital artery.

A. Infraorbital artery
B. Maxillary artery
C. Major palatine artery
D. Sphenopalatine artery
E. Orbital artery
F. External ethmoid artery
G. External ophthalmic artery

short time. If hemorrhage persists, the vessel may be ligated without adverse effects (Gelatt et al., 1970). The skin incision is closed in the routine manner.

Interpretation

The number of arteries visualized will vary with the amount of contrast medium injected. A large-volume injection results in radiographic visualization of the arteries arising from the external carotid and internal maxillary arteries. The superficial facial, auricular, mandibular and glossal vessels are usually demonstrated (Figs. 14–33 and 14–34). Arteries of the orbital floor and choroid are also seen.

The detection of displacement of the large vessels and abnormal vascularization may be diagnostically useful in defining masses in the orbital region.

Sialography

Sialography is the radiographic examination of the salivary ducts and glands after the introduction of a radiopaque medium.

INDICATIONS

Sialography is useful in the diagnosis of disease involving the salivary ducts and glands. In the dog, sialography has helped to definitively locate salivary mucoceles and to elucidate their mechanism of formation (Harvey, 1969). In any fluid-containing swelling that is suspected of being congenital, sialography is useful in eliminating lesions of the salivary gland and ducts. Parotid sialography should be a routine part of the diagnostic investigation of recurrent swellings of the cheek (Harvey, 1969). In addition, confirmation of diagnoses of neoplasia, abscess, sialolithiasis, sialoangiectasis and sialadenitis has been an indication for sialography in humans (Hettwer and Folsom, 1968; Schulz and Weisberger, 1948).

CONTRAINDICATIONS

No specific contraindications for sialography have been reported. Contraindication for general anesthesia would also constitute a contraindication for sialography, however.

TECHNIQUE

Patient Preparation

Patient preparation consists of routine preanesthetic procedures. General anesthesia is usually required.

Materials

Blunt cannulas made from shortened (1 cm long) 22-, 25-, and 26-gauge hypodermic needles or lacrimal cannulas are used for opaque medium injection. A pair of fine tissue forceps, syringes and a mouth gag are also needed. A 60 per cent suspension of propyliodone in peanut oil (Dionosil Oily, Glaxo Laboratories, Ltd., distributed by Picker Corp.) is used as the medium.

Dosage

A contrast medium dose of 0.1 to 0.3 ml is used for retrograde injection into the salivary ducts.

Procedure

Parotid Duct. Precontrast radiographs of the skull in the lateral and VD projections are produced. The parotid salivary duct opens into the mouth on a papilla located on the labial oral mucosa opposite the upper fourth premolar (carnassial) tooth (Fig. 14–35). The parotid duct enters the mouth perpendicularly to the oral mucosa and bends caudally 90 degrees immediately beneath the duct papilla (Miller et al., 1964). Cannulation of the duct may be simplified by straightening the distal portion of the duct by grasping the oral mucosa caudal to the duct papilla with a fine tissue forceps and retracting it rostromedially (Harvey, 1969). A 22-gauge needle (smaller for small dogs) is then directed into the duct opening and gently pushed caudally (Figure 14–35). This procedure should require very little force. The cannula is then inserted to the hub and the contrast medium injected. Lateral and VD radiographs are then produced. Generally, the lateral view has the most diagnostic information and should be produced first.

Zygomatic Duct. Precontrast radiographs of the skull are made in the lateral and V20°R-DCdO oblique (open mouth) projection (see p. 246). The zygomatic salivary

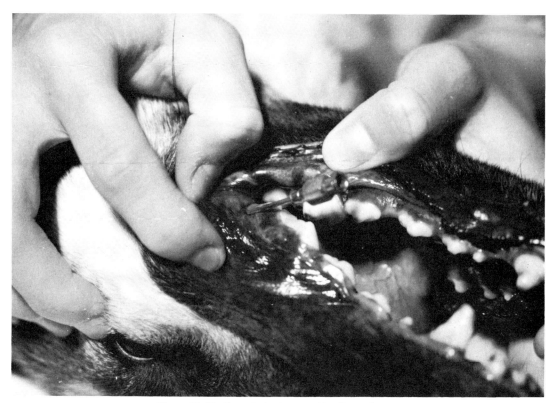

Figure 14–35. Cannula in the parotid salivary duct.

gland has one major duct and two to four minor ducts. The major duct opens into the mouth approximately 1 cm caudal and slightly dorsal to the parotid duct papilla (Fig. 14–36). It lies on a mucosal ridge that runs lateral to the last upper molar tooth. The duct is approximately one half the size of the parotid duct. Fine tissue forceps are used to steady the oral mucosa next to the major duct opening, and a 25- to 26-gauge cannula is directed into the duct opening and passed gently dorsocaudally.

The methods of injection of contrast medium and radiography are the same as those used for parotid duct sialography. Radiographs are then produced.

Mandibular and Sublingual Ducts. Precontrast radiographs of the skull in lateral and VD views are produced. The mandibular salivary duct opens on the lateral surface of the lingual caruncles (Fig. 14–37). The duct opening is a slit-like orifice approximately 1 mm long. The sublingual duct enters the mouth 1 to 2 mm caudal to the mandibular duct opening and appears as a small red dot in approximately two thirds of dogs (Fig. 14–

38). In approximately one third of dogs, the sublingual and mandibular ducts join and enter the mouth at a common opening (Miller et al., 1964). This variation may be bilateral or unilateral. Careful inspection of the lateral surfaces of the caruncles should be performed prior to excessive manipulation or application of forceps since marks left on the oral mucosa may resemble a duct opening (Harvey, 1969).

A 22- or 25-gauge cannula may be used to enter the mandibular duct. A 26-gauge cannula is used for the sublingual duct. Forceps are utilized to retract the lingual caruncle rostrally. The mandibular duct is entered by placing the cannula tip just rostral to the opening and sliding the cannula caudally. Cannulation should be to the cannula hub. If both ducts open into the mouth at a single orifice, the mandibular duct may be entered by sliding the cannula directly caudal from the common opening. A 26-gauge cannula is then inserted at the dorsomedial edge of the opening, and an attempt is made to locate the sublingual duct by gently probing in a medial and dorsal direction from the mandibular duct (Harvey, 1969).

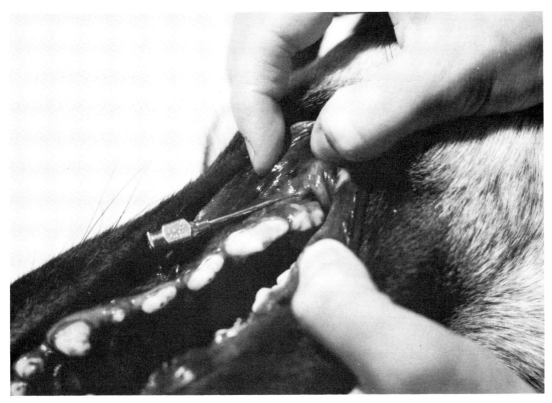

Figure 14–36. Cannula in the zygomatic salivary duct.

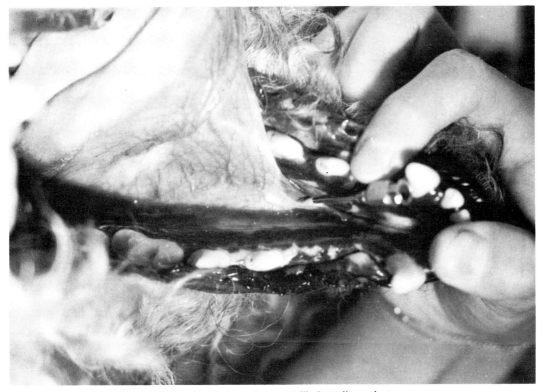

Figure 14–37. Cannula in mandibular salivary duct.

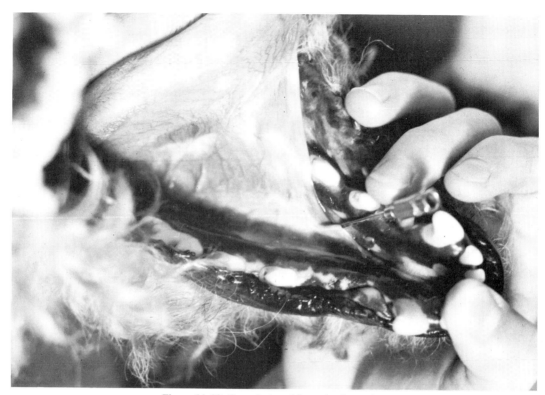

Figure 14–38. Cannula in sublingual salivary duct.

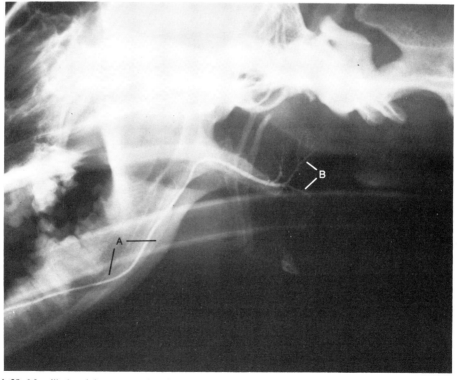

Figure 14–39. Mandibular sialogram, canine, lateral view. Radiograph produced after retrograde injection of contrast medium into the mandibular duct.
A. Mandibular salivary duct
B. Ductules of the mandibular salivary gland

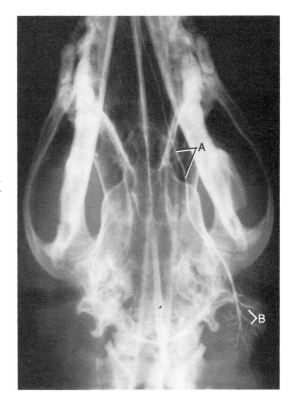

Figure 14–40. Mandibular sialogram, canine, VD view. Radiograph produced after retrograde injection of contrast medium into the mandibular duct.
  A. Mandibular salivary duct
  B. Ductules of the mandibular salivary gland

The method of injection of contrast medium and radiography is the same as that used for parotid duct sialography.

Figures 14–39 and 14–40 illustrate the normal radiographic anatomy of a canine mandibular sialogram, showing the normal appearance of the salivary duct and salivary gland ductules.

Interpretation

Parotid Duct and Gland. The parotid duct course varies with the degree of mouth opening. Decreased mouth opening causes the duct to arc slightly ventrally (Harvey, 1969). The duct should be smooth in outline and course to the angle of the jaw, where it divides into several small ductules before entering the gland. The intraglandular ductules show progressive bifurcation, producing a tree-branch pattern. The parotid gland is an irregular, lobulated structure that lies lateroventral to the external auditory meatus.

Zygomatic Duct and Gland. The main zygomatic duct is short and courses in a dorsocaudal direction. The intraglandular ductules show progressive bifurcation, producing a tree-branch pattern. The gland is a small, single-lobed structure located ventral to the rostral end of the zygomatic arch.

Mandibular Duct and Gland. The mandibular duct courses caudally and parallel to the ramus of the mandible to the angle of the jaw and twists slightly before coursing ventrally to the gland (Fig. 14–39). The intraglandular ductules show progressive bifurcation, producing a tree-branch pattern (Fig. 14–40). The mandibular gland is smooth and single-lobed. The hyoid bones may be superimposed in the region of the gland on the lateral view and should not be mistaken for extravasation of contrast medium from the duct or gland.

Sublingual Duct and Gland. The sublingual duct courses caudally in a manner similar to that of the mandibular duct. Superimposed upon the duct are several lobules, which vary in size and position. A small, isolated lobule is located cranial to the first lower molar tooth, and a collection of small lobules is located at the level of or caudal to this tooth. The main section of the gland is located at the level of the second molar tooth and courses caudoventrally. This area of the gland consists of two parts: a bilobed cranial part, and a caudal part, which is located caudoventral to the cranial part. The intraglandular ductules show progressive bifurcation, producing a tree-branch pattern.

Dacryocystorhinography

Dacryocystorhinography is a radiographic examination of the nasolacrimal duct after the introduction of a positive contrast agent into the punctum lacrimale.

INDICATIONS

Contrast examination of the lacrimal drainage system is indicated in cases of chronic recurring or intractable conjunctivitis, dacryocystitis (Yakely and Alexander, 1971) and neoplasia of the lacrimal duct or periductal tissue (Gelatt et al., 1970).

CONTRAINDICATIONS

Contraindications for dacryocystorhinography are limited to those that might prevent the administration of anesthesia or profound sedation.

TECHNIQUE

Dacryocystorhinography is best performed on anesthetized patients. Precontrast radiographs of the rostral aspect of the skull are then produced in the V20°R-DCdO (open mouth) views (see p. 246). The patient is placed in lateral recumbency with the diseased side up. The superior punctum is then cannulated with a 17- to 22-gauge beveled polyethylene intravenous catheter (I.V. Catheter Placement Unit, Jelco Laboratories), which is then taped to the side of the head to prevent dislodging during subsequent positioning maneuvers (Fig. 14–41). The inferior punctum is occluded with fixation forceps (Graeff Fixation Forceps, Milten Instrument Co.) and the system is flushed with physiologic saline solution. A 50 to 60 per cent solution of water-soluble iodine-based contrast medium (Hypaque 50%, Winthrop Laboratories, or Renografin-60, Squibb & Sons) or an oily medium (Dionosil Oily, Glaxo Laboratories, Ltd., distributed by Picker Corp.) is then injected continuously until several drops are emitted from the nose. Moderate digital pressure applied to the medial canthus will prevent spillage of medium into the conjunctival sac. Placing the nose close to the table during injection and lateral recumbent radiography will prevent excessive retrograde flow of the medium into the nasal turbinates, where it may overlie the course of the lacrimal duct and obscure adequate visualization.

After the injection, the patient is placed with the side to be examined closest to the film, and a lateral recumbent radiograph is produced, using an exposure that is slightly greater than that used for the precontrast radiographic technique (add 5 to 7 kv). The V20°R-DCdO (open mouth) view is then produced.

Interpretation

The lacrimal drainage system in the dog is devoid of a distinct lacrimal sac (Miller et al., 1964). The duct is seen as a smooth, well-delineated structure joining the second canaliculus and continuing rostroventrally and slightly medially through the lacrimal bone into the maxilla, where it opens ventral to the maxilloturbinate crest (caudal to the external nares on the lateral floor of the nasal cavity) (Figs. 14–42 and 14–43). The medial wall of the canal may be thin and incomplete in the maxilla and may protrude into the maxillary sinus (Miller et al., 1964).

There should be no alterations in luminal size nor in the course of the duct. The periductal osseous structures should not show changes in the normal trabecular pattern.

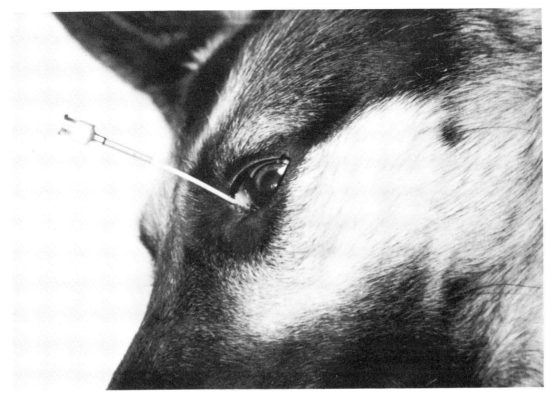

Figure 14–41. Catheter placed in the superior punctum for dacryocystorhinography.

Figure 14–42. Dacryocystorhinography, canine left-right lateral view.
A. Contrast medium in nasal passage
B. Nasolacrimal duct
C. Superior and inferior canaliculi

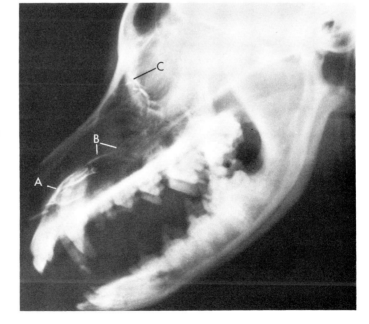

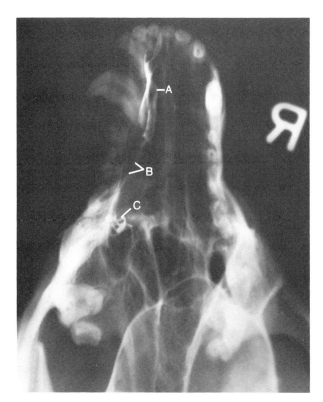

Figure 14–43. Dacryocystorhinography, canine, moderately oblique ventral 20 degree rostral— dorsal oblique (open mouth) view.
A. Contrast medium in nasal passage
B. Nasolacrimal duct
C. Superior and inferior canaliculi

REFERENCES

Gillette, E. L., Thrall, D. E., and Lebel, J. L.: Carlson's Veterinary Radiology. 3rd ed. Philadelphia, Lea & Febiger, 1977.

Douglas, S. W., and Williamson, H. D.: Principles of Veterinary Radiography. 3rd ed. Baltimore, Williams & Wilkins Co., 1980.

Gaskell, C. J.: The radiographic anatomy of the pharynx and larynx of the dog. J. Sm. Anim. Pract., *14*:89, 1974.

Gelatt, K. N., Guffy, M. M., and Boggess, T. S.: Radiographic contrast techniques for detecting orbital and nasolacrimal tumors in dogs. J.A.V.M.A., *156*:741, 1970.

Harvey, C. E.: Sialography in the dog. Am. J. Vet. Radiol. Soc., *10*:18, 1969.

Hettwer, K. J., and Folsom, T. C.: The normal sialogram. Oral Surg., Oral Med. and Oral Path., *26*:790, 1960.

Lombardi, G.: Radiology in Neuro-ophthalmology. Baltimore, Williams & Wilkins Co., 1967.

Miller, M. E., Christensen, G. C., and Evans, H. E.: Anatomy of the Dog. Philadelphia, W. B. Saunders Co., 1964.

O'Brien, J. A., Harvey, C. E., and Tucker, J. A.: The larynx of the dog: Its normal radiographic anatomy. Am. J. Vet. Radiol. Soc., *10*:38, 1969.

Rubin, L. F., and Patterson, D. F.: Arteriovenous fistula of the orbit in a dog. Cornell Vet., *55*:471, 1965.

Schebitz, H., and Wilkins, H.: Atlas of Radiographic Anatomy of Dog and Cat. Berlin, Paul Parley, 1978.

Schulz, M. D., and Weisberger, D.: Sialography, its value in diagnosis of swelling about the salivary glands. Oral. Surg., Oral Med. and Oral Path., *1*:233, 1948.

Spreull, J. S. A., and Archibald, J.: Glands of the head and neck. *In* Archibald, J. (Ed.): Canine Surgery, First Archibald Edition. Santa Barbara, Calif., American Veterinary Publications, Inc., 1965.

Yakeley, W. L., and Alexander, J. E.: Dacryocystorhinography in the dog. J.A.V.M.A., *159*:1417, 1971.

15

Thorax

Thoracic radiography provides an opportunity to examine a body cavity that is relatively inaccessible by other methods. When properly produced, thoracic radiographs can provide valuable diagnostic information, but when inadequately produced, they may be misleading. Exact positioning and exposure factors must be observed to prevent the introduction of misleading artifacts.

Generally, exposure times must be less than 1/20 second to ensure that imperceptible respiratory movements do not result in a loss of radiographic detail. This requires x-ray equipment with milliamperage capabilities of 100 or more for most canine patients (see Chap. 6).

A grid should be used to reduce fog-producing scatter radiation in normal patients with thoracic thicknesses of 15 cm or greater. Patients with thoracic contents that have densities similar to the abdomen (patients with extensive pleural or pulmonary parenchymal fluid, masses or diaphragmatic hernia) require the use of a grid when the thoracic measurement exceeds 9 cm.

Thoracic radiographs are usually produced during the height of the inspiratory pause to enhance the contrast between radiolucent and radiodense structures. An exception to this procedure is made when patients are examined for signs of minimal or moderate pneumothorax, in which case increased density of the visceral pleural surface and pulmonary parenchyma may be accomplished by producing the radiograph during the expiratory pause (Fraser and Paré, 1970). This results in a relative collapse of the pulmonary parenchyma and pleura without changing the pleural air density, thereby increasing the contrast between these regions and aiding the diagnostic quality of the radiographs.

The thorax is examined with a minimum of two views. Survey radiographs should include the right-left or left-right lateral and DV views. VD views may be indicated when it is not possible to position the patient in DV view or when pleural fluid is present. Standing lateral, erect and VD views using a horizontal x-ray beam may be useful in some patients.

The x-ray beam should be collimated to include the entire thorax from 2 cm cranial to the first rib to a point just caudal to the first lumbar vertebra (Ettinger and Suter, 1970). In patients with serious cough, the caudal cervical trachea should be included on the lateral view. A separate lateral view of the cervical trachea should be produced if clinical signs suggest tracheal disorders (Ettinger and Ticer, 1983).

PROCEDURE

Left-Right Lateral (Le-RtL) View. The patient is positioned in right lateral recumbency and the forelegs are pulled cranially so that most of the triceps musculature is displaced from the cranial aspect of the thorax (Fig. 15–1). The sternum is elevated to a level above the x-ray table equal to that of the thoracic vertebrae to prevent rotation. The neck is extended and the occipital-atlantal joint is allowed to flex approximately 45 degrees to avoid displacement of the trachea. The x-ray beam is centered at the fifth intercostal space (approximately the caudal border of the scapula). The radiograph is produced at the inspiratory pause.

Figure 15–2 illustrates the normal radiographic anatomy of the canine thorax in Le-RtL view.

Right-Left Lateral (Rt-LeL) View. The patient is positioned in lateral recumbency and the forelegs are pulled cranially so that most of the triceps musculature is displaced from the cranial aspect of the thorax (Fig. 15–3). The sternum is elevated to a level above the x-ray table equal to that of the

Text continued on page 281

275

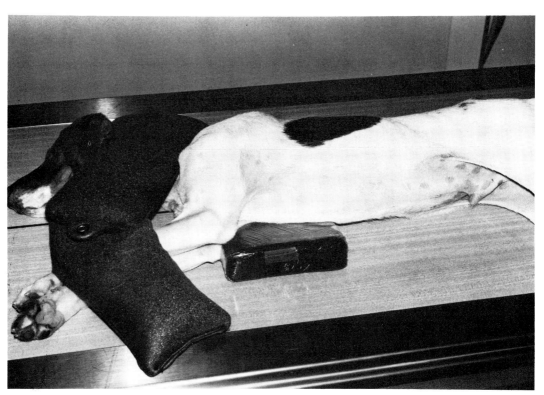

Figure 15–1. Position for left-right lateral view of the thorax.

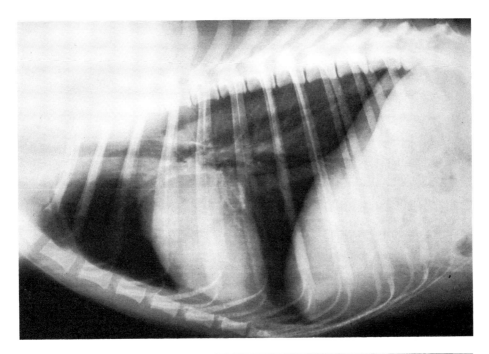

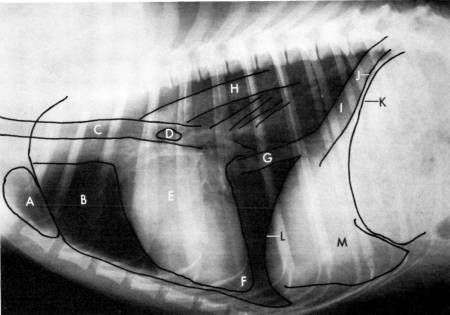

Figure 15–2. Left-right lateral view of the canine thorax. Note that the apex of the heart (*F*) is more conically shaped than in the right-left lateral view (Fig. 15–4). The dependent (right) crus is cranially displaced (*I*):

A. Cranial aspect of the left cranial lung lobe viewed end on
B. Cranial lung lobes superimposed
C. Trachea
D. Origin of the right cranial lobar bronchus viewed end on
E. Cardiac silhouette
F. Cardiac apex

G. Caudal vena cava
H. Descending aorta
I. Right diaphragmatic crus
J. Left diaphragmatic crus
K. Stomach wall
L. Diaphragmatic cupula
M. Liver

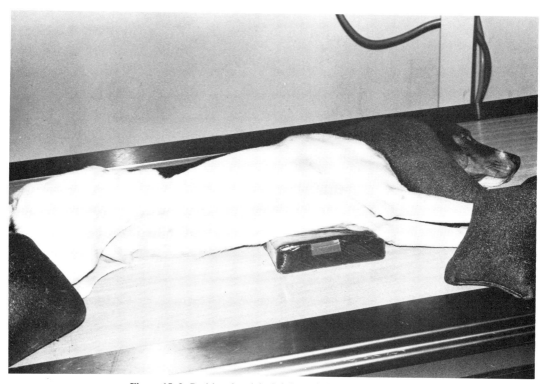

Figure 15–3. Position for right-left lateral view of the thorax.

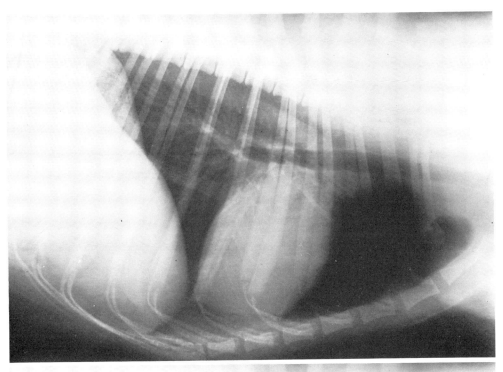

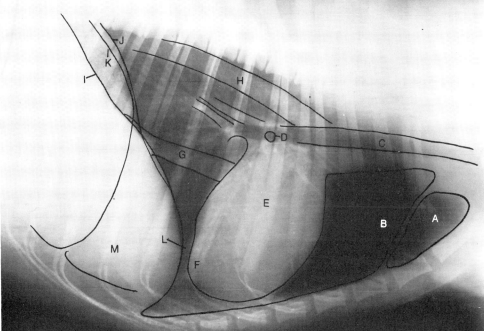

Figure 15–4. Right-left lateral view of the canine thorax. Note that the apex of the heart (F) is allowed to change position when compared with the left-right lateral view (Fig. 15–2), giving a rounded appearance. The left diaphragmatic crus, which is in direct contact with the fundus of the stomach, is displaced cranially (J).

A. Cranial aspect of the left cranial lung lobe viewed end on
B. Cranial lung lobes superimposed
C. Trachea
D. Origin of the right cranial lobar bronchus viewed end on
E. Cardiac silhouette
F. Cardiac apex

G. Caudal vena cava
H. Descending aorta
I. Right diaphragmatic crus
J. Left diaphragmatic crus
K. Stomach wall
L. Diaphragmatic cupula
M. Liver

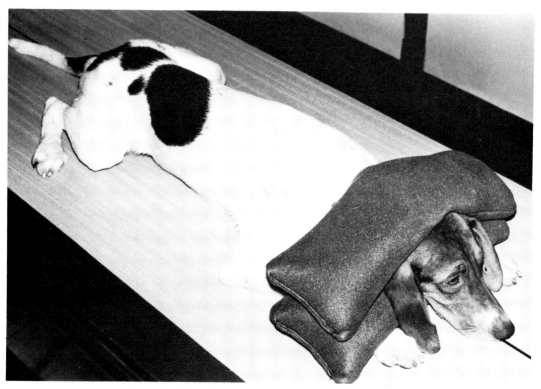

Figure 15–5. Position for the dorsoventral view of the thorax.

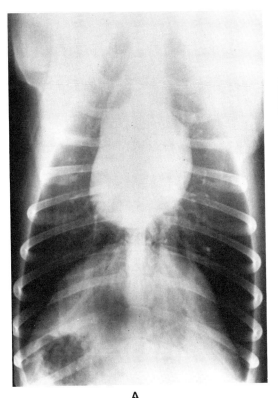 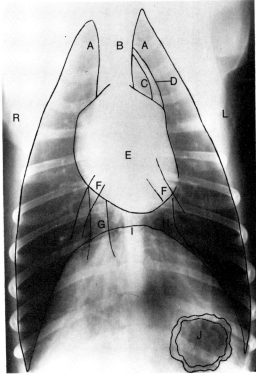

A   B

Figure 15–6. Dorsoventral view of the canine thorax.
A. Cranial lung lobes
B. Cranial mediastinum
C. Ventral aspect of the right cranial lung lobe
D. Ventral aspect of the cranial mediastinum displaced
    to the left
E. Cardiac silhouette
F. Caudal lobar pulmonary arteries
G. Caudal vena cava
H. Ventral aspect of caudal mediastinum (between the
    accessory lobe and the left caudal lobe)
I. Diaphragmatic cupula
J. Air-filled fundus of the stomach

thoracic vertebrae to prevent rotation. The neck is extended and the occipital-atlantal joint is allowed to flex approximately 45 degrees to avoid displacement of the trachea. The x-ray beam is centered at the fifth intercostal space (approximately the caudal border of the scapula). The radiograph is produced at the inspiratory pause.

Figure 15–4 illustrates the normal radiographic anatomy of the canine thorax in Rt-LeL view.

Dorsoventral (DV) View. The patient is placed in ventral recumbency with the thoracic vertebrae superimposed over the sternum. The forelegs are pulled slightly forward and the elbows are rotated outward (abducted), so that the shoulders are displaced

craniomedially and the scapulae are shifted laterally away from the cranial lung field (Fig. 15–5). The rear limbs are allowed to flex in a crouching position, and the head is lowered between the forelimbs to decrease the thickness of the caudal cervical musculature over the cranial lung fields.

The x-ray beam is centered over the fifth intercostal space, which is usually located at the level of the caudal aspect of the scapulae. The radiograph is produced at the inspiratory pause.

Figure 15–6 illustrates the normal radiographic anatomy of the canine thorax in DV view.

Ventrodorsal (VD) View. The patient is placed in dorsal recumbency and the fore-

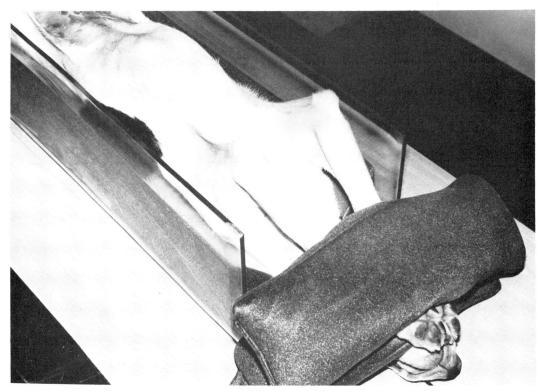

Figure 15–7. Position for ventrodorsal view of the thorax.

limbs are pulled forward (Fig. 15–7). The sternum should be superimposed over the thoracic vertebrae to avoid rotation in the sagittal plane.

The x-ray beam is centered over the fifth intercostal space, which is located at the junction of the cranial two thirds to the caudal one third of the sternum. The radiograph is produced at the inspiratory pause.

Figure 15–8 illustrates the normal radiographic anatomy of the canine thorax in VD view.

Horizontal X-ray Beam Radiographs. Radiographs using a horizontal x-ray beam may be indicated when the diagnosis of pleural fluid is equivocal on survey radiographs. The standing lateral or erect (patient suspended by forelimbs) positions may cause gravitation of fluid to the dependent portions of the pleural space and enhance visualization. Usually, however, clinically significant quantities of pleural fluid may be detected on radiographs produced in the VD view using a routine vertical x-ray beam. The VD view is also useful in allowing the postural drainage of pleural fluid to the dorsocaudal aspects of the pleural space, thus allowing better visu-

alization of the mediastinal structure, heart, lung and diaphragm than with the DV view in patients with moderate to large amounts of pleural fluid (Groves and Ticer, in press).

INTERPRETATION

The position and appearance of the normal thoracic viscera vary, depending on postural relationships, phases of the respiratory cycle, pathophysiologic states, body types and x-ray beam geometry. Generally the most variable appearance is observed in the shape of the cardiac silhouette and diaphragm and in the appearance of the pulmonary parenchyma.

Heart

There is considerable variation in the cardiac silhouette among the different breeds of dogs. Dogs with a deep thorax, such as setters, sight hounds and collies, have a cardiac silhouette that is more upright than that of dogs with a wide, shallow thorax, such as beagles and Boston terriers (Ettinger and

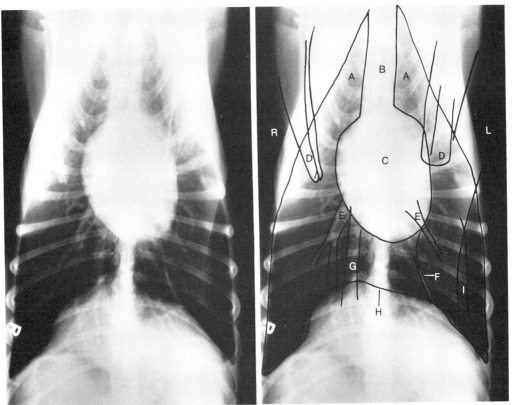

Figure 15–8. Ventrodorsal view of the canine thorax. Note the scapular overlay of the cranial thorax and the increased prominence of the axillary skin folds (I) compared with the dorsoventral view (Fig. 12–6).

    A. Cranial lung lobes
    B. Cranial mediastinum
    C. Cardiac silhouette
    D. Scapulae
    E. Caudal lobar pulmonary arteries
    F. Ventral aspect of caudal mediastinum (between the accessory lobe and the left caudal lobe)
    G. Caudal vena cava
    H. Diaphragmatic cupula
    I. Axillary skin folds

Suter, 1970). In dogs with a deep thorax, the heart occupies a relatively smaller proportion of the thoracic cavity compared with the relatively greater volume and wider appearance of the heart in dogs with a wide, shallow thorax. Animals approximately three months of age or younger have a relatively rounder heart than adult animals (Ettinger and Suter, 1970). In some breeds of dogs, such as the borzoi, Irish wolfhound and Irish setter, the cardiac apex may not reach the sternum in the lateral view, and this sign should not be mistaken for pneumothorax.

Exposures of 1/20 sec or less may demonstrate differences between systole and diastole on the shape and position of the heart (Ettinger and Suter, 1970). The left border may look straighter and the pulmonary artery larger, and the heart may appear slightly smaller and more sharply delineated at the end of systole than during diastole.

Near the end of ventricular systole, the ventricular area is small, and the atrial borders bulge outward and appear well rounded. Near the end of diastole the ventricles are large and rounded, and the atria are not visualized (Suter and Gomez, 1981). The largest variation in size between systole and diastole occurs in the dorsal third of the right and left ventricular borders in lateral views and in the pulmonary artery segment and the atria in DV view (Suter and Gomez, 1981).

Exposures of 1/10 sec or longer usually show the heart in diastole because the slightly enlarged diastolic heart effectively absorbs the x-ray beam, preventing visualization of the smaller cardiac silhouette of systole. The change in cardiac size during exposure accounts for the relative loss of radiographic detail on radiographs produced with long exposures.

Inappropriate cranial displacement of the central x-ray beam will result in a shortening of the cardiac silhouette in the DV view.

The apparent size of the cardiac silhouette varies considerably with the phase of the respiratory cycle. Although the absolute change is a few millimeters, expiration causes the cardiac size to be perceived as enlarged. This is due to increased cranial border-sternal contact, increased diaphragmatic contact and, in general, a decrease in the size of the poorly-inflated thorax.

The description of the normal radiographic appearance is made difficult by the great variety of heart shapes, sizes and positions among different breeds; different phases of the respiratory and cardiac cycles; different degrees of obesity; and differences in position while being radiographed. There are therefore many similarities between the appearance of the normal and diseased heart (Suter and Gomez, 1981). Baseline thoracic radiographs produced in DV and left-right lateral views while the patient is free of disease are a real asset for comparison with future examinations.

Lateral Views. In the lateral thoracic view, most normal dogs have a cranial cardiac border that is located near the third rib, and the caudal border extends to about the eighth rib. The cranial border consists of the right ventricular wall and right auricle. The dorsal portion of the cranial border joins the ventral outline of the cranial vena cava. In some patients, the dorsal aspect of the cranial border is composed of the aortic arch and the conus arteriosus of the main pulmonary artery. Where the cranial vena cava joins the atrium, there may be a slight indentation, which is called the cranial waist. The angle of the cranial waist varies with the inclination of the heart. This angle is more acute in dogs with upright hearts and more obtuse in dogs with greater inclination of the heart.

The curve of the cranial border usually runs parallel to the sternum for various distances, depending upon the cardiac axis inclination. Increased sternal contact is normal in dogs with a wide thorax. Retrosternal fat

accumulates around the cardiac apex and may obscure the junction of the cranial border and apex, especially in right-left lateral view, because the apex shifts in the dependent direction (Spencer et al., 1981) and may appear to be elevated dorsal to the sternum. For this reason lateral radiographs produced for cardiac evaluation should be made in left-right lateral view (Spencer et al., 1981).

The caudal cardiac border is formed by the left ventricle and atrium. The caudal border may merge with or overlie the diaphragmatic cupula, especially in dogs with a wide and short thorax. The distance between the cardiac apex and the diaphragmatic cupula varies with the respiratory cycle. The left ventricular border usually curves inward at the base of the heart to form the caudal waist as it meets the left atrium. The caudal waist corresponds to the atrioventricular groove. The angle of the caudal waist is most acute in hearts with increased inclination. The left atrial border extends caudodorsally to join the pulmonary veins. The caudal vena cava joins the cardiac silhouette just ventral to the atrioventricular groove.

In the lateral view, the dorsal aspect of the cardiac silhouette is obscured by the main pulmonary arteries and veins, lymph nodes and other mediastinal structures.

The main pulmonary artery contributes to the cranial border of the heart only rarely (Ettinger and Suter, 1970) and usually becomes visible only after it bifurcates into the right and left branches immediately cranial to the carina. The left caudal lobar artery passes over the radiographically lucent oval structure of the origin of the right cranial lobar bronchus (Burk et al., 1978) and may be seen for a variable distance into the pulmonary parenchyma. The right pulmonary artery crosses from left to right under the carina and may be seen end on as a dense, round structure at the cardiac base. This normal structure should not be mistaken for an enlarged hilar lymph node (Suter and Gomez, 1981). The right caudal lobar artery is superimposed on the left atrium toward the periphery, making it difficult to distinguish this artery from the pulmonary veins. The pulmonary veins are normally less dense than the arteries, as they converge before joining the left atrium.

The aorta may be seen leaving the cardiac silhouette in a variety of positions, depending on the thoracic conformation. In dogs with a deep thorax, the aortic arch extends farther cranially and emerges more ventrally from the area of the right auricle. The aorta is well delineated only after it crosses the trachea and courses dorsocaudally between the trachea and the thoracic vertebrae.

Dorsoventral View. Moderate rotation of the thorax about the sagittal plane can cause marked change in the shape and size of the lateral borders of the cardiac silhouette (Ettinger and Suter, 1970). If the thorax is rotated, the diaphragmatic cupula and the cardiac border appear closer to the thoracic wall than normal. The lateral borders of the heart appear rounder. This should not be mistaken for ventricular enlargement.

In the true DV view, the cardiac silhouette has been described as a "lopsided egg" (Wyburn and Lawson, 1967). The cranial and right borders are rounded and the left border almost straight, which makes its appearance lopsided. This appearance is most easily reproduced in DV view, making it preferable to the VD view for cardiac examinations (Ettinger and Suter, 1970; Suter and Gomez, 1981).

The cardiac silhouette usually extends from the third to about the eighth rib in the DV view but may vary greatly, depending upon the thoracic conformation. In dogs with a deep thorax, the distance is decreased and the silhouette appears rounder because of the more nearly upright position of the heart as it is suspended in the thoracic cavity. When compared with the VD view, the longitudinal dimension of the heart is decreased (Ruehl and Thrall, 1981). In the DV view the base of the heart lies on the midline, and the apex is directed toward the left side. In breeds with a wide thorax, the apex is directed more toward the left side than in breeds with a narrow thorax, in which the longitudinal axis of the heart almost parallels the midsagittal plane of the thorax. In some brachycephalic breeds, the cardiac apex may lie on the right side.

The right cranial quadrant of the cardiac silhouette is formed by the right atrium. Caudally, the atrial border merges with the right ventricle and right pulmonary artery. The vena cava interrupts the right ventricular border as it courses caudomedially. The right ventricle usually ends immediately to the right of the cardiac apex and may be demarcated by a notch at the interventricular septum.

A structure formerly considered to be the cardiophrenic ligament extends as a thin band of tissue from the cardiac apex to the diaphragm. This line is now known to be the ventral aspect of the caudal mediastinum, where the accessory and left caudal lung lobes meet (Burk, 1976). The entire apex and most of the left cardiac border are formed by the left ventricle. The cranial aspect of the left cardiac border is created by the pulmonary artery and the right ventricular outflow tract. The left auricle, which lies between the pulmonary artery and the left ventricle, seldom extends beyond the left cranial cardiac border in normal dogs, but its appearance may be modified by the phase of the cardiac cycle (see p. 284).

Mediastinum

In lateral views, the cranial mediastinal structures are demarcated ventrally by the ventral border of the cranial vena cava. The tracheal lumen is usually the only structure visualized within the cranial mediastinum except when air or ingesta are present in the esophageal lumen. Usually the esophageal lumen is air-filled only during anesthesia or during severely depressing disease states.

In the DV and VD views, the right cranial mediastinal border is formed by the cranial vena cava. The left subclavian artery forms the left mediastinal border.

The trachea enters the thoracic cavity at the midline or slightly to the right and courses caudally with a slight right lateral curve. The trachea ends by bifurcating to form the main bronchi, which is referred to as the carina.

The width of the mediastinum varies greatly and tends to be increased in brachycephalic breeds and in obesity.

Lungs

The vascular markings are the most prominent structures of the lungs. The air-filled alveoli provide an excellent contrast medium against the dense pulmonary vasculature. The degree of contrast between these structures varies greatly with the respiratory cycle, position, age of the patient and radiographic technique (Ettinger and Suter 1970; Spencer et al., 1981; Groves and Ticer, in press; Ruehl and Thrall, 1981). Older patients usually have denser pulmonary structures caused by nodular or linear markings of interstitial origin (Reif and Rhodes, 1966). Overexposure of lung fields tends to simulate decreased density compared with properly exposed lungs in radiographs produced during the same phase of the respiratory cycle (Fig. 15–9).

The intrapulmonary vasculature may be divided into three zones for purposes of description (Ettinger and Suter, 1970): (1) the central or hilar zone; (2) the middle zone,

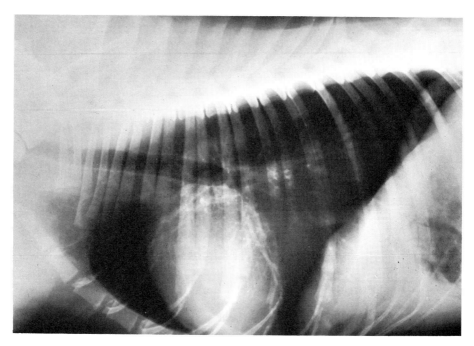

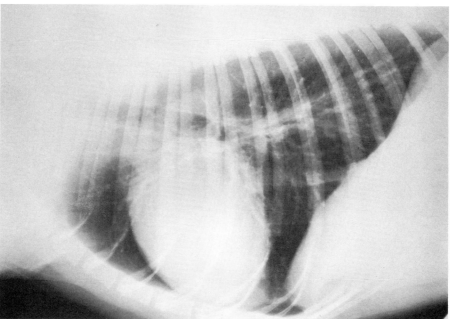

Figure 15–9. *Top,* Left-right lateral view of a canine thorax produced with moderate overexposure, resulting in a relatively decreased density of the lung fields. *Bottom,* Left-right lateral view of a canine thorax (same patient as in top) produced with proper exposure. Notice the visualization of the bronchovascular markings throughout the entire lung field.

which contrains the large bronchial and vascular branches; and (3) the peripheral zone, which is composed of pulmonary parenchyma. The pulmonary vasculature is best evaluated in the middle zone. The peripheral zone usually contains relatively few visible vascular or bronchial markings. The caudal lobe pulmonary vasculature is better visualized in DV view than in VD view (Ruehl and Thrall, 1981; Spencer et al., 1981; Groves and Ticer, in press). This phenomenon has been reported to be the result of magnification and more perpendicular relationship of the diverging indirect x-ray beam with the caudal lobe vessels (Ruehl and Thrall, 1981). Better aeration of this nondependent portion of the lungs in DV view probably also accounts for some of the increased visualization (Spencer et al., 1981).

In the DV and VD views the caudal lobar pulmonary arteries are usually visible lateral to the caudal lobar bronchus, and the vein is located medially.

In lateral view, structures in the nondependent lung are better visualized than those in the dependent lung. This is due to compression on the dependent side and increased aeration on the nondependent side (Grundage, 1978; Spencer et al., 1981). The air-filled lung provides contrast with dense structures such as vessels, bronchi, infiltrates, and masses; therefore, the lung with suspected lesions should be placed on the nondependent side when radiographs are produced in lateral recumbency (Spencer et al., 1981).

In radiographs of patients that have been in prolonged lateral recumbency, especially while anesthetized, the lung that has been dependent can be expected to be partially atelectatic (Suter and Gomez, 1981) (see Fig. 15–10). Reinflation should be attempted prior to radiographing the thorax by placing the patient in the opposite lateral recumbency for a few minutes or, if the patient is anesthetized, by compressing the rebreathing bag a few times.

The lateral view may show the cranial aspect of the left cranial lobe end-on as it courses medially in front of the right cranial lobe (Figs. 15–2 and 15–4).

The retrosternal fat pad may appear as a moderately dense structure that may elevate the lung lobes and cardiac silhouette dorsally from the sternum in obese patients. The magnitude of this elevation decreases on inhalation and increases on expiration (Fig. 15–11). The normal retrosternal fat pad should not be mistaken for pleural fluid. Fat has less radiographic density than fluid.

When pleural fluid is suggested on clinical examination or on survey radiographs, both the VD and DV views are useful in defining

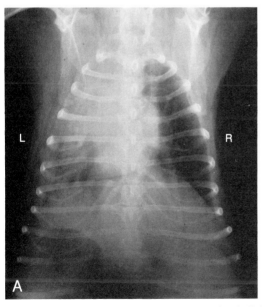 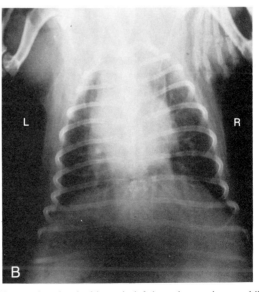

Figure 15–10. Dorsoventral view of an 8-year-old male Pekingese dog that had been in left lateral recumbency while anesthetized, showing an atelectatic left lung and left mediastinal shift (*A*). Same patient after compressing the rebreathing bag a few times, showing reexpansion of the left lung and recovery from the mediastinal shift (*B*).

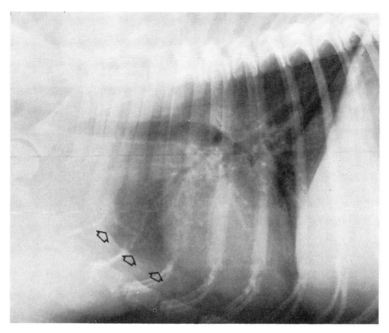

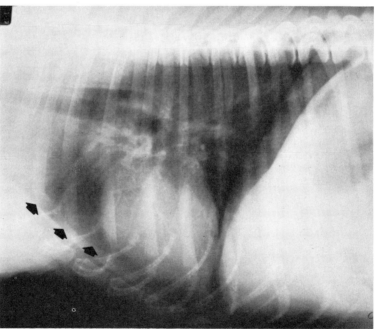

Figure 15–11. *Top,* Left-right lateral view of a canine thorax produced during expiration (note the position of the diaphragm), illustrating the relative increased thickness of the retrosternal fat pad (arrows) when compared with an inhalation radiograph of the same patient (*bottom*). *Bottom,* Left-right lateral view of a canine thorax produced during inspiration (note the position of the diaphragm), illustrating the relative decreased thickness of the retrosternal fat pad when compared with an exhalation radiograph of the same patient (*top*).

the presence and distribution of the fluids (Groves and Ticer, in press). In the DV view (ventral recumbency), the heart, cranial mediastinum, cranial lung lobes and ventral aspect of the diaphragm are submersed in fluid, resulting in a loss of radiographically detect-able margins. In the VD view (dorsal recumbency), there is an improved visualization of these structures owing to movement of the pleural fluid to the dependent caudodorsal aspect of the thorax. The more ventrally located heart, cranial mediastinum and cranial and right middle lung lobes show the most improvement in visualization in the VD view (Groves and Ticer, in press) (Fig. 15–12). This improved visualization may result in identification of the lesion responsible for the pleural fluid production. The fluid moves caudodorsally in the VD projection because of the dorsally sloping caudal aspect of the thoracic cavity that is created by the increased length of the dorsal spinous processes of the cranial thoracic vertebrae. Additionally, the dorsal thoracic cavity has relatively more volume than the ventral thorax, which results in a decreased height of the free pleural fluid column (Groves and Ticer, in press).

The decision to place a dyspneic patient in dorsal recumbency (VD) should be made only after careful assessment of the clinical status. At times, it is more rational to remove some of the pleural fluid and to stabilize the patient's clinical status prior to producing the VD view.

Table 15–1 lists the preferred view for

Table 15–1. PREFERRED VIEW FOR THORACIC RADIOGRAPHIC EXAMINATION IN PATIENTS WITH PLEURAL FLUID

Structure(s)	Ventrodorsal View	Dorsoventral View
Heart	X	
Pulmonary Parenchyma		
Cranial lobes	X	
Right middle lobe	X	
Caudal lobes		X
Pulmonary Vasculature		X
Hilar Structures		X
Cranial Mediastinum	X	

After Groves and Ticer, in press.

thoracic radiographs when examining patients with pleural fluid.

Some patients, especially dogs with a deep thorax, show extensive visualization of the

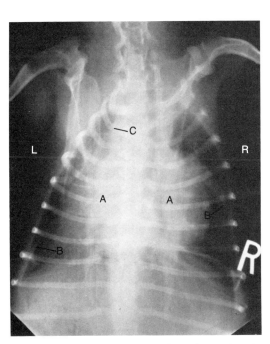

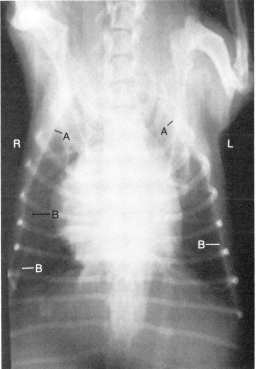

Figure 15–12. *Left,* Dorsoventral view of a canine thorax with pleural effusion, showing collection of the fluid ventrally around the cardiac silhouette (A). Fluid may also be seen in the interlobar fissures (B) and around the cranial mediastinum (C), causing an artifactual widening. *Right,* ventrodorsal view of a canine thorax with pleural effusion (same patient as on the right), showing redistribution of fluid away from the heart and cranial mediastinum. Moderate cranial lobe atelectasis with fluid between the visceral and parietal pleural (A) and interlobar fissure fluid (B) may be seen as evidence of the pleural fluid.

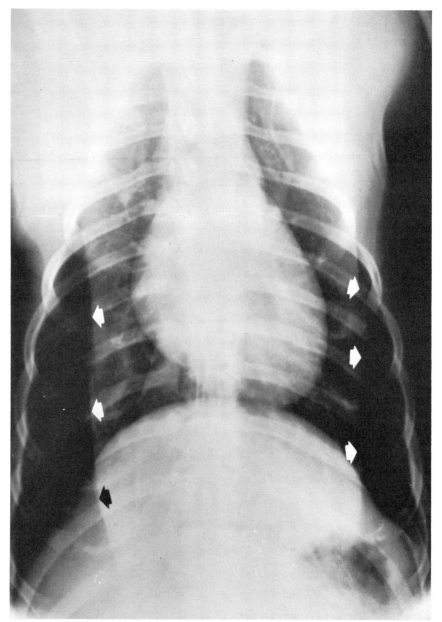

Figure 15–13. Dorsoventral view of a two-year-old female boxer, showing the appearance of the axillary skin folds (arrows) that are seen in some dogs with a deep thorax.

axillary skin folds in the DV and VD positions (Fig. 15–13). These shadows should not be considered pathologic.

Diaphragm

The radiographic appearance of the diaphragm varies markedly with body conformation and phase of the respiratory cycle. In patients with a deep thorax, the VD view shows the distinct outline of the left and right crura and the medially located cupula (Grandage, 1974). Patients with a wide, shallow thorax have a single-lobed diaphragmatic outline with a slightly right lateral cranial location. The cupula may have contact with the cardiac apex and show a slight depression at the point of contact.

In the lateral view, the dependent crus is located cranial to the contralateral crus in most patients (Grandage, 1974; Spencer et al., 1981).

The crus normally intersects the ventral border of the vertebral column between T11 and T13, although it may attach as far forward as T9 and as far back as L1 in normal dogs. The position of the diaphragm may vary as much as two vertebral body lengths. Quietly breathing dogs may show a diaphragmatic excursion of less than one vertebral body length.

Ribs and Sternum

The ribs usually arch laterally from the vertebral column, then course medially to the costochondral junction. In some breeds of dogs, such as the basset hound and some dachshunds, the ribs may invaginate at the costochondral junction, producing a longitudinal indentation on the sides of the thorax in apparently normal animals. The DV or VD view shows this invagination as an undulating longitudinal density on the lateral aspect of the thoracic cavity (Fig. 15–14). This structure should not be mistaken for pleural fluid or thickened pleural margins.

The costal cartilages may become mineralized at a relatively young age in apparently normal dogs. Early in the stages of mineralization, the densities may appear mottled.

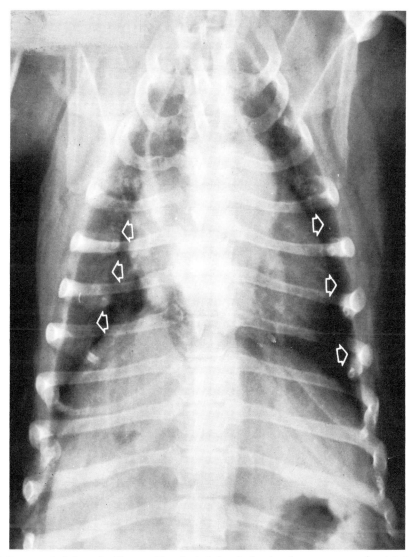

Figure 15–14. Dorsoventral view of a 15-year-old male dachshund, showing the appearance of undulating longitudinal density produced by an invagination of the ribs and pleura at the costochondral junctions (arrows). This structure should not be mistaken for pleural fluid or thickened pleural margins.

The caudal aspect of the sternum may show rather a bizarre structure in the lateral view in apparently normal animals. These deformities should not be mistaken for pathologic processes.

REFERENCES

Burk, R. L.: Radiographic definition of the phrenicopericardiac ligament. J. Amer. Vet. Radiol. Soc., *17*:216–218, 1976.

Burk, R. L., Corwin, L. A., Bahr, R. J., Corley, E. A., and Jones, B. D.: The cranial lung lobe bronchus of the dog: Its identification in lateral chest radiographs. J. Amer. Vet. Radiol. Soc., *19*(6):210–212, 1978.

Douglas, S. W., and Williamson, H. D.: Principles of Veterinary Radiography. 3rd ed. Baltimore, Williams & Wilkins Co., 1980.

Ettinger, S. J., and Suter, P. F.: Canine Cardiology. Philadelphia, W. B. Saunders Co., 1970.

Ettinger, S. J.: Pericardiocentesis. Vet. Clin. N. Amer. *4*:403, 1974.

Ettinger, S. J., and Ticer, J. W.: Tracheal Diseases. *In* Ettinger, S. J. (Ed.): A Textbook of Veterinary Internal Medicine: Diseases of Dog and Cat. 2nd ed. Philadelphia, W. B. Saunders Co., 1980.

Fraser, R. G., and Paré, J. A. P.: Diagnosis of Diseases of the Chest. Vol. II. Philadelphia, W. B. Saunders Co., 1970.

Gillette, E. L., Thrall, D. E., and Lebel, J. R.: Carlson's Veterinary Radiology. 3rd ed. Philadelphia, Lea & Febiger, 1977.

Grandage, J.: The radiology of the dog's diaphragm. J. Small Anim. Pract., *15*:1, 1974.

Groves, T. F., and Ticer, J. W.: Pleural fluid translocation: A comparison of ventral and dorsal recumbent radiographic projections. Vet. Radiol. (in press).

Miller, M. E., Christensen, G. C., and Evans, H. E.: Anatomy of the dog. Philadelphia, W. B. Saunders Co., 1964.

Reed, J. R., Thomas, W. P., and Suter, P. F.: Pneumopericardiography in the normal dog. Vet. Radiol. (in press).

Reif, J. S., and Rhodes, W. H.: The lungs of aged dogs: A radiographic-morphologic correlation. J. Amer. Vet. Radiol. Soc., *7*:5, 1966.

Ruehl, W. W., Jr., and Thrall, D. E.: The effect of dorsal versus ventral recumbency on the radiographic appearance of the canine thorax. Vet. Radiol. *22*(1):10–16, 1981.

Schebitz, H., and Wilkens, H.: Atlas of Radiographic Anatomy of Dog and Cat. Berlin, Paul Parey, 1978.

Spencer, C. P., Ackerman, N., and Burt, J. K.: The canine lateral thoracic radiograph. Vet. Radiol., *22*(6):262–266, 1981.

Suter, P. F., and Chan, K. F.: Disseminated pulmonary disease in small animals: A radiographic approach to diagnosis. J. Amer. Vet. Radiol. Soc., *9*:67, 1968.

Suter, P. F., and Gomez, J. A.: Diseases of the Thorax: Radiographic Diagnosis. Davis, CA, Venture Press, 1981.

Thomas, W. P.: Pericardial Disease. *In* Ettinger, S. J. (Ed.): Textbook of Veterinary Internal Medicine. 2nd ed. Philadelphia, W. B. Saunders Co., 1983.

Wyburn, R. S., and Lawson, D. D.: Simple radiography as an aid to the diagnosis of heart disease in the dog. J. Small Anim. Pract., *8*:163, 1967.

Pneumopericardiography

Pneumopericardiography is a negative contrast radiographic examination of the pericardial sac.

INDICATIONS

Pneumopericardiography is indicated when a complete evaluation of the etiology of pericardial fluid cannot be determined from conventional methods of examination.

CONTRAINDICATIONS

When a diagnosis of pericardial fluid has been positively established on the basis of available clinical data, the only contraindication for pneumopericardiography is congestive heart failure (Ettinger, 1974). In patients with congestive heart failure, the stress of lateral recumbent posture may be an indication to modify the procedure to allow a ventral recumbent posture using a horizontally directed x-ray beam. Patients with pericardial effusion secondary to congestive heart failure usually respond well to digitalization and diuretic therapy. These animals should generally not be subjected to the procedure unless the usual therapeutic agents fail to resolve the problem. In the latter case, pericardiocentesis is in order and pneumopericardiography may then be performed.

TECHNIQUE

Patient Preparation

Prior to performing pericardiocentesis, a clinical diagnosis of pericardial fluid must be made. Clinical, radiographic, electrocardiographic and clinical pathologic evidence must strongly indicate a diagnosis of pericardial fluid accumulation (Ettinger and Suter, 1970; Ettinger, 1974). Patients with severe congestive heart failure, signs of pulmonary edema, cyanosis and respiratory distress are poor candidates for pneumopericardiography. Rapid digitalization and administration of diuretic and narcotic sedatives may be indicated prior to performing the procedure. In apprehensive patients, tranquilizers aid in restraint during the relatively long procedure of fluid drainage. When not contraindicated because of age or disease status, a ketamine-diazepam (Valium) cocktail given intravenously will produce good sedation for this procedure.

The left ventral thorax is clipped and scrubbed.

Materials

A large syringe, 16-gauge Venocath set (Venocath, Abbott Laboratories), three-way stopcock and lidocaine for local anesthesia are needed to perform the pericardiocentesis, fluid drainage and air injection. Fluid collection and sterile culture tubes are required for pericardial fluid analysis.

Use of the same ancillary equipment but a larger needle allows for more rapid removal of the fluid. The Angiocath (Deseret Co) 16-gauge over-the-needle Teflon catheter has worked well in our hands.

Procedure

The site for pericardiocentesis is determined from the survey radiographs. Usually the left fourth to sixth intercostal spaces near the junction of the lower and middle thirds of the thorax provide the most convenient sites. The patient is placed in right lateral recumbency and electrocardiographic leads are attached in a normal manner. Lidocaine is used to infiltrate the skin and intercostal musculature at the site of the needle entry.

A sample of venous blood should be withdrawn to compare with the pericardial fluid. Its color and clotting time are noted prior to the procedure. The needle from the Venocath or Angiocath unit is attached to a large syringe. The needle and syringe are held at an angle of approximately 45 degrees to the intercostal space, and the needle is inserted through the thoracic wall in a mediodorsal direction. When using the Angiocath method, it is wise to make a small nick in the skin with a scalpel blade to allow the Teflon catheter to pass through readily. As the needle touches the pericardium, it is thrust into the pericardial sac.

Electrocardiographic monitoring will show no disturbance in cardiac rhythm if the needle is scratching the pericardial sac or has passed through it. If the needle touches the epicardium or enters the myocardium, one or more premature contractions will be noted (Ettinger, 1974). This suggests that pericardial fluid is not present or that the needle is within the sac and is touching and irritating the epicardial surface. Epicardial contact through the needle and syringe has a scratching-like sensation. Since coronary vessels could be lacerated, the needle should immediately be pulled back.

Twenty-five to 30 ml of fluid are then withdrawn for comparison with the previously drawn peripheral venous blood and for laboratory samples. If the fluid has the appearance of blood, no additional fluid is withdrawn until a comparison with clotting has been made. If clotting occurs readily, it is assumed that the sample is whole blood, which indicates that the procedure should be stopped. This usually requires a waiting period of from 5 to 10 minutes.

The Venocath catheter and wire guide are inserted into the pericardial sac through the needle. The catheter is advanced, while the wire guide is held in place just within the pericardial sac. The needle is then retracted from the thorax and the plastic guards around it are folded into place. A three-way stopcock and syringe are then attached to the catheter. If the sample is not whole blood, the withdrawal of fluid is then started. Since the catheter lumen is small, the entire procedure may require 30 to 60 minutes or more. If the Angiocath technique is used, the needle is immediately withdrawn and the teflon catheter is advanced into the sac. Fluid withdrawal is usually performed in only a few minutes. The patient is rotated about the

sagittal plane of the thorax to assist in complete drainage. After fluid collection is completed, the total volume of fluid is noted and a like amount of air is injected into the pericardial sac.

Dorsoventral and right and left lateral recumbent radiographs are then produced (Reed et al., in press). At times, a standing lateral view using a horizontal x-ray beam is produced to visualize the dorsal aspect of the pericardial sac when a residual amount of fluid makes delineation of these structures difficult.

Upon completion of fluid removal and radiographic procedures, the catheter is withdrawn. The patient may require antibiotic therapy for several days. Digitalis and diuretics may also be necessary to assist in mobilization of other body fluids and to improve cardiac function if failure has been evident (Ettinger, 1974).

The air in the pericardium will be resorbed in a period of 24 to 96 hours. The patient should be reradiographed 48 hours following the procedure to determine the degree or recurrence of pericardial fluid.

Figure 15–15 is a thoracic radiograph of a seven year old male German shorthaired pointer with idiopathic pericardial effusion. Figure 15–16 shows this same patient after pericardial drainage and the production of a pneumopericardiogram. This pneumopericardiogram shows normal cardiac conformation. The cranioventral aspect of the cardiac silhouette is composed of a smoothly marginated right auricular appendage, which is not visualized to this degree in a normal heart that is covered by pericardium. Figure 15–17 shows a nine year old female springer spaniel with a heart-base tumor that is visualized with a pneumopericardiogram. The right auricular appendage is displaced caudoventrally by the mass, which shows a roughened marginal outline.

COMPLICATIONS

Rupture of a coronary vessel may lead to fatal hemorrhage. Excessive irritation of the epicardium may result in ventricular premature contractions which may develop into life-threatening arrhythmia. Neither of these complications is common and therefore should not present a contraindication for the procedure if it is performed correctly.

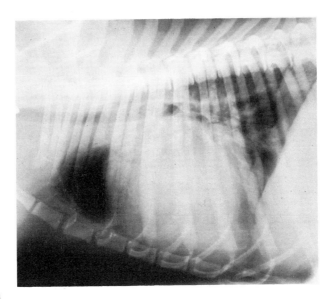

Figure 15–15. *Top,* Left-right lateral view of a seven year old male German shorthaired pointer with a markedly enlarged cardiac silhouette due to pericardial fluid that was secondary to benign pericardial effusion. *Bottom,* Dorsoventral view of the same patient.

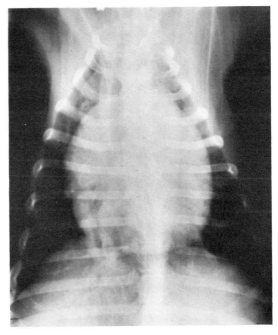

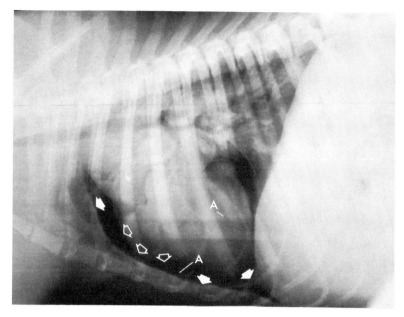

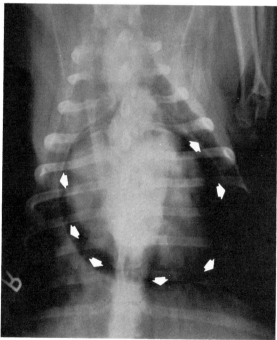

Figure 15–16. Left-right lateral and dorsoventral views of a pneumopericardiogram of a seven year old male German shorthaired pointer with a markedly enlarged pericardium due to pericardial fluid that was secondary to benign pericardial effusion (same patient as in Fig. 15–15). Note the outline of the parietal pericardium as it is contrasted with the pericardial air (arrows). The radiopaque catheter may be seen within the pericardial sac (*A*). The normal right auricular appendage is seen on the cranioventral aspect of the cardiac silhouette (open arrows).

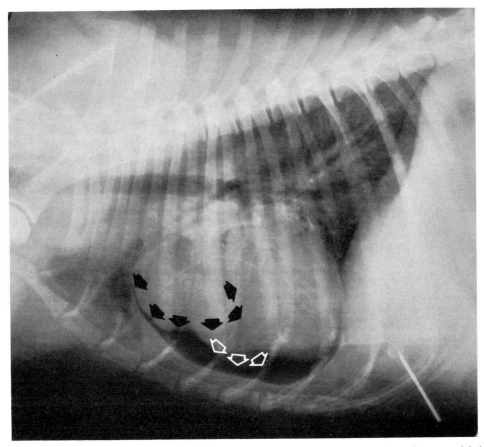

Figure 15–17. Left-right lateral view of a pneumopericardiogram of a nine year old female springer spaniel showing the outline of heart-based tumor (arrows). The right auricular appendage (open arrows) is partially hidden by the tumor mass. Note the lack of smooth margination shown by the tumor silhouette.

REFERENCES

Gillette, E. L., Thrall, D. E., and Lebel, J. L.: Carlson's Veterinary Radiology. 3rd ed. Philadelphia, Lea & Febiger, 1977.

Douglas, S. W., and Williamson, H. D.: Principles of Veterinary Radiography. 3rd ed. Baltimore, Williams & Wilkins Co., 1980.

Ettinger, S. J., and Suter, P. F.: Canine Cardiology. Philadelphia, W. B. Saunders Co., 1970.

Ettinger, S. J.: Pericardiocentesis. Vet. Clin. N. Amer., 4:403, 1974.

Fraser, R. G., and Paré, J. A. P.: Diagnosis of Diseases of the Chest. Vol. II. Philadelphia, W. B. Saunders Co., 1970.

Miller, M. E., Christensen, G. C., and Evans, H. E.: Anatomy of the Dog. Philadelphia, W. B. Saunders Co., 1964.

Reed, J. R., Thomas, W. P., and Suter, P. F.: Pneumopericardiography in the normal dog. Vet. Radiol. (in press).

Schebitz, H., and Wilkens, H.: Atlas of Radiographic Anatomy of Dog and Cat. Berlin, Paul Parey, 1978.

Thomas, W. P.: Pericardial Disease. In Ettinger, S. J. (Ed.): Textbook of Veterinary Internal Medicine. 2nd ed. Philadelphia, W. B. Saunders Co., 1983.

G. L. Wood, S. J. Ettinger, and
E. A. Rhode

Angiocardiography

INTRODUCTION

Angiocardiography refers to the production of radiographs by exposing a sequence of films during the circulation of contrast medium through the heart and blood vessels. This valuable diagnostic tool is utilized primarily by veterinarians in large practices or institutions. Because of the specialized equipment required, angiocardiography usually is not a procedure utilized by the general practitioner. Angiocardiography can provide information relevant to the diagnosis and prognosis of most congenital and some acquired cardiac diseases.

Before contrast radiography is done, it is imperative that a complete cardiovascular examination be performed. Such a work-up should include a complete physical examination, an electrocardiogram, thoracic radiographs and routine blood tests. Special procedures such as phonocardiograms, echocardiograms, or blood gas studies may also be indicated. This section describes the indications, contraindications, procedures and results of angiocardiography.

INDICATIONS

Selective angiocardiography involves placing the catheter as close as possible to a suspected lesion in the heart or great vessels for delivering contrast medium. Its indications are threefold: (1) to obtain a specific diagnosis when routine methods have failed, (2) to better define a known lesion, or (3) to provide information complementary to hemodynamic studies. These indications occur most often with congenital heart defects. Nonselective angiocardiography involves injecting contrast medium in a peripheral or central vein. Its result may be inconsistent; however, it may be very useful in certain disease conditions.

Noninvasive diagnostic methods often do not prove a specific diagnosis in congenital heart lesions. For example, the diagnosis of ventricular septal defect, a valvular insufficiency or a combination of heart defects may be confusing, but can be positively identified by selective angiocardiography. Less often selective contrast studies are indicated for the diagnosis of an acquired disease in veterinary medicine.

Sometimes, although the diagnosis is known, the lesion may be more accurately defined through angiocardiography. For the potential surgical patient, selective contrast radiography can demonstrate the exact morphology of the defect. It may also reveal additional complicating lesions.

Selective angiocardiography used as an adjunct to other cardiovascular studies is usually confined to a research situation. As an example, it may be used to follow the pathogenesis of experimentally produced heart defects in animals.

Non-selective angiocardiography may be helpful in differentiating cardiomyopathies in cats. In such procedures one hopes to demonstrate either a very dilated left ventricular cavity, as in congestive cardiomyopathy, or a very diminished left ventricular cavity, perhaps with filling defects of large papillary muscles, as in hypertrophic cardiomyopathy. In addition, sometimes nonselective procedures can help define right atrial or ventricular masses by demonstrating filling defects, or pericardial disease by showing increased distance between the endocardium and the pericardium.

In congenital heart disease, although the exact nature of the defect may be missed, nonselective studies may demonstrate the presence of a right-to-left shunt by early opacification of the left ventricle or aorta without prior opacification of "upstream" structures such as pulmonary veins. Single right-sided heart defects such as pulmonic stenosis may be demonstrated by nonselective studies. However, the utility of nonselective angiocardiography in congenital disease is limited by the significant chance of multiple defects in individual patients and by the difficulty of demonstrating left-sided heart defects, left-to-right shunts and complicated defects.

CONTRAINDICATIONS

There are six relative contraindications to angiocardiography: (1) inadequate indication, (2) congestive heart failure, (3) serious respiratory disease, (4) life-threatening arrhythmias, (5) foci of infection (especially cardiovascular or respiratory) and (6) hypersensitivity to any agents to be used. Some are relative contraindications because they may be controlled by appropriate therapy. For example, heart failure due to a congenital defect may be temporarily controllable with digitalis, diuretics and a low-sodium diet. Arrhythmias and infections may likewise be controlled medically. Prior to angiocardiography, all patients must be carefully evaluated with a complete medical and cardiovascular examination.

EQUIPMENT

Zimmerman (1966) describes four kinds of equipment used in angiocardiography: (1) that for preparing and catheterizing the patient, (2) that for monitoring the patient, (3) that for producing the image, and (4) that for handling emergencies. In addition, in veterinary medicine, preparation of the patient for selective catheterization usually includes general anesthesia.

Equipment for preparing and catheterizing the patient includes instruments and equipment necessary to perform aseptic vascular surgery. An ample and varied supply of catheters and guide wires is a prerequisite. Some instruments and catheters used by Ettinger and Suter (1970) are listed in Tables 15–2 and 15–3.

The patient parameters monitored or recorded during cardiac catheterization include the electrocardiogram, arterial blood pressure, pressure at the catheter tip and blood oxygen tension. A multichannel medical recorder adapted for electrocardiography and blood pressure measurements, special trans-ducers and blood gas analyzers are part of the basic equipment needed.

The apparatus for producing the image is sophisticated and varies considerably among institutions. The expense of such equipment is one of the main reasons that angiocardiography is limited to large institutions. At a minimum, it requires a conventional x-ray machine and fluoroscopic equipment with image intensification. If the image is recorded on conventional x-ray film, a rapid film changer is used. Such changers are designed for either cut film or roll film. These films are exposed in either a single or biplane manner. If the image is recorded as a moving picture, a cinefluoroscopic unit or video tape recorder may be used. An automatic programmed high powered injector is needed to infuse the contrast medium through the catheter into the heart or vessel. Usually the contrast medium selected is a sodium or methylglucamine diatrizoate (Hypaque, 50%, Hypaque-M, 75%, Renovist, 69%, or Renografin, 76%).

The equipment necessary for handling cardiovascular emergencies includes a direct current defibrillator and an adequate supply of emergency drugs (see Table 15–4).

Proper anesthetic management of patients with cardiovascular disease requires inhalation equipment, whether or not inhalation

Table 15–2. INSTRUMENTS USED FOR CARDIAC CATHETERIZATION

Operating scissors
Curved Iris scissors
Straight Iris scissors
Scalpel handle and blades
Collier needleholder
2 Bulldog clamps
Iris forceps (more than 2)
Iris dressing forceps (2 or 3)
4 Backhaus clamps
4 Straight Halstead mosquito forceps
4 Curved Halstead mosquito forceps
Vessel dilator
Sponge bowl
Saline bowl
Assorted tapered and cutting edge needles
4 × 4 Gauze sponges
5–0 Silk with taper cardiovascular needle
3–0 Medium chromic gut
2–0 Nonabsorbable suture
Umbilical tape
Rubber bands
4 Surgical towels
Assorted glass and plastic syringes

Table 15–3. CATHETERS USED FOR CARDIAC CATHETERIZATION AND ANGIOCARDIOGRAPHY IN THE DOG

Type	Sizes	Description and Tip Styles	Use
NIH (National Institutes of Health)	5F–8F	Closed distal tip with 6 round openings within the first cm. Pediatric types preferred for small and medium-sized dogs	Angiocardiography, mainly aorta and left ventricle.
Odman-Ledin (Kifa)	Red–1 Green–2 (Yellow-3 and Grey–4 not used in dogs)	Tubing bought in coils. Length, curves, and tips are shaped according to the proposed procedure. Requires flange or fittings. Thermoplastic (Polyethylene).	Tapered end for percutaneous catheterization. End-hole for measuring of pulmonary wedge pressure. End- and side-holes for pressure recordings and left and right ventricular angiocardiography. For contrast injections, tip should be tapered.
Goodale-Lubin	5F to 8F	One pair of side-holes close to the open tip. Flexible catheter.	Pressure recordings, angiocardiography, and angiography. Widely used for metabolic studies.
Cournand		End-hole only	Pressure recordings, withdrawal of blood, determination of pulmonary capillary wedge pressure.
Lehman Ventriculography	5F to 8F	Thin, flexible blind tip designed to bend at the aortic valve and then to snap into the ventricle. Closed end, 4 side-holes.	Retrograde aortic catheterization and left ventricular angiocardiography. Long tip might keep the holes in the vicinity of the aortic valve cusps.
Swan-Ganz	4, 5, 7F	Flexible catheter with an inflatable balloon tip to help carry the catheter through the right heart into the pulmonary artery. End-hole or side-hole.	Pulmonary artery blood samples and pressures, wedge pressures and angiography.

agents are the primary anesthetic. In addition, respiration assist apparatus should be available. Anesthetic programs may vary widely but must be carefully designed to minimize the dose of cardiotoxic agents.

Equipment necessary for nonselective procedures is less sophisticated. Although best results are obtained using the same radiographic equipment as that used for selective procedures, adequate results may sometimes be obtained with simple "tunnel"-style film changing techniques and routine radiographic apparatus as described by Owens and Twedt (1977).

CATHETERIZATION PROCEDURE

A team of skilled, experienced personnel is necessary to perform angiocardiography safely. Catheterization teams vary considerably; however, a basic team includes a catheterizer (ideally with an assistant), an anesthetist, a physiologic monitor and a radiologist or radiographic technician.

The patient is prepared for general anesthesia in the usual manner. After anesthesia has been accomplished, the skin over the common carotid artery and jugular vein or femoral artery and vein is prepared for aseptic surgery. Direct cardiac puncture should be reserved only for those patients in whom selective approach through a vessel is impossible. Generally, a cut-down is performed on the desired pair of vessels, which are gently isolated and occluded. Using a fluoroscopic image and pressure tracings as a guide to catheter placement, the catheter is passed along the vessel to the desired position. An-

Table 15–4. DRUGS FOR CARDIAC EMERGENCIES

Cardiovascular Support and Cardiac Arrhythmia

Isoproterenol HCl (Isuprel)—Dilute 1 mg in 250 ml of dextrose and water solution. Use intravenous drip to maintain heart rate between 80 and 140 beats/minute.

Epinephrine HCl (1:10,000)—Administer 1 cc intracardiac to convert cardiac standstill to coarse ventricular fibrillation, or weak bradycardia to rapid stronger beat. Coarse ventricular fibrillation may be converted by DC shock.

Lidocaine HCl (Xylocaine)—This preparation is without epinephrine in a 20 mg/cc strength. To control ventricular arrhythmias, give 2 to 4 mg/lb by slow IV bolus and follow with quinidine sulfate, administered orally if indicated.

Fluid Retention and Pulmonary Parenchymal Fluid
Diuretics
Lasix—½ to 1 mg/lb IV, IM, SC, or orally.
Hydrodiuril—1 mg/lb every 12 hours orally.
Bronchodilators
Aminophylline—250 mg/cc; give 2 to 4 mg/lb IM.

Analgesia
Demerol—1 to 5 mg/lb IM: if shock is present, give 1 mg/lb IM.
Morphine—1 mg/lb IM or SC in dogs. 0.1 mg/lb IM or SC in cats.

Tranquilizers
Acepromazine—1 mg/20 lb IM or IV. It may cause vasodilation; therefore, do not use in shock states.
Chlorpromazine (Thorazine)—¼ to ½ mg/lb IM. If necessary, it can be used when shock is present because it functions as an α-blocker. It can be given after 15 cc/lb of lactated Ringer solution has been given IV.

Supplemental O₂
Administer by mask, intubation, tracheostomy, or in a modified O₂ cage (Kirschner).

Intravenous Fluids
Ringer's lactate—Use 7 cc sodium bicarbonate (44.6 mEq/50 cc) per 250 ml to neutralize; use 10 to 12 cc/250 ml if treating shock. Use 20 to 40 ml/lb, monitoring central venous pressure as the fluids are administered.
Saline—Use 7 cc sodium bicarbonate to neutralize.
Dextrose and saline.
Whole fresh blood.

Antibiotics
Broad-spectrum antibiotics should be given to all injured animals.
Shock States
Crystalline sodium penicillin—1 to 5 million units in initial IV drip. Give IM penicillin and streptomycin simultaneously.
Chloromycetin IV—10 to 25 mg/lb initially.
Intravenous Liquamycin—25 mg/lb.
Nonshock States
Crystalline penicillin—SC or IM, 10,000 units/lb twice daily.
Penicillin—streptomycin IM.
Liquamycin—25 mg/lb.
Chloromycetin IV—10 to 25 mg/lb initially; then orally, 10 mg/lb qid for follow up.

Sodium Bicarbonate (44.6 mEq/50 cc)
Give ½ to 1 cc/10 lb of body weight for shock and acidosis. Give in IV drip unless emergency such as cardiac arrest dictates that it be given directly. Often it is given as part of the IV drip solution as outlined above.

Corticosteroids (for shock)
Dexamethasone (Azium)—1 to 5 mg/lb IV in association with 20 to 40 cc/lb of IV fluids for the first hour depending on cardiopulmonary function and urine output.
Hydrocortisone sodium succinate (Solu-Cortef)—10 to 20 mg/lb IV.

For Strengthening Myocardial Contraction and Increasing Myocardial Excitability
Calcium gluconate—10 per cent solution, 3 to 10 cc intravenously or intracardially.
Calcium chloride—1 to 2 cc intravenously or intracardially.

From Ticer, J. W., and Brown, S. G.: Thoracic trauma. *In* Ettinger, S. J.: Textbook of Veterinary Internal Medicine: Diseases of the Dog and Cat. Philadelphia, W. B. Saunders Co., 1975.

ticoagulant flushes are used frequently. Some of the patients are treated with systemic anticoagulants.

If arrhythmias occur, slight catheter withdrawal will usually result in a return to normal rhythm. These are most often single atrial or ventricular premature contractions. If arrhythmias persist or advance to more serious disturbances (e.g., ventricular tachycardia), additional steps should be taken. Reducing the anesthetic level and increasing oxygen flow are imperative. Short-acting antiarrhythmic drugs such as lidocaine may be indicated. Ventricular fibrillation requires immediate corrective measures, including external cardiac massage and direct current defibrillation, as detailed by Kirk and Bistner (1981).

Once the catheterization of the heart or vessel has been performed, the physiologic data are collected. Pressures and blood gases from all locations catheterized and dye dilution studies may substantiate the diagnosis

without the use of contrast medium injections. Ettinger and Suter (1970) have given examples of such data and have summarized the findings of others.

When physiologic data collection is completed, the contrast medium is injected at selected locations. Its flow is followed by several radiographs or cinefluoroscopic film. Special care must be taken to choose the proper dose, pressure and duration of injection and appropriate film sequence to demonstrate the suspected lesion. The films are developed (preferably in an automatic processor) and studied for completeness. Before removing the catheters and closing the surgical site, it is important to ensure that all desired information has been collected. The patient is monitored while recovering from anesthesia. All equipment is serviced properly to avoid damage to sensitive transducers or clotting within the catheter and stopcocks.

See Owens and Twedt (1977) for nonselective angiocardiography procedures.

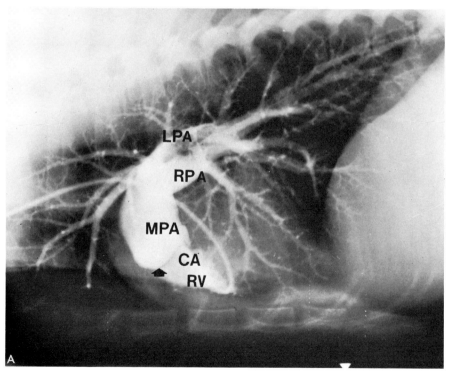

Figure 15–18. Lateral and dorsoventral angiocardiograms exposed simultaneously using a biplane roll-film changer. Selective right ventricular injection of a normal, 3 year old male dog of mixed breed.

A, Lateral angiocardiogram. The dog was placed in a prone position, and a horizontal beam was used. The angiocardiogram demonstrates that the details of the right ventricle (RV) and the main pulmonary artery (MPA) can be outlined much better with a selective than with a nonselective technique. The catheter was inserted into the right ventricle via the jugular vein. The pulmonic valve (arrow) separates the funnel-shaped conus arteriosus (CA) from the main pulmonary artery (MPA). Notice the slight curve of the normally branching peripheral pulmonary arteries. (Courtesy of Ettinger, S. J., and Suter, P. F.: *Canine Cardiology.* Philadelphia, W. B. Saunders Co., 1970.)

RESULTS

To diagnose cardiac lesions by angiocardiography one must first be familiar with the normal angiocardiogram. The easiest way to acquire this understanding is to follow the circulation of contrast medium through each side of the heart. Refer to Figures 15–18 through 15–21 for an understanding of the normal circulatory pattern.

Contrast medium injected into the right ventricle outlines its irregular cavity (Figs. 15–18 and 15–20). Next the contrast medium is seen in the conus arteriosus of the ventricle. It crosses the pulmonic valve, entering the main pulmonary artery. This vessel branches immediately into the left and right pulmonary arteries. Contrast material then outlines the respective arteries of each lung lobe. In many studies, circulation of contrast medium through the lungs presents enough of a bolus to the pulmonary veins to produce reasonable opacification of the left heart circulation. However, the clarity needed for diagnostic films of the left side must usually come from selective injection there. For the same rea-

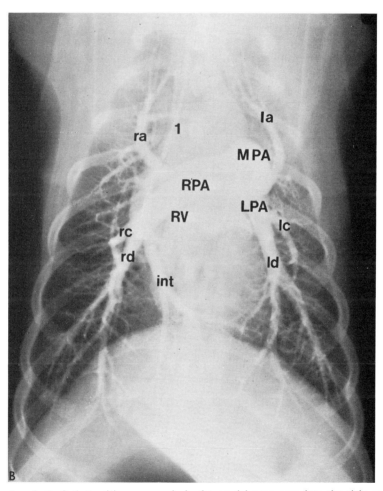

Figure 15–18 *Continued. B,* Catheter (1) was passed via the cranial vena cava into the right atrium and curves medially into the right ventricle (RV). The right pulmonary artery (RPA) is superimposed on the right ventricle; it branches into the right cranial lobar artery (ra), the right middle lobar artery (rc), the right caudal lobar artery (rd), and the artery to the intermediate or azygos lobe (int). Because the exposure was made at the end of systole, the main pulmonary artery (MPA) is very large. The bulge caused by the main pulmonary artery is also referred to as the pulmonary artery segment of the cardiac silhouette. The left pulmonary artery (LPA) branches into the left cranial lobar artery (la), the left middle lobar artery (lc), and the left caudal lobar artery (ld). Notice the slight curvature of the small arterial branches in the caudal lobar area. In addition, notice that the inclination of the heart can also be seen in this view. Normally, the right ventricle would be nearly completely obscured by the right pulmonary artery. (Courtesy of Ettinger, S. J., and Suter, P. F.: *Canine Cardiology.* Philadelphia, W. B. Saunders Co., 1970.)

son, nonselective studies are usually not diagnostic for specific lesions in the heart or between the two circulations.

If contrast medium is injected in the left atrium (Figs. 15–19 and 15–21), some of the pulmonary veins may be briefly outlined in a retrograde manner. This is followed by rapid filling of the left ventricle as the contrast medium crosses the mitral valve. The normal left ventriculogram is smooth and cone-shaped. Systole ejects the contrast medium across the aortic valve, outlining the three bulging sinuses of the aorta and the ascending and descending aorta. The coronary arteries may be seen just above the aortic sinuses. The contrast medium leaves the vascular structures in the same order in which it enters them, although usually less dramatically because of blood dilution.

In nonselective angiocardiography (Figs.

Text continued on page 310

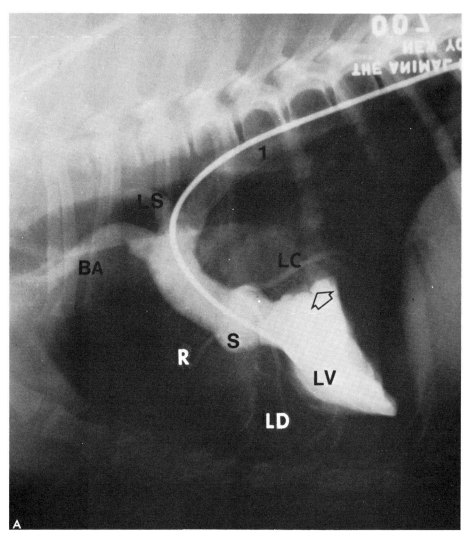

Figure 15–19. *A,* Left lateral angiogram, selective ventricular injection, normal Basset-mixed breed dog of unknown age. Notice the catheter (1) which was advanced retrograde from the femoral artery, through the descending aorta, and into the left ventricle. Both the mitral valve (open arrow) and the aortic valve are closed, and the ventricular outline (LV) is relatively small and well delineated, indicating that the exposure was made at the beginning of diastole (isometric relaxation). The sinuses of the aorta (S) are filled with contrast medium. The right coronary artery (R) leaves the cranial sinus. The left coronary artery, which is about twice the size of the right coronary artery, branches almost immediately into the left circumflex coronary artery (LC), lying in the left coronary sulcus, and the left descending branch (LD), lying in or near the left longitudinal sulcus. At the aortic arch, the origin of the larger brachiocephalic artery (BA) is just ventral to the origin of the smaller left subclavian artery (LS). (Courtesy of Ettinger, S. J., and Suter, P. F.: *Canine Cardiology.* Philadelphia, W. B. Saunders Co., 1970.)

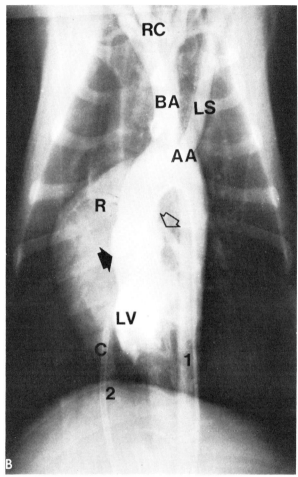

Figure 15–19 *Continued. B,* Ventrodorsal angiocardiogram, selective left ventricular injection, normal male Collie-mixed breed dog approximately 1 year old. Notice the catheter (1) which has been advanced retrograde from the femoral artery into the aorta and the left ventricle. A second catheter (2), introduced via the femoral vein, is seen entering the right atrium from the caudal vena cava (C). Hypaque-M 75% (1 ml/kg body weight) was injected over a period of 1.5 sec. This exposure was made 2 sec after the beginning of the injection. The left ventricle (LV) is in diastole, and the caudal portion of the ventricle has filled with blood containing no contrast medium, which entered from the left atrium. The aortic valve (black arrow) is closed. The left coronary artery (open arrow) originates from the sinuses of the aorta. The right coronary artery (R), which is smaller than the left coronary artery, is barely visible. The brachiocephalic artery (BA) and the left subclavian artery (LS) originate from the aortic arch (AA). The brachiocephalic artery then divides into the right common carotid artery (RC), the left common carotid artery (to the left of RC), and the right subclavian artery (to the right of RC). The heart has rotated to the right side despite the correct positioning of the thorax; this is due to the normal mobility of the heart. The rotation makes the aortic arch wider than usual. (Courtesy of Ettinger, S. J., and Suter, P. F.: *Canine Cardiology,* Philadelphia, W. B. Saunders Co., 1970.)

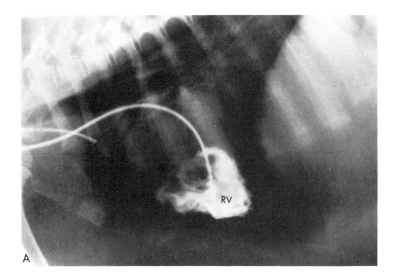

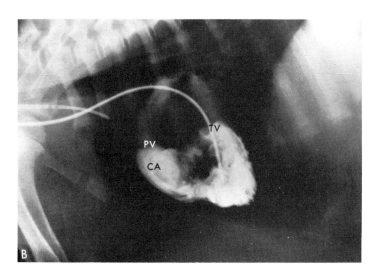

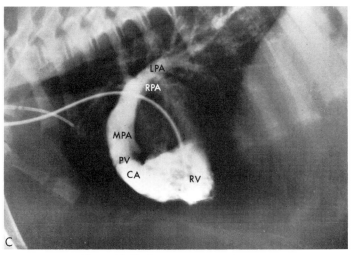

Figure 15–20. *See opposite page for legend.*

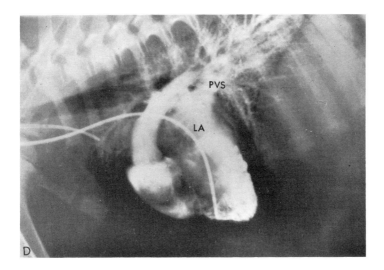

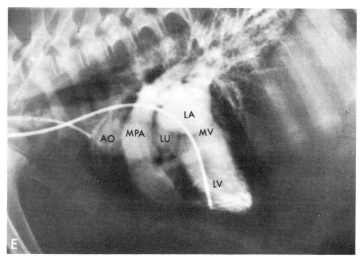

Figure 15–20. Right laterial angiocardiogram, after selective right ventricular injection, of 3 month old Newfoundland female. A 5F Swan-Ganz catheter was passed down the right jugular vein, through the right atrium, and into the right ventricle. (Usually a less flexible side-hole catheter is used for ventricular injections.) A 5F Lehman ventriculography catheter lies in the brachiocephalic artery. Film A was exposed 5/6 sec after beginning an injection of 9 cc Hypaque-M 75% at 150 psi. Film B was exposed 2 sec post injection, film C at 4 sec, film D at 5 sec and film E at 5.5 sec post injection. *A,* The catheter tip is in the right ventricle (RV) whose trabeculae will cause a roughened border. *B,* The right ventricular cavity is more completely filled as contrast medium enters the conus arteriosus (CA). The pulmonic valve (PV) is closed. The level of the tricuspid valve is marked by TV. The ventricle is in diastole. Lucency in the center of the ventricle is caused by unopacified blood entering from the right atrium. *C,* The ventricle is in early systole. The tricuspid valve (TV) is closed across the top of the full ventricle and the pulmonic valve (PV) is beginning to open. An earlier contraction has filled the main pulmonary artery (MPA) and has begun to outline the left and right pulmonary arteries (LPA, RPA). Superimposition of the pulmonary arteries is due to slight rotation of the thorax. Compare with Figure 12–34A. *D,* Contrast medium remains in the previously outlined structures and has entered the pulmonary venous circulation. Pulmonary arteries and veins are seen simultaneously. Contrast medium is approaching the left atrium (LA) through the pulmonary veins (PVS). *E,* The left atrium (LA) is filled, and contrast medium has moved through the mitral valve (MV) to outline the left ventricle (LV). Contrast medium remains in the conus arteriosus and among the trabeculae of the right ventricular wall which wraps around the left ventricle caudally. The left auricle (LU) is seen over the area occupied by the sinuses of the aorta. In addition, the aorta (AO) is seen over the main pulmonary artery (MPA). In nonselective angiocardiography these superimpositions are further complicated by the presence of the cranial vena cava and right auricle, thus making diagnosis of lesions in this area extremely difficult by that method. (Angiocardiogram courtesy of Dr. Richard D. Park.)

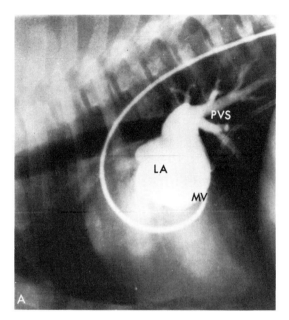

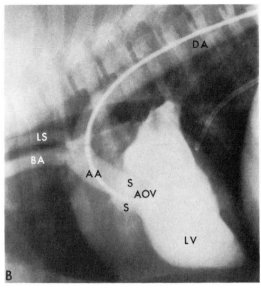

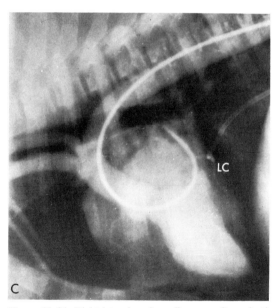

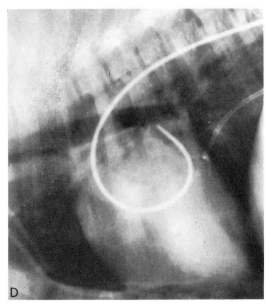

Figure 15–21. Right lateral angiocardiogram, after selective left atrial injection, of female Chesapeake Bay Retriever approximately 10 weeks old. A 5F Kifa catheter was fashioned so that it could be passed from the femoral artery through the aorta, left ventricle, and into the left atrium. Another Kifa catheter lies in the caudal vena cava. Six milliliters of Hypaque-M 75% was injected. Film A was exposed immediately after injection, film B 2 sec later, film C 3 sec, and film D 4 sec after film A. *A,* The left atrium (LA) is filled with contrast medium. It has a smooth wall. The left auricle is not well seen in this series. The pulmonary veins (PVS) are filled briefly in a retrograde manner. The mitral valve (MV) is closed because the ventricle is in systole.

B, The mitral valve has opened and the diastolic left ventricle (LV) is filled. It has a smooth, cone-shaped outline. Contrast medium has been ejected through the aortic valve (AOV), which is now closed. A previous contraction has outlined the sinuses of the aorta (S), the ascending aorta (AA), and descending aorta (DA) with contrast medium. The brachiocephalic artery (BA) and left subclavian artery (LS) branch from the aortic arch.

C, The ventricle is in systole. Its diameter is less. Contrast medium in the left atrium is diluted with fresh blood. The left circumflex coronary artery (LC) is seen; the left descending and right coronary arteries are not well outlined. (See Fig. 15–19*A.*)

D, The left atrium is nearly empty. Contrast medium in the left ventricle and aorta is barely visible, as it has nearly all been carried away with unopacified blood. (Angiogram courtesy of Dr. Peter F. Suter.)

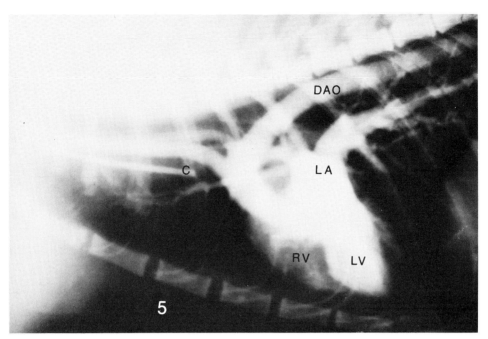

Figure 15–22. Nonselective angiocardiogram of a normal adult cat. This exposure was made 5 seconds after the rapid injection of 3 cc Renografin 76% into the cranial vena cava. The left ventricle has a normal volume and a smooth contour. Compare this figure with Figures 15–23 and 15–24, which show abnormal volume and shape of the left ventricle. The left atrium and aorta are normal size. Unlike selective left-side heart studies, some contrast medium remains in the right ventricle, pulmonary arteries and particularly pulmonary veins. *LV*, left ventricle; *RV*, right ventricle; *LA*, left atrium; *DAO*, descending aorta; *C*, catheter tip in cranial vena cava. (Angiocardiogram courtesy of Dr. Barbara Watrous and Cornell University.)

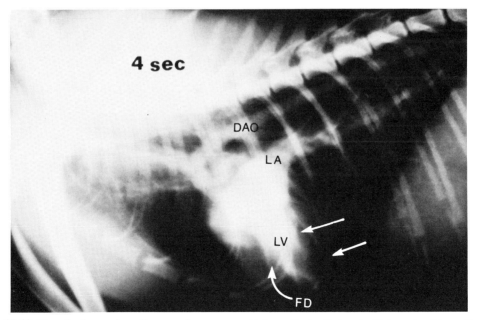

Figure 15–23. Nonselective angiocardiogram of a one-year-old domestic shorthair cat with hypertrophic cardiomyopathy. This exposure was made 4 seconds after rapid injection of 3 cc Renografin 76% into the jugular vein. The left ventricular volume is diminished. Filling defects representing hypertrophied papillary muscles are present. The left ventricular wall is thickened. The left atrial volume is increased. The aorta may be diminished in width, suggesting reduced cardiac output. Contrast medium in the main pulmonary artery obscures detail near the proximal ascending aorta. *FD*, filling defect; straight arrows show thickened caudal left ventricular wall; *LA*, left atrium; *DAO*, descending aorta. (Angiocardiogram courtesy of Dr. Barbara Watrous and Cornell University.)

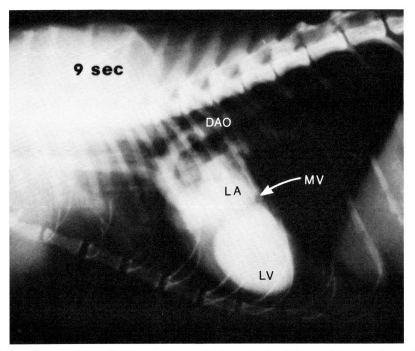

Figure 15–24. Nonselective angiocardiogram of a 7-year-old domestic shorthair cat with congestive cardiomyopathy. This exposure was made 9 seconds after the rapid injection of 3 cc Renografin 76% into the jugular vein. Both the left atrium and left ventricle have increased volume. Even though it has been 9 seconds since the injection, contrast medium is just beginning to adequately opacify the aorta, suggesting reduced cardiac output. Details of the left heart study are somewhat obscured by residual contrast medium in the right heart and pulmonary vessels. *LV*, left ventricle; *MV*, level of the mitral valve; *DAO*, descending aorta. (Angiogram courtesy of Dr. Barbara Watrous and Cornell University.)

15–22 through 15–24), the flow of contrast medium is the same as that used for selective procedures, but structures are usually less well defined. This is because it is usually impossible to get an adequate bolus effect and because diluted contrast medium remaining in the structures opacified early somewhat obscures the structures opacified later. However, if one merely needs to know the relative volume of the ventricle or the distance from pericardium to endocardium, then the results of nonselective angiocardiography may be adequate, particularly in cats (Figs. 15–23 and 15–24).

REFERENCES

Bonagura, J. D., Myer, C. W., Pensinger, R. D.: Angiocardiography. Vet. Clin. N. A. Sm. Anim., 12(2):239, May, 1982.

Buchanan, J. W.: Selective angiography and angiocardiography in dogs with acquired cardiovascular disease. J. Amer. Vet. Radiol. Soc., 6:5, 1965.

Buchanan, J. W., and Patterson, D. F.: Selective angiography and angiocardiography in dogs with congenital cardiovascular disease. J. Amer. Vet. Radiol. Soc., 6:21, 1965.

Detweiler, D. K., Hubben, K., and Patterson, D. F.: Survey on cardiovascular disease in dogs: preliminary report on the first 1000 dogs screened. Amer. J. Vet. Res., 21:329, 1960.

Detweiler, D. K.: Cardiovascular disease in animals. A. Trisala (ed.), *Encyclopedia of the Cardiovascular System*, Vol. 5. New York, McGraw-Hill, 1961.

Ettinger, S. J., and Suter, P. F.: *Canine Cardiology*. Philadelphia, W. B. Saunders Co., 1970.

Fabian, L. W., and Short, C. E.: Anesthesia for the patient with acquired and congenital heart disease. Vet. Clin. N. Amer., 3:33–44, 1973.

Felson, B. (ed.): *Roentgen Techniques in Laboratory Animals*. Philadelphia, W. B. Saunders, 1968.

Grossman, W. (ed.): *Cardiac Catheterization and Angiography*. Philadelphia, Lea and Febiger, 1974.

Hamlin, R. L.: Angiocardiography for the clinical diagnosis of congenital heart disease in small animals. J. Amer. Vet. Med. Assoc. 135:112, 1959.

Hamlin, R. L.: Radiographic anatomy of the heart and great vessels in healthy living dogs. J. Amer. Vet. Med. Assoc., 136:265, 1960.

Hurst, J. W. (ed.): The Heart, Arteries and Veins. 5th Ed. New York, McGraw-Hill, 1982.

Kirk, R. W., and Bistner, S. I.: Handbook of Veterinary

Procedures and Emergency Treatment. Philadelphia, W. B. Saunders Co., 1981.

Knight, D. H.: Principles of catheterization. *In* R. W. Kirk (ed.): *Current Veterinary Therapy V.* Philadelphia, W. B. Saunders, 1971.

Kory, R. C., Tsagans, T. J., and Bustamontc, R. A.: *A Primer of Cardiac Catheterization.* Springfield, Ill. Charles C Thomas, 1965.

Kraner, K. W.: Angiocardiography in acquired heart disease. J. Amer. Anim. Hosp. Assoc., *8*:308, 1972.

Moscovitz, H. L., Donoso, E., Gelb, I. J., and Wilder, R. J.: *An Atlas of Hemodynamics of the Cardiovascular System.* New York, Grune Stratton, 1963.

Owens, J. M., and Twedt, D. C.: Nonselective Angiocardiography in the Cat. Vet. Clin. N. A. 7:309–321, 1977.

Patterson, D. F.: Angiocardiography. J. Amer. Vet. Radiol. Soc., *1*:26, 1961.

Pyle, R. L.: Angiocardiography in congenital cardiovascular diseases of the dog. J. Amer. Anim. Hosp. Assoc., *8*:310, 1972.

Rhodes, W. H., Patterson, D. F., and Detweiler, D. K.: Radiographic anatomy of the canine heart. Part I. J. Amer. Vet. Assoc., *137*:283, 1960.

Rhodes, W. H., Patterson, D. F., and Detweiler, D. K.: Radiographic anatomy of the canine heart. Part II. J. Amer. Vet. Med. Assoc., *143*:137, 1963.

Rising, J. L., and Lewis, R. E.: A technique for arterial catheterization in the dog. Amer. J. Vet. Res., *31*:1309, 1970.

Rushmer, R.: Cardiovascular dynamics. 4th ed. Philadelphia, W. B. Saunders Co., 1976.

Tashjian, R. J., and Albanese, N. M.: A technique of canine angiocardiography. J. Amer. Vet. Med. Assoc., *136*:359, 1960.

Wallace, C.: Cardiac catheterization to aid in diagnosis of cardiovascular disease. Small Anim. Clin., *2*:324, 1962.

Wood, G. L. and Suter, P. F.: Principles of Cardiac Catheterization. *In* R. W. Kirk (ed.): *Current Veterinary Therapy VI.* Philadelphia, W. B. Saunders, 1977.

Zimmerman, H. A. (ed.): *Intravascular Catheterization,* 2nd ed. Springfield, Ill., Charles C Thomas, 1966.

16

Abdomen

Radiographic examination of the abdomen requires careful technique. Excellent radiographic quality is essential for providing accurate diagnostic information.

Patient Preparation

Radiographic visualization of abdominal structures is very difficult, if not impossible, in the presence of a large amount of ingesta within the gastrointestinal tract (Root, 1974a). A 12-hour fast should precede most routine abdominal radiographic examinations. In patients with a history of emesis or anorexia for 12 hours or more, this fasting period may be omitted. Generally, routine examinations do not require that an enema be given. Water may be given during the fasting period, but the patient should not be allowed excessive consumption immediately prior to radiography.

In severely debilitated patients and patients with life-threatening metabolic disorders, such as diabetes mellitus, fasting may be contraindicated. In these cases, a diet of low residue foods, such as baby foods or dietary concentrates (Pet Kalorie, Haver-Lockhart Laboratories; Nutri-cal, EVSCO Pharmaceutical Corp.), may be fed 12 to 24 hours prior to radiographic examination.

Mild cathartics or enemas may be used in the preparation of patients for abdominal radiography, especially if there is a relatively good chance that a special contrast procedure will be performed after the initial radiographs are produced. Generally, gravity flow, isotonic saline (8 tsp table salt per gallon tap water or 45 g table salt per 5 L tap water) enemas are superior to hypertonic enema preparations (Root, 1974a). The enema fluid temperature should be less than that of the body, since this seems to stimulate expulsion of much of the gas that usually remains in the colon after warm enemas (Root, 1974a).

Exposure Technique

Marked loss of radiographic detail occurs if exposures are made during normal diaphragmatic excursions. Exposures are best made during the pause that occurs at the end of expiration. At this point in the respiratory cycle, the diaphragm is cranially displaced and the body wall is relaxed (Root, 1974a). This avoids crowding of abdominal viscera and ensures adequate time to make the exposures so that motion unsharpness produced by diaphragmatic movements is prevented. By producing radiographs of the abdomen during the expiratory pause, there is an added benefit in that there is maximum separation of the kidneys in the lateral projection, thus enhancing visualization (Grandage, 1975).

Measurement for determining exposure technique is usually best made over the caudal rib cage, where the greatest width of the abdomen occurs. This will avoid underexposure of the relatively dense structures of the cranial abdomen. In dogs with an extremely deep thorax, additional radiographs produced with a decreased exposure may be necessary to examine the caudal abdomen.

Procedure

Left-Right Lateral View. The patient is placed in right lateral recumbency, with the

312

sternum elevated to the same height above the x-ray table as the lumbar spine, and the femurs are placed at approximately 120 degrees to the vertebral column (Fig. 16–1). The x-ray beam is centered midabdominally and is collimated to include the region from the xyphoid to the pubis. The radiograph is produced during the expiratory pause.

Figure 16–2 illustrates the normal radiographic anatomy of the canine abdomen in left-right lateral view.

Right-Left Lateral View. The patient is placed in left lateral recumbency, with the sternum elevated to the same height above the x-ray table as the lumbar spine, and the femurs are placed at approximately 120 degrees to the vertebral column (Fig. 16–3). The x-ray beam is centered midabdominally and is collimated to include the region from the xyphoid to the pubis. The radiograph is produced during the expiratory pause.

Figure 16–4 illustrates the normal radiographic anatomy of the canine abdomen in right-left lateral view.

Ventrodorsal View. The patient is placed in dorsal recumbency with the rear limbs in a "frog leg" position (Fig. 16–5). This will prevent stretching of the flank skin folds, thus avoiding the artifacts frequently caused by these structures (Root, 1974a). The x-ray beam is centered at the umbilicus and is collimated to include the region from the xyphoid to the pubis. The radiograph is produced during the expiratory pause.

Figure 16–6 illustrates the normal radiographic anatomy of the canine abdomen in VD view.

Dorsoventral View. The patient is placed in ventral recumbency, with the rear limbs in "frog leg" position (Fig. 16–7). The x-ray beam is centered just caudal to the thirteenth rib arch and collimated to include the region from the xyphoid to the pubis. The radiograph is produced during the expiratory pause.

Figure 16–8 illustrates the normal radiographic anatomy of the canine abdomen in DV view.

Interpretation

The position and appearance of the normal abdominal viscera vary, depending on postural relationships, phase of the respiratory cycle, physiological state, body type, and x-ray beam geometry. Generally the most variable position is observed in the structures of the cranial abdomen: diaphragm, liver, stomach, descending duodenum, spleen and kidneys.

Stomach and Diaphragm

The fundus of the stomach is located on the left side of the midline and is in direct contact with the left hemidiaphragm. In lateral projection, the air- or ingesta-filled stomach may be seen in direct contact with the left diaphragmatic crus. Since the dependent crus sags cranially in lateral recumbency, the left crus and stomach will be projected cranial to the right crus in right-left lateral view (Grandage, 1974; Root, 1974a). The crural lines tend to cross at the intracrural cleft. A line drawn through the fundus, body and pylorus on the lateral recumbent radiograph may be perpendicular to the vertebral column, may run parallel to the ribs or may lie in between these extremes in normality (Root, 1974a).

In the VD view, a line drawn through the fundus to the pylorus is perpendicular to the vertebral column in most patients.

Fluid gastric contents are extremely mobile and tend to move the dependent portions of the stomach during postural changes.

In left-right lateral view, gas is seen in the fundus and body of the stomach, and in right-left lateral view, gas is seen mostly in the pylorus.

Ventrodorsal views of the stomach show air in the fundus, body, and pylorus, while in the DV view, most of the air is in the fundus. The VD abdominal view tends to show the diaphragmatic outline as a single dome-like shadow with the right hemidiaphragm slightly displaced cranially (Grandage, 1974). There may be a distinct cardiac depression seen slightly to the left of the midline, particularly in small dogs with a wide thorax.

In dogs with a deep thorax, the DV abdominal view projects the diaphragm as a trilobed shadow with the right and left crus located lateral to a centrally located cupula.

Spleen

The splenic shadow may vary in location and appearance with postural changes. The head of the spleen is attached to the stomach,

Text continued on page 318.

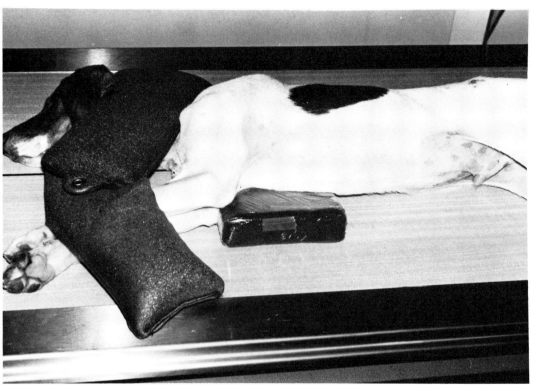

Figure 16–1. Position for left-right lateral view of the abdomen.

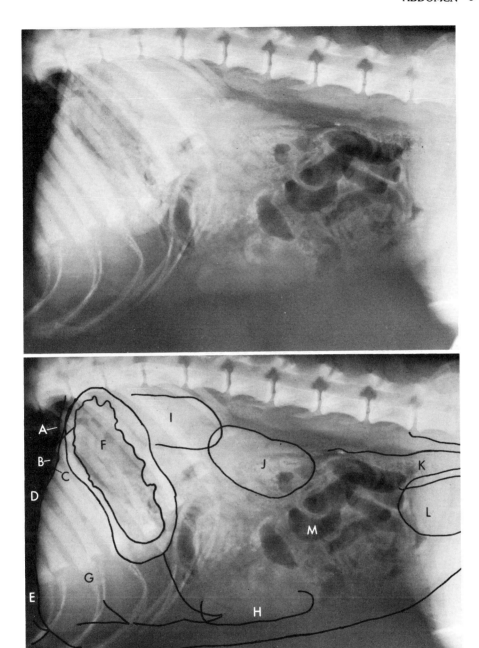

Figure 16–2. Left-right lateral view of the canine abdomen. Note that the right crus *(A)* is cranially displaced and the vena cava *(D)* is more dorsally located compared to the right-left lateral view (Fig. 16–4). The liver *(G)* also appears moderately larger in left-right lateral view. The left kidney is bean-shaped in left-right lateral view (see text). Gas pattern of the stomach outlines the fundus and body *(F)* in the left-right view.

    A. Right diaphragmatic crus
    B. Intercrural cleft
    C. Left diaphragmatic crus
    D. Caudal vena cava
    E. Heart
    F. Fundus and body of the stomach
    G. Liver
    H. Spleen
    I. Right kidney
    J. Left kidney
    K. Descending colon
    L. Urinary bladder
    M. Small bowel

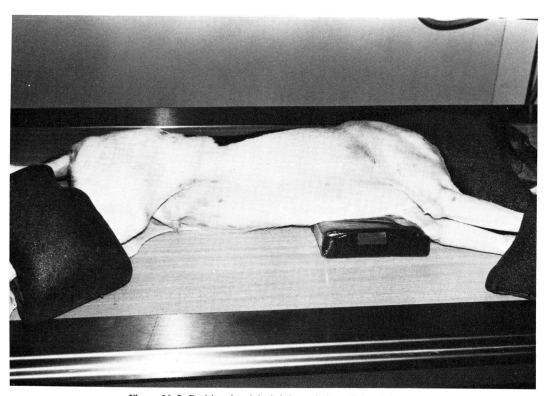

Figure 16–3. Position for right left lateral view of the abdomen.

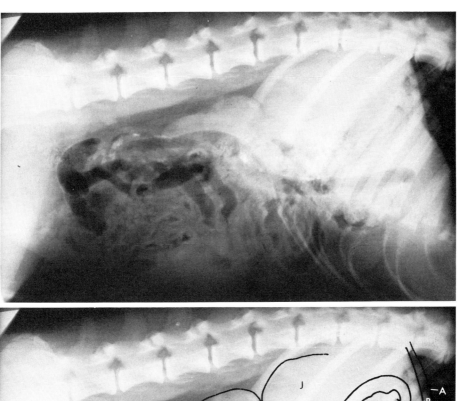

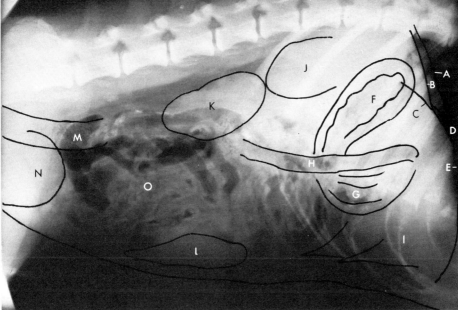

Figure 16–4. Right-left lateral view of the canine abdomen. Note that the left crus *(A)* is cranially displaced and the vena cava *(D)* is more ventrally located compared to the left-right lateral view (Fig. 16–2). The liver *(I)* appears smaller compared to the left-right lateral view. The gas pattern of the stomach shows a decreased volume in the fundus *(F)* and increased volume in the pyloric antrum *(G)* compared to the left-right lateral view (Fig. 16–2).

A. Left diaphragmatic crus
B. Right diaphragmatic crus
C. Intracrural cleft
D. Caudal vena cava
E. Diaphragmatic cupula
F. Fundus of the stomach
G. Pyloric antrum of the stomach
H. Descending duodenum
I. Liver
J. Right kidney
K. Left kidney
L. Spleen
M. Colon
N. Urinary bladder
O. Small bowel

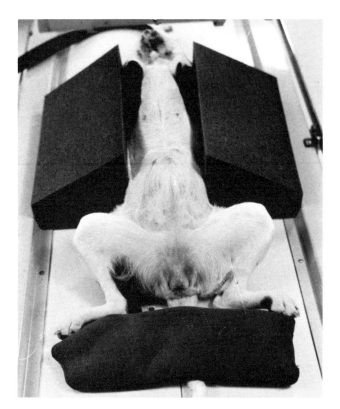

Figure 16–5. Position for the ventrodorsal view of the abdomen.

and the body and tail are very mobile. In right-left lateral view, the entire splenic shadow may be hidden beneath the small intestines and may not be visualized radiographically. In left-right lateral view, a portion of the spleen is usually seen on the ventral abdomen just caudal to the liver margin. The spleen usually appears as a crescent-shaped or curved triangular structure, produced as the x-ray beam is absorbed by a portion of the spleen that is tangential to the central ray. The remaining portion of the spleen is presented with its flat surface to the x-ray beam, thereby not absorbing sufficient x-rays to produce a distinct shadow.

In the VD or DV projection, the spleen appears as a small triangle caudolateral to the stomach fundus.

Liver

The position and size of the liver vary with postural changes and phase of the respiratory cycle. Left-right lateral view allows the left lateral liver lobe to slide caudally, causing the projection of a larger shadow than that seen in right-left lateral view (Grandage, 1974). Moderate rotation of the trunk may allow the increased obliquity of the x-ray

beam to produce a falsely rounded caudoventral margin (Root, 1974a). The fat-laden falciform ligament of the liver appears larger on exhalation and smaller on inhalation.

Kidneys

Kidney size may be estimated by comparing the kidney length to the length of a vertebral body (Kneller, 1974). The normal canine kidney length is roughly three times the length of the second lumbar vertebra (Finco et al., 1971). A range of from 2½ to 3⅓ times the length should be considered within normal limits (Osborn et al., 1972). The normal feline kidney is 2½ to 3 times the length of the L2 (Barrett and Kneller, 1972). Very young kittens and large male cats have relatively large kidneys (Hall and MacGregor, 1937).

The width and shape of the kidney may vary with postural changes. In lateral recumbency, the nondependent kidney will rotate on its longitudinal axis, profiling the hilar notch, and appear bean-shaped (Grandage, 1974). This appearance is due to the relative mobility of the kidney that allows the lateral aspect to fall downward in lateral recumbency.

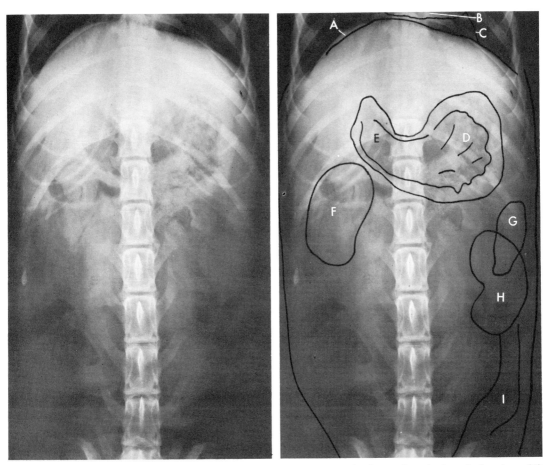

Figure 16–6. Ventrodorsal view of the canine abdomen. Note the increased volume of gas in the pyloric antrum (E) compared to the dorsoventral view (Fig. 16–8).

A. Diaphragm
B. Heart
C. Ventral aspect of caudal mediastinum (between the accessory and left caudal lobes)
D. Fundus of the stomach
E. Pyloric antrum of the stomach
F. Right kidney
G. Spleen
H. Left kidney
 I. Descending colon

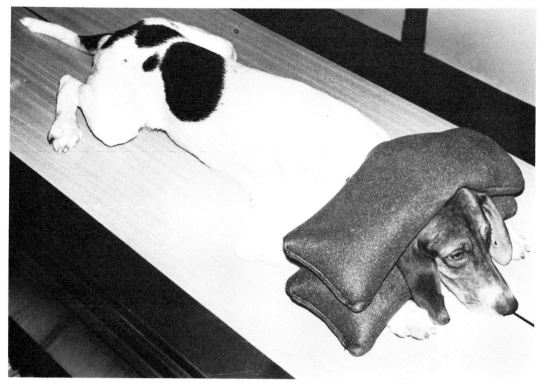

Figure 16–7. Position for the dorsoventral view of the abdomen.

This rotation also allows the region of kidney that is well covered by adipose tissue to be presented tangentially to the x-ray beam, thus allowing better radiographic contrast between the perirenal fat and the kidney capsule. Therefore, when one of the kidneys is of particular interest, it should be nondependent in the lateral recumbent position.

Movement of the diaphragm may allow a shift in the location of the kidneys by 2 cm or more (Grandage, 1974). In left-right lateral view, the right kidney may be displaced cranially ½ to 1 vertebral length when compared with right-left lateral view, because of the cranial displacement of the dependent diaphragmatic crus. The normally staggered arrangement of the kidneys, with the left kidney slightly caudal to the right, is therefore usually accentuated in left-right lateral view and reduced in right-left lateral view (Grandage, 1975). Survey radiographs of the kidneys are best produced in left-right lateral view in order to provide maximum kidney separation.

Small Bowel

The small bowel occupies nearly all of the abdominal space not taken up by the less mobile viscera. Displacement usually indicates the presence of a pathologic process, such as a space-occupying mass or a specific intestinal disorder.

Colon

The ascending colon and cecum are usually located on the right side of the abdomen, and the descending colon is located on the left side when viewed in VD or DV projection. The descending colon may be displaced to the right by a distended urinary bladder. When viewed in lateral projection, the ascending and descending sections of the colon are usually superimposed and located approximately halfway between the vertebral column and the ventral abdomen.

Urinary Bladder and Prostate Gland

A distended urinary bladder may displace abdominal viscera cranially and the descending colon to the right. The prostate gland should be mostly contained in the pelvic canal but may be cranially displaced by benign prostatic hyperplasia without clinical significance.

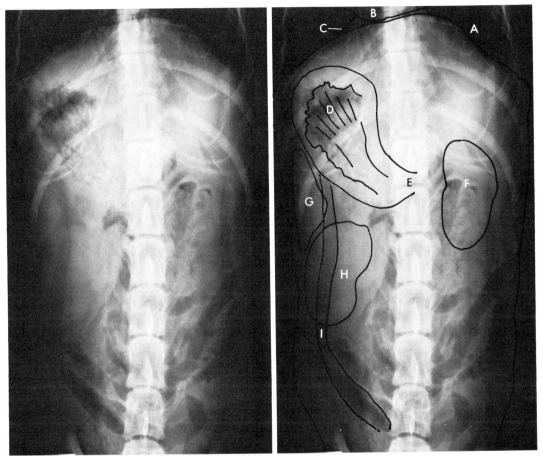

Figure 16–8. Dorsoventral view of the canine abdomen. Note the decreased volume of gas and medial displacement of the pyloric antrum *(E)* compared to the ventrodorsal view (Fig. 16–6).

    A. Diaphragm
    B. Heart
    C. Ventral aspect of caudal mediastinum (between the
        accessory and left caudal lobes)
    D. Fundus of the stomach
    E. Pyloric antrum of the stomach
    F. Right kidney
    G. Spleen
    H. Left kidney
    I. Descending colon

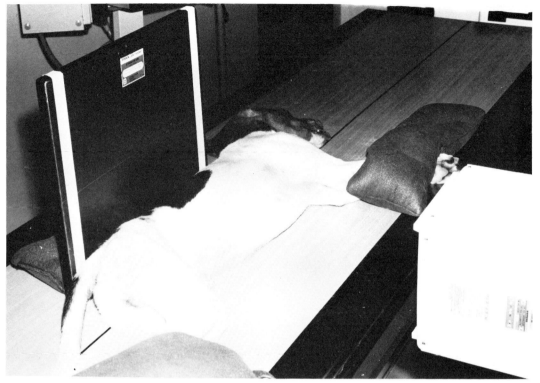

Figure 16–9. Position for ventrodorsal/horizontal view with horizontal x-ray beam.

Other Viscera

Normally the adrenal glands, mesentery, mesenteric lymph nodes, omentum, pancreas, abdominal aorta, abdominal vena cava, gallbladder, ovaries and uterus are not seen radiographically (Root, 1974a).

Left Lateral Recumbent VD View With Horizontal X-ray Beam (VD/Horizontal)

The patient is placed in left lateral recumbency and a horizontal x-ray beam is used to produce a VD view (Fig. 16–9). The x-ray beam is centered at the cranial abdomen and the exposure is made during the expiratory pause.

This examination is indicated when free air is suspected in the peritoneal space because of ruptured viscus.

Figure 16–10 illustrates the appearance of free air in the peritoneal space as a result of a ruptured small bowel segment.

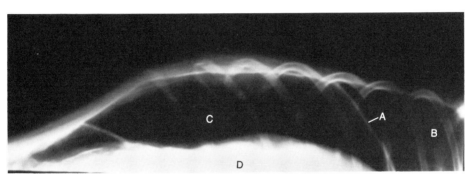

Figure 16–10. Radiograph with left recumbent ventrodorsal/horizontal beam with free gas in the peritoneal space due to a perforated duodenal ulcer.

A. Diaphragm
B. Right lung
C. Free air in the peritoneal space
D. Abdominal viscera

Pneumoperitoneography

Pneumoperitoneography is a negative contrast medium examination of the abdominal cavity after the introduction of a gas into the peritoneal space for the purpose of increasing subject contrast.

Indication

Pneumoperitoneography is indicated when the demonstration of an organ or mass is not possible with routine radiography because of an inherent lack of subject (patient) contrast. These situations exist when there is insufficient abdominal adipose tissue to cause contrast and may also be caused by many physiologic or pathologic states, the most common being an accumulation of excessive peritoneal fluid.

Contraindication

Contraindications for pneumoperitoneography are limited to those that preclude profound sedation or anesthesia and when diaphragmatic hernia is suspected. In some cooperative patients, this contraindication may be overcome by performing the procedure with local anesthesia.

Technique

Patient Preparation

Generally a 12-hour fast and profound sedation or anesthesia are necessary. Local anesthesia at the injection site is sometimes sufficient, but this method should be reserved for those patients for whom chemical restraint is contraindicated.

The midventral abdomen should be clipped and prepared by surgical scrub.

Materials

A large syringe, three-way valve and an 18-gauge indwelling catheter (Sovereign In-

dwelling Catheter, Sherwood Medical; Jelco I.V. Catheter Placement Unit, Jelco Laboratories) are used for patients without peritoneal fluid. Compressed gases (such as oxygen, carbon dioxide, or nitrous oxide) may be used instead of room air, but these must be administered with caution to avoid overdistention of the abdomen. The advantage of carbon dioxide and nitrous oxide is their increased rate of absorption from the peritoneal space.

If peritoneal fluid is present, a small rubber feeding catheter (Brunswick Feeding Catheter) with several previously placed side-holes is used to facilitate drainage prior to air injection.

Dosage

Generally 200 to 1000 cc of gas provides sufficient contrast for most pneumoperitoneograms; however, if gross displacement of mobile viscera is desired for horizontal x-ray beam studies, the volume of gas may be increased until moderate abdominal distention is obtained (Gillette et al., 1977).

Medium Injection

The patient is placed in left lateral recumbency, theoretically to permit any inadvertent vascular gas introduction to be trapped in the right atrium. This is said to allow slow liberation of the air into the pulmonary circulation, preventing air embolism (Root, 1974b). If no peritoneal fluid is present, the indwelling catheter is introduced into the abdomen approximately 1 cm lateral to the umbilicus. To assure that no organ is penetrated, the needle and catheter assembly are directed at a 70 to 90 degree angle to the sagittal plane (vertebral-sternal axis) of the abdomen (Barrett, 1975).

The catheter and needle assembly should just penetrate the parietal peritoneum. The needle is then withdrawn approximately 1 cm from the catheter before the assembly is advanced into the peritoneal space to the full length of the catheter. The needle is then withdrawn fully and a 3-way valve and syringe are attached. The use of the indwelling catheter instead of a needle for medium injection has the advantage of being less traumatic during subsequent manipulations. This technique will also decrease the incidence of medium injection into the falciform ligament, small bowel, spleen or vasculature. Splenic or vascular injection may result in air embolism. Gas is then injected, while respiration is monitored. Simultaneous pneumothorax may be produced in patients with a ruptured diaphragm. Demonstration of a ruptured diaphragm may be accomplished by performing pneumoperitoneography with 10 to 20 cc of air and radiographing in an erect VD view, using a horizontal x-ray beam (Roenigk, 1971; Ticer and Brown, 1975). In the presence of an intact diaphragm, the injected air will accumulate under the diaphragm and allow the liver to fall away in a caudal direction. If diaphragmatic rupture is present, the air will be found at the pleural space cranial to the cranial lung lobes.

A positive contrast peritoneogram may also be performed to diagnose diaphragmatic hernia. A peritoneal injection of sodium and meglumine diatrizoate (Renographin-76, E.R. Squibb & Sons, Inc.), 1.5 ml/kg body weight, warmed to body temperature, is followed rotation of the patient on its longitudinal axis. VD and lateral radiographs are then made (Rendano, 1979).

Excessive peritoneal fluid accumulation necessitates drainage prior to pneumoperitoneography. This is accomplished by the insertion of a catheter into the peritoneum through a small incision made immediately lateral to the umbilicus. This procedure is best accomplished by making a stab incision with a No. 11 blade and introducing the catheter tip through the hole while holding the catheter between the jaws of a small forceps. The forceps is then retracted and the catheter is inserted approximately 3 to 4 cm and fixed in place with a single suture. Drainage of peritoneal fluid will then occur without aspiration. Upon completion of drainage, a sufficient amount of air will have been aspirated into the peritoneal space to impart adequate radiographic contrast to the serosal surfaces. A small additional amount of air (200 to 500 cc) may be injected if desired (Fig. 16–11).

Radiography

Routine VD and lateral views are produced upon completion of medium injection. A DV view may be needed if the structures in the dorsal abdomen are of interest.

Erect, inverted and standing radiographs may be produced using a horizontal x-ray beam if a specific demonstration of a given abdominal region is desired.

Interpretation

Interpretation of pneumoperitoneograms is essentially the same as for routine abdominal radiography. Care should be taken not to mistake normal structures not usually seen on routine radiographs (such as the normal ovarian bursa) for abnormalities.

Figures 16–12 through 16–18 show the normal radiographic anatomy of the canine abdomen seen with pneumoperitoneography.

Text continued on page 334.

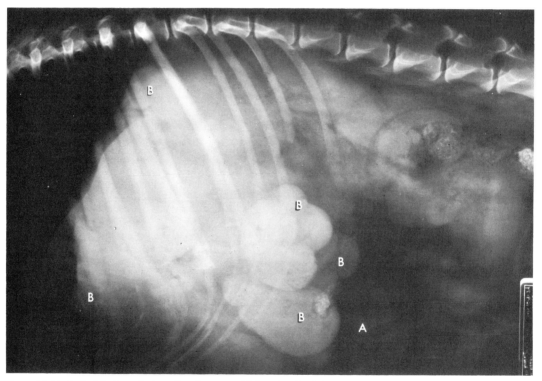

Figure 16–11. Left-right lateral view of a nine-year-old female Airedale terrier abdomen with pneumoperitoneogram produced after drainage of 9 liters of serosanguineous fluid and injection of 1 liter of air via an indwelling catheter *(A)*. Radiographs produced prior to drainage and air injection were undiagnostic because the serosal surfaces were rendered indistinct by the peritoneal fluid. The pneumoperitoneogram shows multiple globular masses on the liver and spleen *(B)*. Histological diagnosis was hemangiosarcoma.

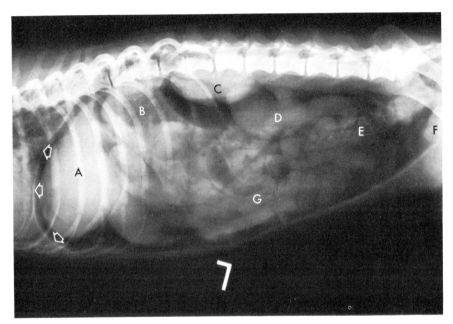

Figure 16–12. Right-left lateral view of a canine pneumoperitoneogram. Arrows indicate diaphragm.

A. Liver
B. Fundus of the stomach
C. Right kidney
D. Left kidney
E. Colon
F. Urinary bladder
G. Small bowel

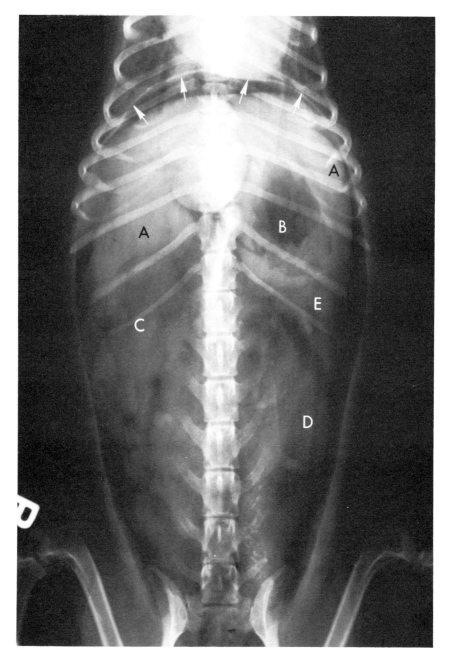

Figure 16–13. Ventrodorsal view of a canine pneumoperitoneogram. Arrows indicate diaphragm.
A. Liver
B. Fundus of the stomach
C. Right kidney
D. Left kidney
E. Spleen

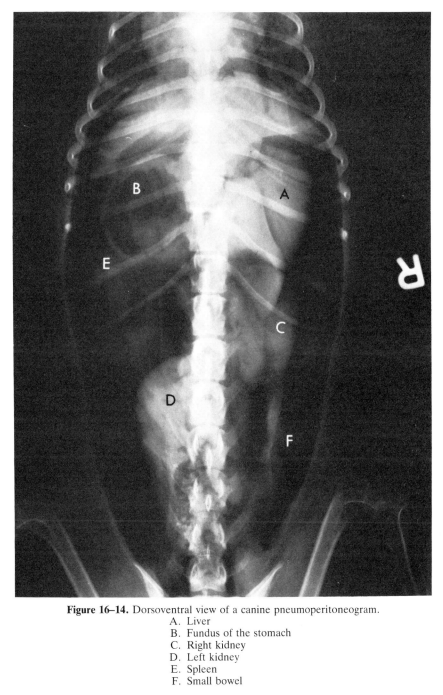

Figure 16–14. Dorsoventral view of a canine pneumoperitoneogram.
A. Liver
B. Fundus of the stomach
C. Right kidney
D. Left kidney
E. Spleen
F. Small bowel

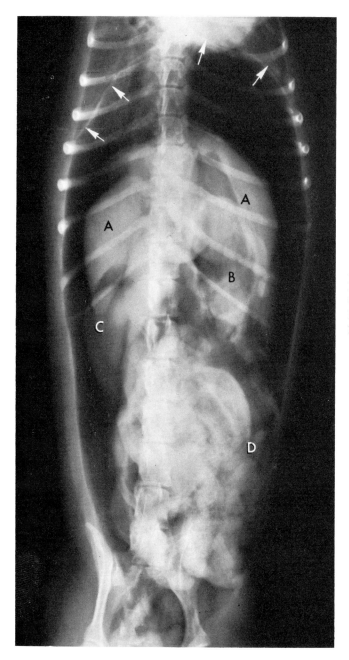

Figure 16–15. Ventrodorsal view of a canine pneumoperitoneogram using an erect posture (patient suspended by forelimbs) and a horizontal x-ray beam. Arrows indicate diaphragm.
- A. Liver
- B. Fundus of the stomach
- C. Right kidney
- D. Small bowel

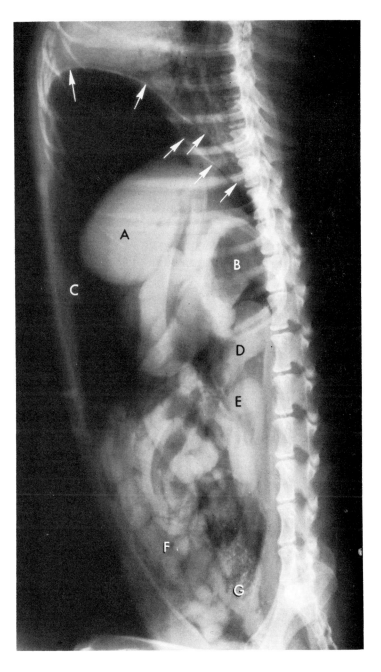

Figure 16–16. Left-right lateral view of a canine pneumoperitoneogram using an erect posture (patient suspended by forelimbs) and a horizontal x-ray beam. Arrows indicate diaphragm.

A. Liver
B. Fundus of the stomach
C. Falciform ligament of the liver
D. Right kidney
E. Left kidney
F. Small bowel
G. Colon

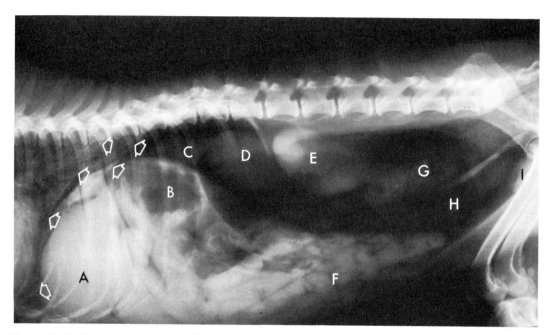

Figure 16–17. Standing left-right lateral view of a canine pneumoperitoneogram using a horizontal x-ray beam. Arrows indicate diaphragm.

A. Liver
B. Fundus of the stomach
C. Caudate lobe of the liver
D. Right kidney
E. Left kidney
F. Small bowel
G. Colon
H. Uterus
I. Urinary bladder

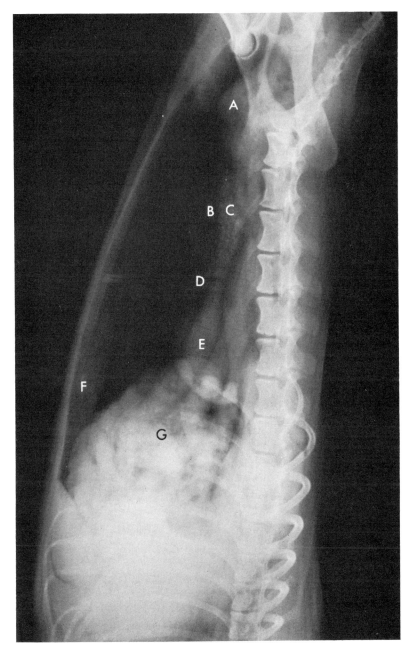

Figure 16–18. Right-left lateral view of a canine pneumoperitoneogram using an inverted posture (patient suspended by rear limbs) and a horizontal x-ray beam.

A. Urinary bladder
B. Uterus
C. Colon
D. Ovary
E. Left kidney
F. Falciform ligament of the liver
G. Small bowel

Cholecystography

Cholecystography is the radiographic examination of the main bile ducts and gallbladder after uptake of a radiodense medium.

Indications

Cholecystography may be indicated to visualize the bile ducts and gallbladder when there is evidence of biliary tract or gallbladder disease, such as cholangiectasis, chole-cystitis, cholelithiasis, or gallbladder or bile duct neoplasia.

Contraindications

The use of meglumine iodipamide is contraindicated in patients with hypersensitivity to organic iodides. This condition is rare in dogs and cats. Administration of the salts of iodipamide are also contraindicated in pa-

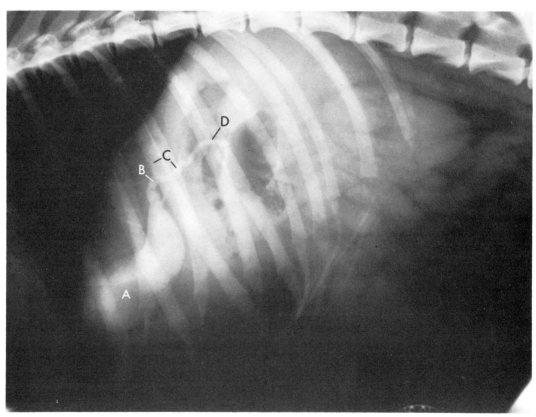

Figure 16–19. Left-right lateral view of a canine cranial abdomen with a cholecystogram. This radiograph was produced 60 minutes after an intravenous injection of 0.2 ml/kg body weight of meglumine iodipamide.

A. Gallbladder
B. Cystic duct
C. Hepatic ducts
D. Common bile duct

tients with severe impairment of renal or liver function or in cases of hyperthyroidism.

Technique

Materials

The preferred medium for cholecystography in the dog and cat is meglumine iodipamide U.S.P. (Cholografin Meglumine, Squibb and Sons), injected intravenously.

Dosage

An intravenous dose of 0.2 ml/kg body weight is usually adequate.

Procedure

Survey radiographs of the cranial abdomen are produced in at least the lateral and VD projections. The medium is injected into the cephalic vein over a period of approximately 3 minutes. Rapid injection may produce discomfort and retching. Radiographs of the cranial abdomen are then produced at approximately 30 minutes, 60 minutes, and, if necessary, 90 minutes after injection.

If post-emptying study of the gallbladder is desired, a small fatty meal may be fed and radiographs produced in approximately 15 minutes.

Interpretation

The main bile ducts and gallbladder should be well opacified by the contrast medium (Fig. 16–19). Alterations in margination or content should be considered signs of disease. The radiographic appearance of bile duct and gallbladder disease has not been adequately described in dogs and cats; however, this should not discourage the use of the technique.

REFERENCES

Amberg, J. R., and Roenigk, W. J.: In Felson, B. (Ed.): Roentgen Techniques in Laboratory Animals: Radiography of the Dog and Other Experimental Animals. Philadelphia, W. B. Saunders Co., 1968.

Barrett, R. B.: A new method of abdominal and thoracic pericentesis in the dog and cat. Vet. Med./Sm. Anim. Clin., 70:76, 1975.

Barrett, R. B., and Kneller, S. K.: Feline kidney measuration. Acta Radiol. Suppl., 319:279, 1972.

Douglas, S. W., and Williamson, H. D.: Principles of Veterinary Radiography. 3rd ed. Baltimore, Williams & Wilkins Co., 1980.

Finco, D. R., Stiles, N. S., and Kneller, S. K.: Radiologic estimation of kidney size of the dog. J. Amer. Vet. Med. Ass., 159:995, 1971.

Gillette, E. L., Thrall, D. E., and Lebel, J. L.: Carlson's Veterinary Radiology, 3rd ed. Philadelphia, Lea & Febiger, 1977.

Grandage, J.: The radiology of the dog's diaphragm. J. Small Anim. Pract., 15:1, 1974.

Grandage, J.: Some effects of posture on the radiographic appearance of the kidney of the dog. J. Amer. Vet. Med. Ass., 166:165, 1975.

Hall, V. E., and MacGregor, W. W.: Relation of kidney weight to body weight in the cat. Anat. Rec., 69:319, 1937.

Kneller, S. K.: Role of the excretory urogram in diagnosis of renal and ureteral disease. Vet. Clin. N. Amer., 4:843, 1974.

Miller, M. E., Christensen, G. C., and Evans, H. E.: Anatomy of the Dog. Philadelphia, W. B. Saunders Co., 1964.

Osborne, C. A., Low, D. G., and Finco, D. R.: Canine and Feline Urology. Philadelphia, W. B. Saunders Co., 1972.

Rendano, V. T.: Positive contrast peritoneography: An aid in the radiographic diagnosis of diaphragmatic hernia. J. Amer. Vet. Radiol. Soc., 20(2):67, 1979.

Roenigk, W. J.: Injuries to the Thorax. J. Amer. Anim. Hosp. Assoc., 7:266, 1971.

Root, C. R.: Interpretation of Abdominal Survey Radiographs. Vet. Clin. N. Amer., 4:763, 1974a.

Root, C. R.: Abdominal masses: The radiographic differential diagnosis. J. Amer. Vet. Radiol. Soc., 15:26, 1974b.

Schebitz, H., and Wilkins, H.: Atlas of Radiographic Anatomy of Dog and Horse. Berlin, Paul Parey, 1968.

Ticer, J. W., and Brown, S. G.: Thoracic trauma. In Ettinger, S. J. (Ed.): Textbook of Veterinary Internal Medicine; Diseases of Dog and Cat. Philadelphia, W. B. Saunders Co., 1975.

Contrast Radiography of the Alimentary Tract

Few practicing veterinarians have access to equipment that will permit clinical evaluation of the dynamics of the alimentary tract. Fluoroscopy or its modern counterpart, image-intensified fluoroscopy, enables one to thoroughly evaluate the upper gastrointestinal tract (esophagus, stomach and small bowel) with respect to peristalsis, transit time, mucosal integrity, and luminal size, shape and content. Of these factors, only peristalsis cannot be satisfactorily evaluated by routine radiography. The type of equipment necessary for appreciation of the dynamics of the gastrointestinal tract is expensive and usually is found only in teaching institutions, large private practices or specialty practices. Therefore, the following discussion of contrast radiography of the alimentary tract will not include the use of fluoroscopy or image intensification. The emphasis will be upon screening studies or those procedures most likely to yield a large amount of information. Special studies using barium-impregnated food or variations in concentration of barium will not be discussed.

ESOPHAGRAM (BARIUM SWALLOW)

Indications

In general, the esophagus should be evaluated every time barium sulfate suspension is administered. In most instances this is not done, making examination of the upper alimentary tract technically incomplete.

Specific indications for esophageal contrast studies include regurgitation of undigested food, persistent gagging or vomiting, and suspected esophageal foreign bodies (Douglas and Williamson, 1970, 1972; Morgan, 1964). Breed and age predisposition for megaesophagus should be borne in mind,

especially if the clinical history specifically includes regurgitation rather than vomiting. Gagging, as an independent sign, often accompanies pharyngeal or tracheal disease. However, when gagging is accompanied by swallowing motions or excessive salivation or both, esophageal lesions are more likely. Positive history of the ingestion of any type of foreign body, accompanied by compatible signs, such as mild to severe dysphagia, salivation, gagging, hematemesis or anxiety, provides ample justification for contrast radiography of the esophagus. Contrast radiography of the esophagus has been used in the assessment of esophageal neoplasia (Ridgway and Suter, 1979), reflux esophagitis (Pearson et al., 1978a), esophageal deviation (Woods et al., 1978), esophageal diverticula (Pearson et al., 1978b), and esophageal foreign bodies (VanStee et al., 1980). Delay in clinical detection of an esophageal lesion or detection of such a lesion at necropsy cannot be excused for economic reasons, either those of the client or those of the veterinarian.

True vomiting, which is not responsive to symptomatic treatment, is often indicative of lesions in the stomach or in the orad portion of the small bowel. However, even when the stomach and intestinal tract are the organs of primary interest, an esophageal study may demonstrate contributory, secondary, or simultaneous lesions.

Contraindications

Barium sulfate contrast radiography of the esophagus has not been recommended if there is reason to suspect rupture or perforation. However, it has been shown that neither barium sulfate nor organic iodides adversely affect existent periesophageal mediastinitis (Vessal, 1973). The presence of bronchoesophageal or similar fistulae is also

336

a contraindication for esophageal contrast study. A small amount of pure barium sulfate suspension is well tolerated by normal lungs and bronchi (Dunbar, 1959; Nelson et al., 1964; Nice, 1964; Shook and Felson, 1970), but if introduced into diseased lung tissue, it may not be cleared normally. Another major contraindication for contrast radiography of the esophagus in practice is the inability to swallow, since the danger of aspiration is increased when a large amount of barium is present in the caudal pharynx. Profound dysphagia should be evaluated with cineradiography (Watrous and Suter, 1979), a technique that permits the use of smaller volumes of contrast material and detailed retrospective assessment of all phases of the act of swallowing. This type of study can only be done at suitably-equipped teaching institutions, large private practices, or referral clinics.

Preparation of Patient

The animal should be fasted for at least 12 hours before the administration of contrast material. Fasting permits the esophagus to empty, should it contain ingesta, which is often seen on survey films of the thorax in patients with one of the various forms of congenital or acquired megaesophagus. Fasting is advised even when esophageal dilation is not suspected, to reduce the possibility of artifacts caused by adherence of a small amount of ingesta to luminal masses or mucosal defects.

Survey radiographs should be made in VD and lateral projections immediately before the contrast material is administered. Films made one to two days before giving the opaque agent will not suffice, since lesions may change significantly in the interim.

Materials

No specific special equipment is required for esophageal contrast studies, but a large syringe facilitates administration of the contrast material. Esophageal contrast materials are supplied commercially in many forms, including BaSO₄ U.S.P., and micropulverized BaSO₄ powder (Micropaque, Barium Sulfate Powder, Picker Corp.), suspension (Novopaque, Barium Sulfate Suspension, Picker Corp.) and paste (Esophotrast, Barium Sulfate Esophageal Cream, Barnes-Hind Diag-

nostics). If the esophageal study is part of a complete upper gastrointestinal series, one of the liquid suspensions is preferred. Thick paste alone is not satisfactory for upper G.I. series and mixes poorly with the additional thin suspension necessary for the study of the stomach and small bowel. If, however, the study is specifically for opacification of the esophagus, one of the thicker suspensions or one of the esophageal pastes is recommended. Such preparations tend to coat the esophageal mucosa better than the thin or watery media (Douglas and Williamson, 1970). It is the author's opinion that $BaSO_4$ U.S.P. (Gillette et al., 1977; Crago, 1960; Seward, 1951) is worthless for any meaningful contrast study and should not be used, despite the fact that it is cheap. Barium-impregnated food should be given only if a routine esophagram is negative and clinical signs are strongly suggestive of an esophageal lesion.

Dosage of Contrast Material. If the study is being done at the beginning of an upper G.I. series, the dose is not important. The dose necessary for opacification of the stomach and small bowel will coat the mucosal surface of the esophagus sufficiently for radiographic evaluation. In instances in which a specific study of the esophagus is desired, enough esophageal paste or thick barium sulfate suspension should be administered to distend or completely coat the esophagus. Since megaesophagus requires more contrast material than a normal esophagus, and since it is impossible to overdistend the normal esophagus, it is best to give enough barium suspension to distend the esophagus if it will distend. A rough guide appears to be 2 to 6 ml of contrast medium per kilogram of body weight. Passage of this amount of contrast material will surely coat the mucosal surface if distention does not occur. If the first radiographs show incomplete distention of the esophagus, give more contrast medium and repeat the study. Much more contrast material may be required for adequate demonstration of the degree of dilation and for evaluation of the terminal portion of the esophagus in animals with long-standing achalasia.

Procedure (Table 16–1)

The contrast material is slowly administered orally, via the buccal pouch, with a large syringe. Even the thickest of pastes may be successfully given in this way. Rapid de-

Table 16–1. SUMMARY OF PROCEDURE FOR ESOPHAGEAL CONTRAST STUDIES

1. Fast the animal for at least 12 hours.
2. Obtain current survey radiographs of the thorax.
3. If the purpose of the study is to delineate only the esophagus:
   a. Slowly administer enough barium sulfate paste or similar thick barium suspension orally via the buccal pouch to distend or coat the esophagus. The dosage is extremely variable; unless extreme esophageal dilation is present, 2 to 6 ml per kg of body weight is usually satisfactory.
   b. Make lateral, VD and right VD oblique radiographs of the thorax.
4. If the study is made as part of an upper G.I. series:
   a. Administer 6 to 12 ml of the liquid barium suspension orally per kg of body weight.
   b. Immediately make lateral and VD or V30°Le-DRtO (right VD oblique) radiographs of the thorax.

livery of the contrast material should be avoided, since aspiration of the agent may lead to coughing, anxiety and delayed administration time. Thick barium paste may be given with a tongue depressor or similar object, but delivery time is slow.

As the last of the contrast medium is being swallowed, radiographs of the thorax are made in both projections. If the study is to be specifically of the esophagus, a ventral right-dorsal left (V30°Rt-DLeO) (formerly right VD oblique) radiograph of the thorax is also made. This view projects the esophagus away from the spine, upon which it is normally superimposed in the VD view. This oblique view also may be performed in conjunction with the upper G.I. series, but it is usually not considered necessary unless the esophagus is of primary interest. If lesions are demonstrated in such films, an esophagram should be done with esophageal paste for better visualization.

Complications

Aspiration of contrast material is most often due to hasty administration. This is usually not disastrous if only a small amount of the medium is inhaled, but a large amount can result in death if alveolar flooding occurs.

Extraluminal deposition of barium sulfate may occur if the esophagus is ruptured or perforated. However, animals with such ruptures or perforations die from infection rather than from the ectopic barium (Vessal, 1973). In the presence of bronchoesophageal fistulae (which are admittedly rare) barium sulfate may be cleared slowly and further aggravate a seriously diseased lung lobe.

Normal Findings

Barium sulfate suspension or paste coats the esophagus and appears radiographically as a series of regular, parallel lines of nearly uniform width (Gillette et al., 1977; Douglas and Williamson, 1970, 1972), which correspond to longitudinal crypts between folds of the esophageal mucosa (Fig. 16–20). This appearance is better appreciated if one recalls that the surface area of the mucosa of the esophagus greatly exceeds that of the serosa. Further, the muscular wall of the esophagus can stretch to accommodate a bolus of food, while the epithelial lining, relatively much less capable of stretching, allows passage of boluses by passive flattening of its multiple redundant longitudinal folds. At the thoracic inlet, the esophagus may be transiently roughened and irregular, probably because of slight delay in bolus passage of that site. In cats, the caudal third of the esophagus usually is transversely striated (Kneller and Lewis, 1973), in addition to having longitudinal folds. This produces a striking "herringbone" or "burlap" pattern (Fig. 16–21), which often has been mistaken for a cloth foreign body or a fish skeleton within the caudal esophagus.

GASTROGRAPHY (NEGATIVE CONTRAST GASTROGRAPHY, POSITIVE CONTRAST GASTROGRAPHY, DOUBLE CONTRAST GASTROGRAPHY)

Indications

Specific radiographic study of the stomach is indicated when there is strong suspicion of mural or luminal gastric masses or when there is likelihood of radiolucent gastric foreign bodies. This type of study is often done for further evaluation of the stomach after suspicious or equivocal gastric findings are noted during a complete upper gastrointestinal series, but contrast radiography of the stomach

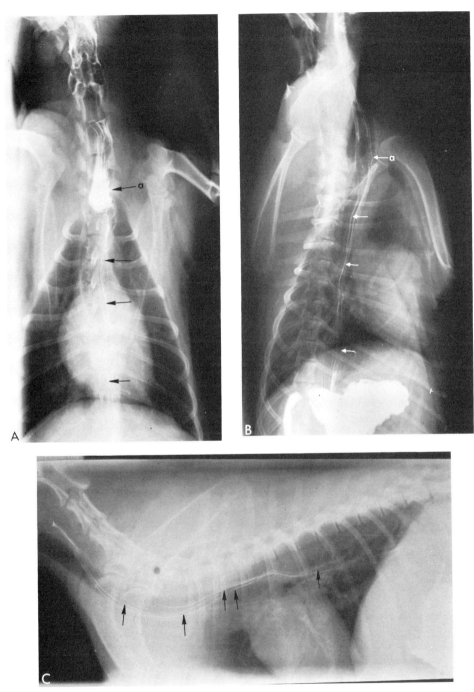

Figure 16–20. Normal esophagram (dog). *A*, VD; *B*, ventral right-dorsal left oblique; and *C*, lateral views of a normal canine thorax after administration of barium sulfate paste. Notice the parallel opaque lines (arrows) formed by barium collected between multiple longitudinal mucosal folds. At the thoracic inlet, the esophageal mucosa may be transiently roughened and irregular (*A*). The oblique view allows visualization of the esophagus without interference by the spine.

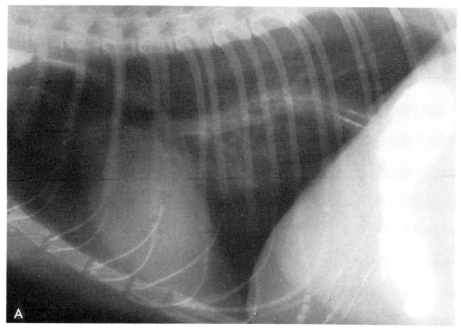

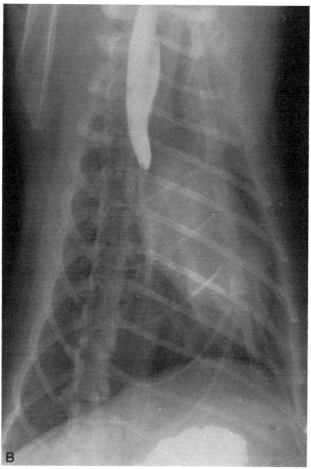

Figure 16–21. Normal esophagram (cat). *A*, lateral and *B*, ventral right–dorsal left oblique (formerly right VD oblique) views of a normal feline thorax after administration of barium sulfate paste. A bolus of contrast material is entering the cranial thoracic esophagus and parallel opaque lines show the linear striations of the normal esophageal mucosal pattern over the base of the heart. The caudal esophagus is only faintly opacified, and the longitudinal parallel lines are interrupted by transverse striations. *(Legend and illustration continued on opposite page)*

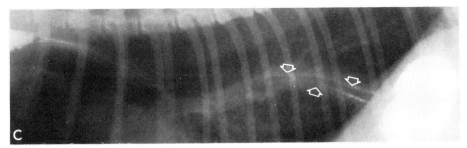

Figure 16–21 *Continued. C*, close-up of the caudal esophagus in the lateral projection showing the normal transverse striations (arrows) creating a "herringbone" or "burlap" pattern.

may be performed as an independent study if clinically indicated (Morgan, 1964; Schnelle, 1950; Evans and Laufer, 1981). Double contrast gastrography has the advantage over both positive contrast gastrography and pneumogastrography, in that lesions need not be presented tangentially to be fully appreciated (Evans and Laufer, 1981).

Double contrast gastrography may be inconclusive if simultaneous mucosal coating and gastric distension are precluded by normal or accelerated gastrointestinal motility. A pharmacoradiographic procedure has been described in which double contrast gastrography is performed after parenteral induction of gastrointestinal hypomotility (Evans and Laufer, 1981).

Contraindications

Gastrography (using positive contrast material, room air, or both) is contraindicated in the presence of ingesta or fluid. Also, if the animal has diarrhea, probably more information will be gained by performing a complete upper gastrointestinal series.

Double contrast gastrography preceded by parenteral administration of glucagon is contraindicated in patients with diabetes mellitus or suspected pheochromocytoma (Evans and Laufer, 1981). The procedure may be done without induction of hypomotility, but gastric emptying with resultant loss of negative contrast or superimposition of opacified bowel may render the procedure inconclusive (Laufer, 1975).

Preparation of Patient

A 12-hour fast and recent survey radiographs of the abdomen should precede any of the three types of gastrography.

Definitive double contrast gastrography (Evans and Laufer, 1981) requires previous gastric paralysis with intravenous glucagon (Glucagon, Eli Lilly and Co.) or Pro-Banthine (Propantheline Bromide, Searle Laboratories). The dosage for glucagon depends upon the size of the patient. The following glucagon dosage scale produces satisfactory hypomotility for approximately 15 minutes:

below 8 kg	0.10 mg
8 to 20 kg	0.20 mg
20 to 40 kg	0.30 mg
over 40 kg	0.35 mg

The dose can be repeated if longer gastric hypotony is necessary, but the maximum dose of glucagon should not exceed 1.0 mg. Alternatively, propantheline bromide may be administered orally at a dosage of 7.5 to 30.0 mg (Kinsell and Swick, 1981). Unfortunately, the drug is available in the tablet form only and must be given orally. In man, peak plasma concentration occurs approximately 6 hours after oral administration, suggesting that oral administration in dogs should precede double contrast gastrography by several hours.

Materials

The necessary materials for gastric contrast radiography depend upon the type of study to be done.

Negative Contrast Gastrography (Pneumogastrography). The simplest contrast study of the stomach is performed with room air. With this method, a stomach tube, a three-way valve, a mouth gag, and a large syringe are needed. However, carbonated beverages or various commercially available effervescent agents (E-Z-Gas Effervescent Granules, E-Z-EM Corp.; Sparkles Effervescent Tablcts, Lafayette Pharmacal, Inc.) may be employed to distend the stomach with gas. In the author's experience, the effervescent tablets are much slower than the gas-producing granules in producing satisfactory gastric distention; further, the granules are difficult to administer to companion pets. Therefore the effervescent agents are considered inferior to the other methods of purposeful gaseous gastric distension in animals. Oral administration of a highly carbonated beverage, on the other hand, is a satisfactory method of introducing gas into the stomach. Realize, however, that the use of a carbonated beverage also adds fluid to the stomach. Fortunately, the volume of gas liberated usually far exceeds the volume of fluid introduced, allowing satisfactory visualization of the tangential surfaces of the gastric lumen.

Positive Contrast Gastrography. Barium sulfate suspension or aqueous organic iodide solution may be used to distend the stomach. If barium sulfate suspension is employed, only the micropulverized agents (Barosperse, Barium Sulfate U.S.P. Formulation, Mallinckrodt Pharmaceuticals; Micropaque, Barium Sulfate Powder, Picker Corp.) should be used, since plain barium sulfate (non-micropulverized, no suspending or coating agent added) will flocculate and will not coat the mucosal surface (Root and Morgan, 1969). If one of the water-soluble organic iodide preparations (Gastrografin, Meglumine Diatrizoate Oral Solution, Squibb and Sons; Oral Hypaque, Sodium Diatrizoate Liquid, Winthrop Laboratories) is used, one should recognize that they are bitter-tasting and hyperosmolaric (Allan et al., 1979). Further, they may be partially absorbed into the bloodstream and excreted by the kidneys (Allan et al., 1979), are somewhat irritating, and may induce hypermotility. In cats, however, pylorospasm (instead of hypermotility) may result, causing prolonged gastric retention and ultimate vomiting. Presumably, this is due to pyloric irritation and hyperosmolaric increase in gastric volume.

Regardless of the type of positive contrast material employed, the concentration is critical. Mural and luminal masses may be hidden if the material is too dense. If barium sulfate is used, the concentration should not exceed 15 per cent (W/W). If organic iodide is used, its concentration should be no greater than a 10 per cent diatrizoate solution (W/V). Gastrografin contains 367 mg meglumine diatrizoate per ml while Oral Hypaque Liquid contains 50 g sodium diatrizoate per 120 ml. Both of these concentrations approximate 40 per cent diatrizoate (W/V). Therefore, 1 volume of either diluted to 4 volumes with water approximates a 10 per cent W/V diatrizoate solution. These concentrations of barium sulfate and organic iodide will insure mural and luminal detail, even when the stomach is satisfactorily distended.

Double Contrast Gastrogram. The materials used for double contrast radiography of the stomach depend upon the chosen method.

If the study is performed during the early phases of an otherwise conventional upper G.I. series, after barium has exited the stomach leaving a contrast-coated mucosal surface, only a source of gas need be provided. A stomach tube, a three-way valve, a mouth gag, and a large syringe may be used to introduce room air. Alternatively, carbonated beverage may be administered or one of the commercial effervescing agents may be given.

If optimum information is desired, however, double contrast gastrography should be done as a specific procedure (Evans and Laufer, 1981). This requires an agent to induce gastric hypotony (Glucagon, Eli Lilly and Co.; Pro-Banthine, Propantheline Bromide, Searle Laboratories), a high-density micropulverized barium sulfate suspension (Polibar Barium Suspension, E-Z-EM Corp.), a stomach tube, a mouth gag, a three-way valve, and a large syringe. Room air, a carbonated beverage, or an effervescent agent may be used to provide the gas. Room air delivered via stomach tube is the simplest and most reliable method for gaseous gastric distention (Evans and Laufer, 1981; O'Brien, 1978).

Dosage of Contrast Material. The amount of contrast material depends upon the method selected for gastric contrast radiography.

For pneumogastrography or for double contrast gastrography during an upper G.I. series, room air should be given via stomach tube at the dosage of 6 to 12 ml per kilogram body weight. Alternatively, 30 to 60 ml of a carbonated beverage may be given orally, depending on the size of the patient, or enough effervescent material may be given to liberate 6 to 12 ml of gas per kilogram of body weight. When using one of the effervescent products, the manufacturer's instructions will specify the quantity of material necessary to produce a given quantity of gas. These materials cannot be pre-mixed with liquid and delivered with a syringe, since the liberated gas builds up pressure and makes it impossible to control the delivery rate.

Positive contrast gastrography requires the administration of 6 to 12 ml diluted (15% W/W maximum) micropulverized barium sulfate suspension (Micropaque Barium Sulfate Powder, Picker Corp.; Barosperse, Barium Sulfate U.S.P. Formulation, Mallinckrodt Pharmaceuticals; Novopaque Barium Sulfate Suspension, Picker Corp.) per kilogram of body weight, or 6 to 12 ml per kilogram body weight of diluted (10 per cent W/V maximum) water-soluble organic iodide solution (Gastrografin, Meglumine Diatrizoate Oral Solution, Squibb and Sons; Oral Hypaque, Sodium Diatrizoate Liquid, Winthrop Laboratories).

Double contrast gastrography, if done during an otherwise conventional upper G.I. series, requires no modification of the recommended dose (6 to 12 ml/kg) or concentration (20% W/W) of barium sulfate suspension, but gastric mucosal detail may be suboptimal. Double contrast cannot be achieved if organic iodide is used instead of barium, since water-soluble agents do not adhere to viable mucosal surfaces.

Definitive double contrast gastrography, after temporary gastric paralysis (Evans and Laufer, 1981), requires high density barium sulfate (Polibar Barium Sulfate Suspension, E-Z-EM Corp.). It is administered at dosages of 3.0 ml/kg up to 8 kg, 2.0 ml/kg between 8 and 40 kg, and 1.5 ml/kg over 40 kg. This is followed by gastric insufflation with 20 ml/kg room air. It should be noted that high density barium preparations have a relatively large average particle size (Gelfund, 1979). They are, therefore, considered unsuitable for routine upper G.I. radiography in small animals, since they flocculate and since they do not render fine mucosal detail of the small bowel.

Procedure (Table 16–2)

Negative Contrast Gastrography (Pneumogastrography. If a carbonated beverage is used, it is administered with a large syringe into the buccal pouch, rather than by a stomach tube. The swallowing action of the patient permits most of the gas to be liberated by the time the carbonated beverage reaches the stomach. Four standard projections are made of the cranial abdomen (ventrodorsal, dorsoventral, right-left lateral and left-right lateral).

If air is the chosen medium, a gastric tube is introduced and the calculated volume of air is introduced (6 to 12 ml/kg). After the air is introduced, the tube is removed and the gastric region is radiographed in the four standard projections.

Effervescent granules (mixed with water) should be administered into the buccal pouch

Table 16–2. SUMMARY OF GASTROGRAPHIC PROCEDURES

1. Fast the animal for 12 to 24 hours.
2. Obtain current survey radiographs of the abdomen.
3. *Negative contrast gastrography (pneumogastrography):*
   Administer 6 to 12 ml of air per kg of body weight via stomach tube *or*
   Give (orally) enough effervescent material (according to the manufacturer's instructions) to liberate 6 to 12 ml gas per kg of body weight *or*
   Give 30 to 60 ml of a highly carbonated beverage via the buccal pouch.
4. *Positive contrast gastrography:*
   Administer 6 to 12 ml of 15% (W/W) micropulverized barium sulfate suspension or 10% (W/V) diatrizoate solution per kg of body weight via a stomach tube.
5. *Double contrast gastrography:*
   a. As part of an otherwise standard upper G.I. series, after most of the contrast material has exited the stomach, perform one of the procedures listed above for negative contrast gastrography.
   b. As an independent study, assisted by gastric paralysis:
      1) Induce gastric hypomotility with glucagon (see text for contraindications):

up to 8 kg	0.10 mg
8–40 kg	0.20 mg
20–40 kg	0.30 mg
over 40 kg	0.35 mg

      2) Administer high density, low viscosity barium sulfate suspension:

up to 8 kg	3.0 ml/kg
8–40 kg	2.0 ml/kg
over 40 kg	1.5 ml/kg

      3) Insufflate the stomach with room air, 20 ml/kg.
6. Immediately make VD, DV, left-right lateral, right-left lateral, and (if needed) positional radiographs of the cranial abdomen.

from an open container rather than from a large syringe, because the effervescence may become uncontrolled in the relatively enclosed syringe barrel, resulting in loss of much of the foaming solution before it can be administered.

Positive Contrast Gastrography. If either barium sulfate suspension or organic iodide solution is used, it should be properly diluted and administered by gastric intubation. After the proper volume (6 to 12 ml/kg) of contrast material has been instilled in the gastric lumen, the stomach tube is removed and the cranial abdomen is radiographed in ventrodorsal, dorsoventral, right-left lateral and left-right lateral projections. These radiographs should be obtained as quickly as possible to permit visualization of the stomach while it is optimally distended with contrast material. Remember that barium sulfate suspension and organic iodine solution, in concentrations greater than 15 per cent W/W and 10 per cent W/V, respectively, are likely to obscure luminal and non-tangential mural detail.

Double Contrast Gastrography. A double contrast study of the stomach may be performed in several ways. First, room air, a carbonated beverage, or effervescent agents may be used to distend the stomach during the early phases of conventional contrast radiography of the upper G.I. tract. After most of the barium has exited the stomach, room air (6 to 12 ml/kg) may be introduced with a stomach tube, 30 to 90 ml (depending on the size of the patient) of a carbonated beverage may be introduced via the buccal pouch, or enough effervescent material to liberate 6 to 12 ml gas per kg may be administered in a small amount of water, orally or with a stomach tube.

Superior visualization of the gastric mucosal surface is afforded, however, if double contrast gastrography is preceded by gastric paralysis, performed with high-density barium sulfate suspension, and followed by gastric distention with room air (Evans and Laufer, 1981). After administration of barium, the patient is rolled or rotated about its spinal axis several times to facilitate complete coating of gastric mucosa with adherent barium. Oral administration of a mixture of barium sulfate suspension and an effervescent agent has been advocated in humans (Gelfand and Hachiya, 1969), but this method has not reliably produced satisfactory gastric distension in animals. In humans, administra-

tion of the gas-producing agent may precede administration of positive contrast material (Laufer, 1975) or vice versa (Freeny, 1979); either technique results in satisfactory double contrast gastrography. Satisfactory mucosal coating seems easier to accomplish in companion animals if the stomach is distended with gas after the barium sulfate suspension has been given. Then multiple radiographic projections of the cranial abdomen are made (ventrodorsal, dorsoventral, right-left lateral and left-right lateral), bearing in mind the gravitational changes in contrast interfaces (Grandage, 1974). Multiple oblique views of the stomach may be helpful as well. Erect lateral, erect ventrodorsal, standing lateral, and other horizontal x-ray beam projections may be employed if necessary.

Complications

No adverse effects have been noted by the author with these procedures to date. The risks of, and contraindications for, administering gastric hypotonicity agents should be borne in mind, and the inconclusive results obtained when using undiluted contrast material for positive contrast gastrography must be avoided by proper dilution of contrast agents.

Normal Findings

The stomach should be uniformly and evenly distended with gas, and the width of the crypts between rugae should be at least as wide as the rugae themselves (Figs. 16–22 and 16–23). The wall and rugal folds should not be distorted, either intrinsically or extrinsically. The lumen should be free of filling defects, and the gastric wall should be of uniform thickness. Better visualization of the wall of the distended stomach occurs with double contrast gastrography (Fig. 16–23) than with either negative or positive contrast gastrography.

UPPER GASTROINTESTINAL SERIES (BARIUM SERIES, SMALL BOWEL SERIES)

Indications

The major indications for performing contrast radiography of the upper G.I. tract are

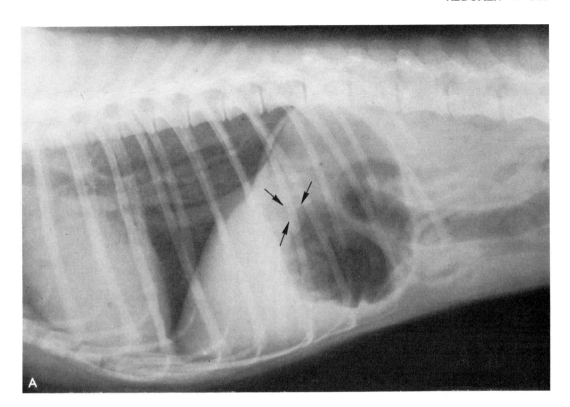

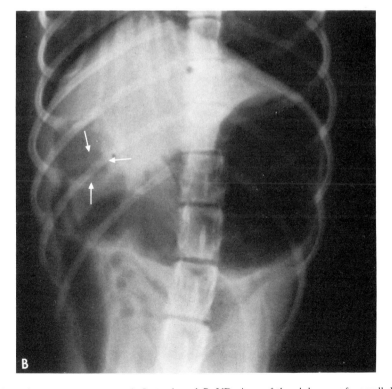

Figure 16–22. Normal pneumogastrogram. *A,* Lateral, and *B,* VD views of the abdomen of a small dog given 30 ml of a highly carbonated beverage. The rugal folds are regular, even, smooth, and nearly parallel. The crypts between adjacent rugal folds in the distended stomach are normally at least as wide as the rugal folds. The gastric wall is uniform in thickness. The pylorus (arrows) is entirely to the right of the midline in the VD view and is superimposed upon the midportion of the fundus in the lateral view.

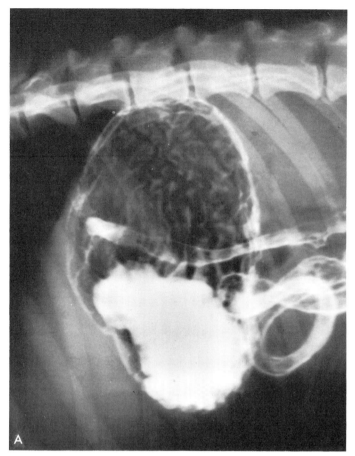

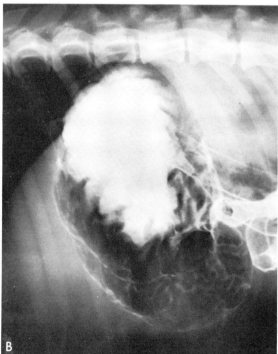

Figure 16–23. Normal double contrast gastrogram. *A*, Left-right; *B*, Right-left lateral.

(Legend and illustration continued on opposite page)

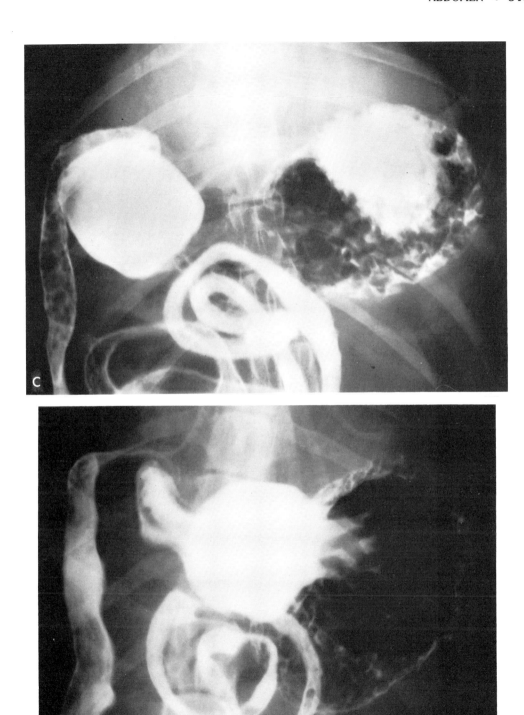

Figure 16–23 *Continued. C,* VD; and *D,* DV views of the abdomen of a dog given 6 ml/kg of room air via gastric intubation 10 to 15 minutes after being given 6 ml/kg micropulverized barium sulfate suspension. Superior visualization of the gastric mucosal surface results from this technique, as the stomach is not only coated with barium but also is distended with gas. Under the influence of gravity, the barium remaining in the lumen of the stomach changes location in each view.

recurrent or nonresponsive vomiting, refractory or recurrent diarrhea, hematemesis, suspected gastric or enteric foreign bodies or neoplasms, suspected intestinal obstruction, the need for assistance in localization and identification of certain abdominal masses, or confirmation of various types of herniae (Barrett, 1968; Douglas and Williamson, 1970; Gomez, 1974; Morgan, 1964; Morgan, 1977; Schnelle, 1950).

In the instances in which the dog or cat is vomiting or has diarrhea, and has not responded to rigorous symptomatic treatment, contrast radiography of the stomach and small bowel is indicated.

Hematemesis is rare in dogs and cats. When it does occur, contrast radiography of the upper G.I. tract is definitely indicated. Ulcerated gastric or duodenal neoplasms are sometimes found, and radiographic assessment of such lesions is a rapid and direct approach.

Suspected radiolucent foreign bodies, partial obstructions or early complete obstructions of the gastrointestinal tract justify performing an upper G.I. series. In these situations, the rapid appraisal of the gastrointestinal tract provided by enteric contrast studies can mean the difference between life and death.

Abdominal masses which cannot readily be separated from the gut on the basis of survey radiographs may be better appreciated after the intestinal tract is opacified (Morgan, 1964). This use of the upper G.I. series should be limited to cases with special medical problems, such as severe pneumonia or lesions leading to respiratory distress which preclude the use of pneumoperitonography (a study which is more likely to yield information about several organ systems).

Various forms of herniae can be confirmed by contrast radiography of the gut if portions of the bowel have passed through the hernial ring but have not strangulated. Examples are diaphragmatic, ventral, umbilical, inguinal and perineal herniae in which the gut is involved.

Contraindications

Barium contrast radiography of the upper G.I. tract should be avoided in patients suspected of having perforation or rupture of the stomach or gut, since barium sulfate in the peritoneal cavity may lead to the formation of granulomata. Without concomitant sepsis, however, extravasated barium sulfate is rarely fatal. Water soluble contrast media, such as the oral diatrizoates, may be used without fear of producing granulomata when there is suspicion of ruptures or perforations of the stomach or small bowel.

Contrast radiography should not be performed if there are clinical or radiographic signs of obstructive ileus or small bowel atony, especially in weakened, depressed, or debilitated patients, since satisfactory progressive opacification of the gut will not occur. The time lost in attempting to perform such a procedure and the additional stress to the patient are not justifiable in light of the very remote possibility of learning something new or significant about the condition of the patient. Such patients should be surgically explored as soon as possible. If bowel hypotony is suspected, as occurs with some foreign bodies and most neoplasms, one should be aware that the small bowel transit time, and thus the timely demonstration of the lesion, will be delayed. This is true even when the patient is not dramatically sick.

It has long been recommended that barium sulfate suspension not be administered when there is a strong indication of obstruction of the lower bowel. This has largely been refuted by research in dogs and observations in humans with partial and complete obstructions of the colon (Grossman et al., 1980). Severe debility is a contraindication for use of any of the oral diatrizoates because of their hyperosmolality and consequent dehydrating effect (Nelson et al., 1965; Allan et al., 1979). These agents also become progressively diluted as they pass through the intestinal tract, and are usually of little value in demonstrating lesions of the lower jejunum and ileum.

Preparation of Patient

The animal should be fasted for 24 hours prior to the administration of contrast material. A thorough flushing enema with tepid (not warm) salt solution (8 tsp table salt per gallon of tap water or 45 g table salt per 5 L tap water) should be given until clear fluid returns. Warm, soapy enemas are usually inadequate because the surfactant agent causes coalescence of gas that is not expelled with the solid fecal material. The various hypertonic commercial enema preparations are inadequate because they tend to cause evacuation of only the terminal portion of the colon. As in all other contrast procedures of the abdominal viscera, current survey radiographs should be made in VD and lateral projections. Unless absolutely necessary, no tranquilizers or sedatives should be given prior to upper G.I. radiography, as these drugs modify gastrointestinal activity (Zontine, 1973; Bargai, 1982) and therefore may alter small bowel transit time. Anticholinergic drugs should not have been administered within 24 hours of the radiographic examination.

Materials

Types of contrast material for the G.I. tract are numerous. Of the barium sulfate suspensions, one of the micropulverized preparations is preferred. These are supplied in several dry powder forms (Barosperse, Barium Sulfate U.S.P. Formulation, Mallinckrodt Pharmaceuticals; Micropaque, Barium Sulfate Powder, Picker Corp.) or in various concentrations of premixed liquid suspension (Novopaque, Barium Sulfate Suspension, Picker Corp.). Barium sulfate U.S.P. is markedly inferior to the micropulverized products. It does not coat the mucosal surfaces, it flocculates in the gut lumen and its passage through the small bowel is slightly slower than that of the micropulverized media (Root and Morgan, 1969).

If there is reasonable suspicion that the upper G.I. tract is ruptured or perforated, barium products should be avoided (Gomez, 1974). Instead, the organic iodides (Gastrografin, Meglumine Diatrizoate Oral Solution, Squibb and Sons; Oral Hypaque, Sodium Diatrozoate Liquid, Winthrop Laboratories) are recommended (O'Brien, 1978). They are also recommended if it seems imperative to reach a radiographic conclusion quickly, because these agents pass through the small bowel very rapidly.

In addition to the contrast material, the only other items needed are a large syringe with a tapered catheter adapter, a stomach tube, and a mouth gag. Oral, rather than gastric, administration of contrast material requires only a large syringe.

Dosage of Contrast Material. In general, the volume of barium sulfate suspension administered is as important as its concentration. The object in opacification of any hollow visceral structure should be reasonable physiologic distention of its lumen without masking its contents. Contrary to previous recommendations of other authors (Gillette et al., 1977; Douglas and Williamson, 1970, 1972; Morgan, 1964), a small volume of a very concentrated contrast material is considered by this author to be ineffective in evaluation of the stomach and gut. A larger volume of relatively dilute material is much more satisfactory because the lumen of the G.I. tract is adequately distended, and radiolucent luminal filling defects are not obscured. The recommended concentration of barium sulfate preparations is 15 to 20 per cent for G.I. opacification. The dosage should be 6 to 12 ml $BaSO_4$ suspension per kilogram in dogs (Barrett, 1968; Root and Morgan, 1969; Kealy, 1979; O'Brien, 1978), and 12 to 16 ml per kg (Morgan, 1977) in cats.

The water-soluble organic iodine solutions (Gastrografin, Meglumine Diatrizoate Oral Solution, Squibb and Sons; Oral Hypaque, Sodium Diatrozoate Liquid, Winthrop Laboratories), full strength, should be administered at the rate of 2 ml per kilogram of body weight. Their concentrations are usually fixed. Further dilution is ill-advised for study of the intestinal tract, since these solutions lose density as they pass through the G.I. tract (Nelson et al., 1965; Allan et al., 1979).

Procedure (Table 16–3)

Administer the contrast material per os by the buccal pouch or, preferably, through a stomach tube. If using the buccal pouch, allow the patient to swallow slowly in order to avoid aspiration of contrast material into the trachea and lungs. The organic iodide preparations should be administered by stomach tube only, because they are extremely bitter (Allan et al., 1979). Cats seem to find the taste of these latter agents especially unpleasant.

In dogs given barium products, lateral and ventrodorsal radiographs of the abdomen are made immediately, at 15 minutes, at 30 minutes, at 60 minutes and at hourly intervals until the contrast material reaches the colon.

Table 16–3. SUMMARY OF PROCEDURE FOR UPPER G.I. SERIES

1. Fast the animal for 24 hours and give a cleansing tepid saline enema (see text).
2. Obtain current survey radiographs of the abdomen.
3. If barium sulfate suspension is used:
   a. Slowly administer 6 to 12 ml of 20 to 25% (W/V) micropulverized barium sulfate suspension per kg of body weight orally via the buccal pouch.
   b. If screening radiographs of the esophagus are to be omitted, the contrast medium may be administered with a stomach tube.
   c. Make lateral and VD radiographs of the abdomen immediately, at 15 minutes, 30 minutes, 1 hour, 2 hours, 3 hours, etc., until the colon contains contrast material. The immediate and 15 minute radiographs may be DV rather than VD, if desired.
4. If an organic iodide solution is used:
   a. Administer 2 ml of the medium per kg of body weight, by stomach tube.
   b. Radiograph the abdomen at 0, 5, 15, 30 and 60 minutes and every half hour thereafter until the colon is opacified.

If desired, DV rather than VD radiographs may be made immediately and at 15 minutes, theoretically permitting better visualization of the wall of the body of the stomach. (O'Brien, 1978). Additional radiographs may be made at 24 hours if desired. In cats, the recommended filming protocol is lateral and ventrodorsal radiographs immediately, 5 minutes, 30 minutes, and 60 minutes following administration of contrast material, although the immediate radiographs are not recommended by one author (Morgan, 1977), and others recommend the addition of multiple ventral left–dorsal right oblique (V30°Le-DRtO) (formerly left ventrodorsal oblique) views to supplement or replace the conventional ventrodorsal projections (Farrow and Back, 1980). If an organic iodide is administered in dogs, lateral and VD radiographs of the abdomen should be made immediately, at 5 minutes, at 15 minutes, at 30 minutes and every half-hour thereafter until the colon is visualized. The radiographic protocol for diatrizoate gastrointestinal studies in cats probably should be similar to that used for barium contrast radiography, since small bowel transit time of the water-soluble agents in cats is variable (Allan et al., 1979; Allan et al., 1980) but appears to be greater than that reported in the dog (McAlister and Margulis, 1964; Nelson et al., 1964).

Complications

Aspiration of a small amount of pure barium sulfate suspension into the lungs during oral administration is of little serious consequence, as proved by the fact that certain commerical barium sulfate preparations have been used successfully as bronchographic agents (Dunbar, 1959; Nelson et al., 1964; Nice, 1964; Shook and Felson, 1970). However, aspiration of a large amount of any barium sulfate preparation may be fatal, since the alveoli may be flooded. Aspiration of vomited barium, even in small quantities, is potentially a very serious situation, probably owing to the action of acid gastric content upon airway epithelium.

Peritoneal granulomata may be the sequela to leakage of barium through perforated or ruptured G.I. lumen. If leakage of ingesta with concomitant infection is suspected, barium preparations should be avoided. Usually this may be determined by critical examination of the survey radiographs, analysis of the clinical and hematologic findings, or both.

The presence of barium sulfate preparations in the lumen of the G.I. tract might be considered by some to be a contraindication to gastric or intestinal surgery. Peritoneal contamination with barium obscures natural color and interferes with normal texture of the mucosal surface. However, the value of the information obtained from upper G.I. series usually far outweighs the inconvenience, and careful surgical technique minimizes the possibility of peritoneal contamination with barium.

Administration of organic iodides has proved to be deleterious to the patient that is already dehydrated and debilitated (Nelson et al., 1965). Further dehydration can be brought about by the hyperosmolality of these products. Additional loss of body fluids is caused by rapid passage of luminal contents, which results from the irritation caused by this type of contrast medium. As the contrast medium progresses through the G.I. tract, it becomes more dilute because of its hyperosmolality, and its radiopacity is often unsatisfactory by the time it reaches the terminal small bowel. In some animals, especially cats, the irritant property of organic iodides causes severe pylorospasm, which results in gastric retention of the medium until it is vomited.

Normal Findings

The normal small bowel transit time for micropulverized barium sulfate suspensions in dogs (Fig. 16–24) is two to three hours (Barrett, 1968; Root and Morgan, 1969). Barium sulfate U.S.P. requires, on the average, one hour longer to reach the canine colon (Root and Morgan, 1969). In cats, small bowel transit time of micropulverized barium sulfate suspension is normally 30 to 60 minutes (Morgan, 1977, 1981). The organic iodides (McAlister and Margulis, 1964; Nelson et al., 1964) pass through the canine small bowel in 45 minutes to one hour (Fig. 16–25) but do not appear to transit the feline gut proportionately faster than barium preparations (Morgan, 1977; O'Brien, 1978; Allan, 1979).

With both the micropulverized agents and the organic iodides (Figs. 16–24 and 16–25), a smooth halo is seen surrounding the luminal column of contrast material, except in the ileum, where the wall is very smooth. The halo is presumed to be caused by the presence of these contrast agents in the crypts between the intestinal villi (Barrett, 1968; Root and Morgan, 1969). This halo effect is much more pronounced with organic iodide (Fig. 16–25) than with one of the micropulverized barium agents. Barium sulfate U.S.P. is too coarse to produce this effect, and often flocculates rather than causing uniform opacification of the gut lumen (Fig. 16–26).

Regardless of the agent employed in contrast radiography of the G.I. tract, the small bowel should always appear to be evenly dispersed throughout the peritoneal cavity. No extrinsic masses should displace the small bowel.

The rugal folds of the distended stomach should be roughly parallel, and their individual widths should not exceed the distance between adjacent rugae. There should be no gastric or enteric filling defects. The mucosal borders should be uniform, except in the duodenum, where crater-shaped pseudo-ulcers (Fig. 16–24) are often seen along the antemesenteric border (O'Brien et al., 1969).

In cats, early in the upper G.I. series, the normal duodenal pattern has been described as a "string of pearls" (Morgan, 1981; O'Brien, 1978). This finding should suggest neither duodenitis, contrary to a previous report (Root and Lord, 1971), nor linear foreign body. Rhythmic segmentation of the small bowel is responsible for both mixing of bowel contents and slowing the passage of chyme through the normal gut (Strombeck, 1979), appearing radiographically as three to four adjacent constrictions in a short segment of the bowel. This phenomenon normally occurs 17 to 18 times per minute in the duodenum, 15 to 16 times per minute in the jejunum and 12 to 14 times per minute in the ileum (O'Brien, 1978). Although subject to many variables and not documented by a controlled research protocol, fewer than four to five such segmentation regions should be present in the normal small bowel on any one radiograph obtained during conventional contrast radiography of the small intestine, in the author's opinion and except as previously described in the feline duodenum. This type of bowel activity is normally inversely related to small bowel transit time. Paradoxically, many animals with diarrhea have radiologic evidence of enteric hypersegmentation. Perhaps this is due to diminished amplitude of contractions in the diseased gut, or perhaps this finding can be explained by relative volume overload due to hypersecretion into the lumen of the inflamed bowel. Suffice it to say that a certain amount of segmentation is normally present radiographically, but excess segmentation should be viewed with suspicion and should be correlated with other radiographic and clinical signs of bowel disease. In dogs, the total thickness of the two visible walls of the small bowel should be no greater than one fourth to one third the width of the physiologically distended lumen. The lumen of the small bowel should generally be uniform in width, and there should be no extensive regions of luminal narrowing which persist in sequential radiographs. The width of the normal small bowel lumen rarely exceeds 12 mm in cats (Morgan, 1981) but is more variable in dogs owing to the large variation in canine body sizes and conformations. In many dogs, the sphincters of the ileocolonic (Kelly, 1967) and cecocolonic junctional zones may be seen as these regions become opacified (Fig. 16–24F).

Text continued on page 364.

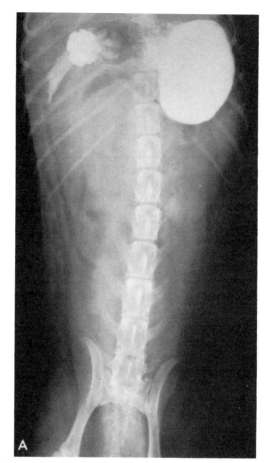

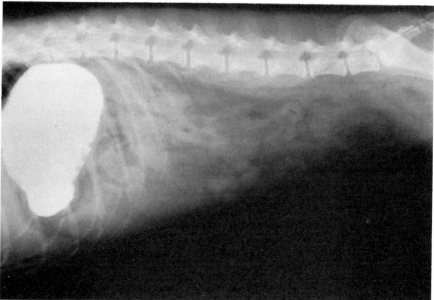

Figure 16–24. Normal upper G.I. series — micropulverized barium sulfate. Lateral and VD radiographs of the abdomen of a normal dog, made immediately (*A*), 15 minutes (*B*), 30 minutes (*C*), 60 minutes (*D*), 2 hours (*E*) and 3 hours (*F*) after oral administration of 6 ml 20% (weight per volume) micropulverized barium sulfate suspension per kg of body weight.

Immediately after administration of contrast material the stomach is distended. Its wall is of uniform thickness and rugal folds are regular, even, smooth and nearly parallel. The crypts between adjacent rugal folds in the distended stomach normally are at least the same width as the rugae. The mucosal surface of the small bowel should be smooth

(Legend and illustration continued on opposite page)

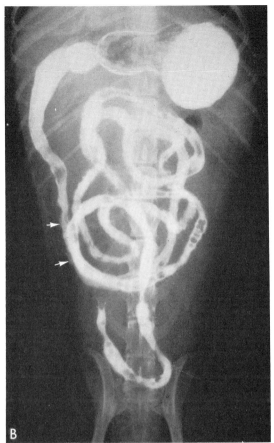

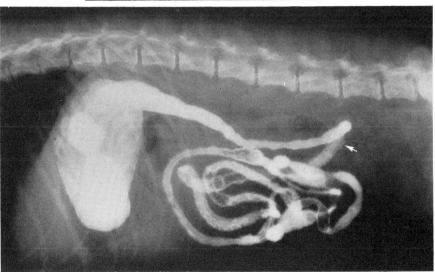

Figure 16–24 *Continued*

and is usually outlined by a faint halo or a slightly roughened edge. There may be ulcer-shaped defects ventrally and laterally in the mucosa of the duodenum (arrows). These are called pseudoulcers and are of no clinical significance.

Between 15 minutes and 2 hours after administration, contrast material should progressively opacify and distend the duodenum, jejunum and ileum. Segmental peristaltic constrictions in the gut are important in mixing and slowing passage of ingesta. There is no definite line of demarcation between jejunum and ileum, but the mucosal surface of the ileum lacks the mucosal halo common to the jejunum. The ileum terminates at the ileocolic valve *(a)* near the cecum *(b)* (page 357). In many animals, approximately 1 hour before the contrast material enters the colon, it collects and appears to become more concentrated in the caudal jejunum and ileum. Normal small bowel transit time is 2 to 3 hours with this type of contrast medium.

(Illustration continued on the following page)

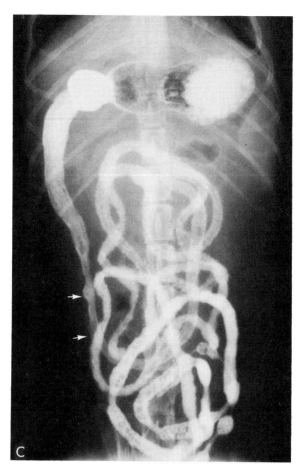

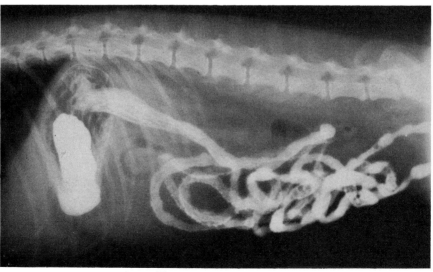

Figure 16–24 *Continued*

(Illustration continued on opposite page)

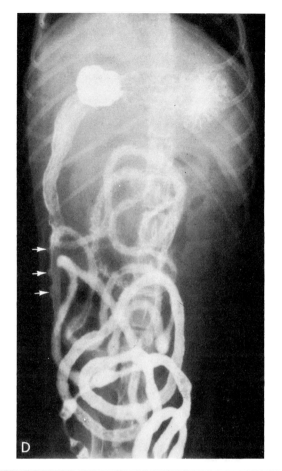

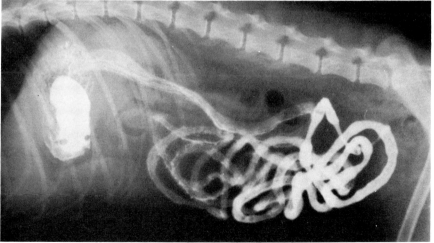

Figure 16–24 *Continued*

(Illustration continued on the following page)

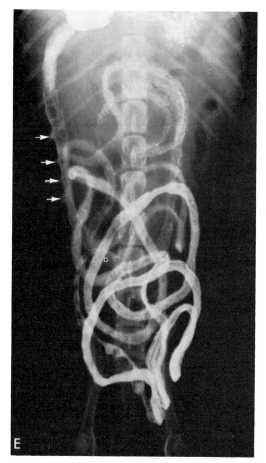

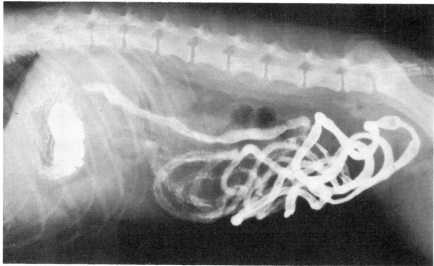

Figure 16–24 *Continued*

(Illustration continued on opposite page)

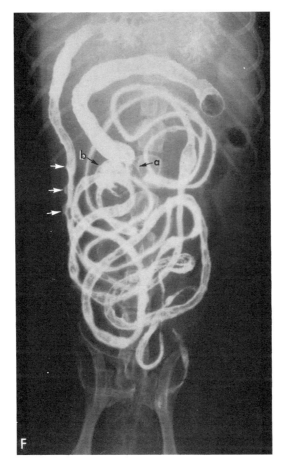

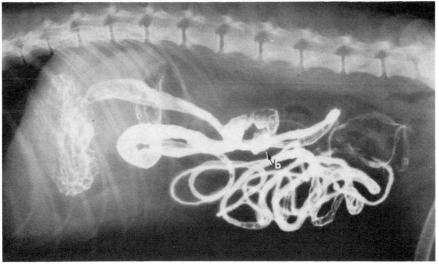

Figure 16–24 *Continued*

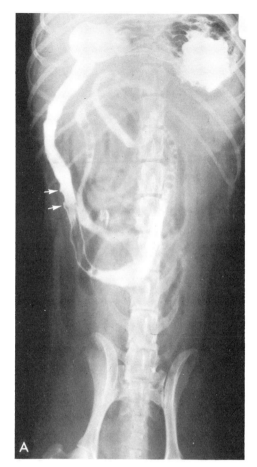

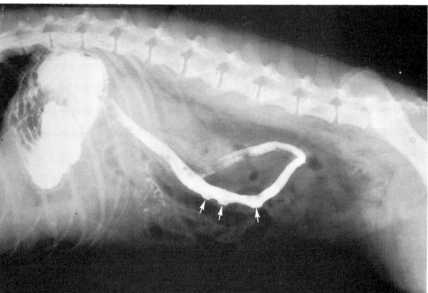

Figure 16–25. Normal upper G.I. series—water-soluble contrast medium. Lateral and VD radiographs of the abdomen of a normal dog, made immediately (*A*), 5 minutes (*B*), 15 minutes (*C*), 30 minutes (*D*), 45 minutes (*E*), and 1 hour (*F*), after gastric administration of 2 ml/kg of a water-soluble gastrointestinal contrast medium. As in Figure 16–24, all the normal anatomic structures and relationships can be appreciated. The periluminal halo and peristaltic segmentation may be much more pronounced when using one of the water-soluble products than when using a barium

(Illustration and legend continued on the opposite page)

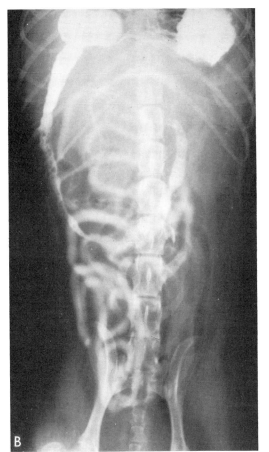

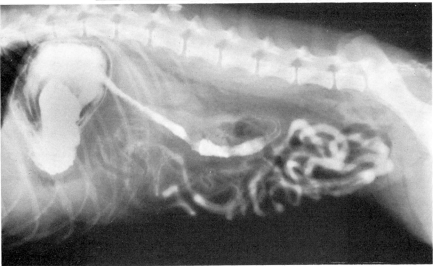

Figure 16–25 *Continued*

sulfate suspension. The contrast material is usually well into the small bowel by 15 minutes. By 30 minutes, it has proceeded into the terminal portion of the small intestine. In the normal animal, this type of medium has usually entered the colon by 45 minutes to 1 hour. By this time, however, its density may have been markedly diminished by dilution due to its hyperosmolality. Pseudoulcers (arrows), the ileocolic valve (a) and the cecum (b) may be seen (page 363). Renal pelvic opacification may be seen in radiographs made near the end of the study.

(Illustration continued on the following page)

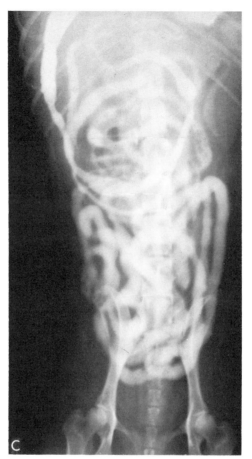

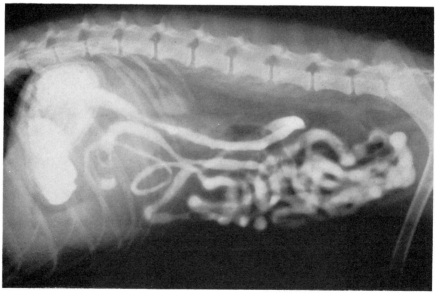

Figure 16–25 *Continued*

(Illustration continued on opposite page)

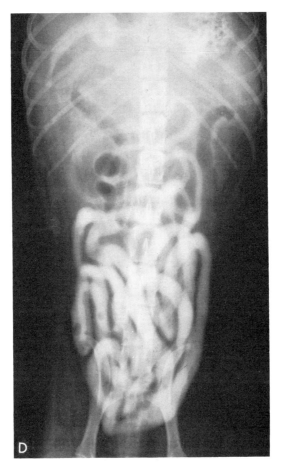

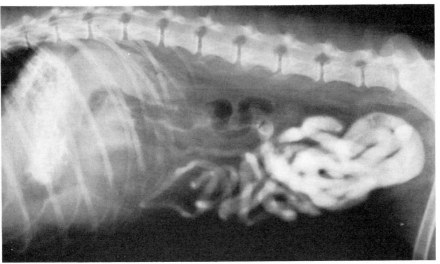

Figure 16–25 *Continued*

(Illustration continued on the following page)

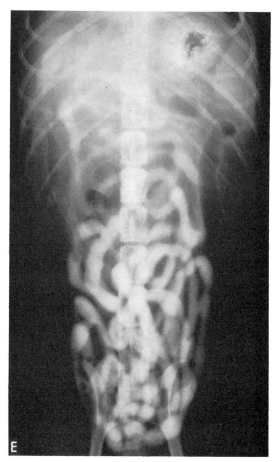

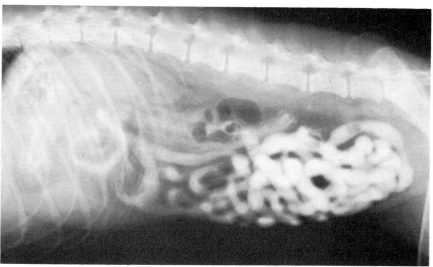

Figure 16–25 *Continued*

(Illustration continued on opposite page)

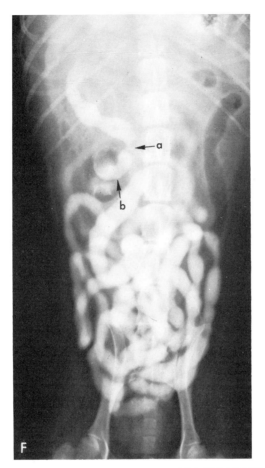

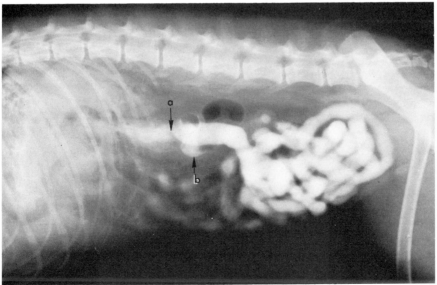

Figure 16–25 *Continued*

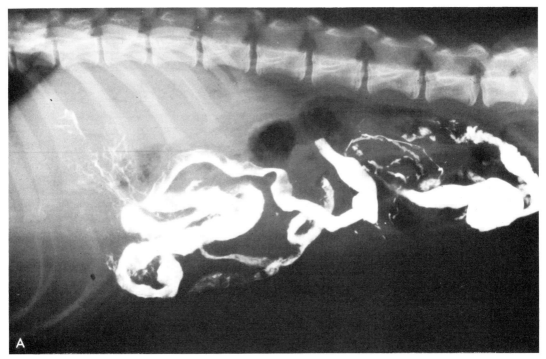

Figure 16–26. Upper G.I. series — barium sulfate U.S.P. Lateral (*A*) and VD (*B*) abdominal radiographs of a young dog 1 hour after oral administration of 6 ml/kg of 30% (weight per volume) barium sulfate U.S.P. This material is an unsatisfactory gastrointestinal contrast medium due to its tendency to flocculate and its inability to outline the normal enteric mucosal pattern.

(Illustration continued on opposite page)

CONTRAST RADIOGRAPHY OF THE COLON (BARIUM ENEMA, LOWER BOWEL SERIES, DOUBLE CONTRAST RADIOGRAPHY OF THE COLON)

Indications

Refractory or recurrent bloody diarrhea probably is the most common indication for performing contrast radiography of the colon. Low volume, high frequency stools, with or without blood, are ample justification for contrast radiology of the colon, especially if unresponsive to rigorous symptomatic therapy. Rectal tenesmus, if severe or chronic, is another common justification for lower bowel studies. Ileocolonic intussusception is thought by some to be best demonstrated by opacification of the large bowel (Gillette et al., 1977, Douglas and Williamson, 1970). However, this lesion commonly can be seen well during contrast radiography of the upper G.I. tract, provided that obstruction of the ileum is incomplete. It is sometimes possible to reduce ileocolonic intussusceptions during inflation of the colon with contrast material. If

reduction occurs, demonstration of the lesion by colonic opacification may be impossible.

Contraindications

Historically, it has been strongly recommended that barium sulfate suspension not be given if obstruction of the colon is suspected (Nelson et al., 1965) and immediate surgery is not contemplated. Inspissation of the barium suspension theoretically leads to severe constipation, resulting in the same type of obstipation caused by ingestion of a large amount of bony material. This potential complication has been proved to be highly overrated, however, both by observations in humans with various types of colonic obstructive lesions and by research involving dogs as experimental subjects (Grossman et al., 1980).

Rupture or perforation of the colon or recent biopsy of the colonic wall also contraindicates retrograde distension of the lower bowel. Rupture or perforation of the lower bowel is more likely to result in sepsis than is rupture or perforation of the stomach

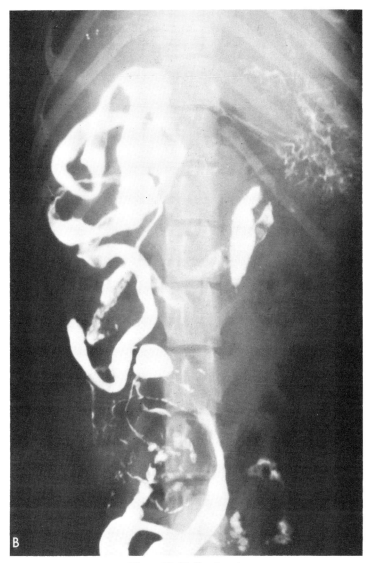

Figure 16–26 *Continued*

or small bowel. If such a lower bowel lesion is suspected, the contrast radiographic study should not be performed.

Contrast radiographic evaluation of lesions that are clinically limited to the rectum or terminal colon should not be attempted, since lesions in this region will be obscured by the inflated cuff of the catheter.

Preparation of Patient

The animal must be fasted for at least 24 hours prior to the contrast study (Watters, 1970; O'Brien, 1978). A mild cathartic should be administered at least 12 hours before the colon is opacified. A flushing enema must be given, using salt solution (8 tsp salt per gallon tap water or 45 g salt per 5 L tap water) at slightly less than body temperature, until the returning fluid is absolutely clear. Tepid, rather than warm, enema solutions are recommended, since they result in more complete evacuation. Commercial hypertonic enema kits are not thorough enough for satisfactory preparation of the patient. Current survey radiographs in both VD and lateral projections are necessary before the colon is opacified.

General anesthesia is required for this study, since inflation of the bulb of the cuffed catheter induces discomfort and stimulates violent tenesmus in the conscious animal.

Materials

The most important item required for contrast radiography of the colon is the catheter through which the contrast material is introduced. Cuffed rectal catheters (Bardex Cuffed Rectal Catheters, 24 to 38 French and Bardex Cuffed Pediatric Rectal Catheter, 18 French, Bard Hospital Division, C. R. Bard, Inc.) have been used successfully in medium-sized and large dogs. Cats and small dogs require smaller catheters. However, any other type of cuffed rectal catheter may be used, provided that the cuff can be distended adequately to occlude the lumen of the rectum. Disposable enema nozzles with removable inflatable cuffs (Dispos-A-Tube Enema Tips and Disposable Cath-Cuffs, Picker Corp.) may be used, but owing to their size, are not suitable for cats and smaller dogs. An adapter and a three-way valve are also required, regardless of the type of catheter used.

The concentration of the contrast medium is as important in opacifying the colon as it is in visualizing the stomach and small intestine. However, because larger volumes of contrast medium are used in studies of the colon, the concentration should be less to prevent obliteration of luminal masses. Dilute barium sulfate suspension may be prepared from powder (Micropaque, Barium Sulfate Powder, Damancy & Co., Ltd.) or may be made from commercially available liquid suspensions (Novopaque Barium Sulfate Suspension, Picker Corp.) or powdered products (Barosperse, Barium Sulfate U.S.P. Formulation, Mallinckrodt Pharmaceuticals). The final concentration of barium sulfate suspension should be 15 to 20 per cent (W/V). Some type of suspended reservoir should be provided for the contrast material. This may be a used intravenous fluid bottle with its attached tubing or merely a standard enema can. If an emptied parenteral fluid bottle is used, a large disposable syringe is necessary for alternate aspiration of the contrast medium from the hanging bottle and injection of the material into the rectal catheter through the three-way valve. If the enema can is used, a clamp should be used to control the speed of gravity flow of the contrast material from the can into the colon. The disadvantage of the latter method is the relatively poor control or estimation of the volume of contrast material instilled into the colon at any time.

Dosage of Contrast Material. The object is to distend the colon to its normal physiologic capacity, but it should not be overfilled. A rough guide for dosage is 20 to 30 ml barium sulfate suspension per kg of body weight. Because the volume needed to fill the colon is extremely variable, the contrast material should be administered in several smaller increments until the desired effect is seen radiographically.

Procedure (Table 16–4)

After the patient is anesthetized, the cuffed catheter or disposable enema nozzle is inserted into the rectum so that the cuff is cranial to the pubis. The cuff should be

Table 16–4. SUMMARY OF PROCEDURE FOR CONTRAST RADIOGRAPHY OF THE COLON

1. Fast the animal for at least 24 hours.
2. Mild catharsis is recommended beginning at least 12 hours before the procedure is performed.
3. Give a flushing enema with tepid saline solution until the returning fluid is clear (see text).
4. Obtain current survey radiographs of the abdomen.
5. Anesthetize the patient.
6. Using an appropriate cuffed rectal catheter or cuffed enema nozzle with the inflated bulb or cuff seated slightly cranial to the anal sphincter:
   a. Slowly instill 10 ml (15 to 20% W/V) dilute micropulverized barium sulfate suspension per kg body weight into the colon, with the animal in right lateral recumbency.
   b. Make a VD radiograph of the abdomen to determine if the colon is adequately distended. If it is not, instill more contrast material and repeat the radiograph.
   c. When the colon is adequately distended, note the total volume of contrast material used and radiograph the abdomen in VD and lateral projections.
   d. Leaving the bulb or cuff of the rectal catheter inflated, remove as much of the contrast material as possible and radiograph the abdomen in both projections.
   e. Replace the recovered contrast material with an equal volume of air and repeat the radiographs of the abdomen.
   f. Deflate the bulb or cuff and remove the catheter or enema nozzle from the rectum.

inflated only enough to occlude the lumen firmly, and the catheter or nozzle should be pulled caudally to seat the inflated cuff against the cranial portion of the anal sphincter.

The colon is then slowly filled with contrast material at body temperature with the patient in right lateral recumbency. At this point, a fluoroscope or an image intensifier is very useful but is rarely available. Without the benefit of such equipment, 10 ml of contrast material per kg of body weight should be instilled slowly and the abdomen radiographed in the VD projection. If the radiograph shows that the colon is not adequately distended, another 10 ml per kg of body weight is instilled, and the abdomen is radiographed again. This procedure must be repeated until the colon and cecum become uniformly distended. The abdomen is then radiographed in both the VD and lateral projections. The total volume of contrast material used should be noted.

Next, the contrast material is removed from the colon via the catheter. An attempt should be made to recover as much of the contrast material as possible. At this point, the importance of proper cleansing of the colon will be appreciated (Zezulin, 1971). If preparation was inadequate, the catheter will become occluded with fecal material and it will be impossible to remove a significant portion of the contrast material. If the colon was properly cleansed, most of the contrast agent may be retrieved by massage, manipulation and positioning of the abdomen to take advantage of the effect of gravity during gentle aspiration. Placing the animal in left lateral recumbency is helpful because it permits most of the contents to gravitate into the descending colon. When the lower bowel is satisfactorily emptied, the abdomen is radiographed in the VD and lateral projection. This is known as the post-evacuation study.

The final step in this procedure is the filling of the colon with a volume of air equal to the amount of contrast material recovered. Ventrodorsal and lateral radiographs of the abdomen are then made. This study provides double contrast opacification of the colon and probably produces the most valuable radiographs in the entire series, because superior visualization of the doubly-contrasted mucosal surface is provided.

At the conclusion of the study, the cuff is deflated and catheter or nozzle is removed.

Complications

The most common "complication" in contrast radiography of the colon, although it is of no significance to the patient, is flooding of the tabletop with contrast material if the cuff is not properly inflated or if the patient expels the cuff because of improper anesthesia.

Another complication is retrograde filling of the ileum and jejunum (see Fig. 16–28), which is also of no serious consequence to the patient. In as many as one third of patients, this filling occurs without overdistention. If this reflux is massive, however, it can obscure visualization of portions of the colon.

It is possible to rupture the colon in several ways if proper care is not taken. The catheter cuff can be overinflated, causing a rent or rupture to occur in the terminal colon or rectum. Rupture can occur anywhere in the colon wall if it is subjected to severe overdistention. This can be avoided by making monitoring radiographs during the filling procedure. Also, the colon can rupture without overdistention if it has been recently biopsied proctoscopically, or if its wall is otherwise weakened by disease or surgery.

Normal Findings

During the positive contrast study (Fig. 16–27A), the colon is uniformly distended and smooth in outline (Barrett, 1968; Morgan, 1964; Watters, 1970). It forms the outline of a question mark or a shepherd's crook in the VD view. In normal animals, the colon usually lies in a plane nearly parallel to the spine in the lateral projection and is located roughly halfway between the spine and the ventral body wall, with the cecum, the ascending colon and the cranial descending colon being superimposed. The colon may be redundant; that is, it may appear to be too long and may have a convoluted appearance (Fig. 16–28). This is a normal variant.

In the post-evacuation radiographs (Fig. 16–27B), the only variations in the appearance of the colon are the lumen size and the appearance of the wall. The lumen narrows and the wall becomes collapsed and irregular.

After the addition of air (Fig. 16–27C), the colon is once again completely distended, but the mucosal surface is doubly contrasted with air and barium. This study is of little value

Text continued on page 372.

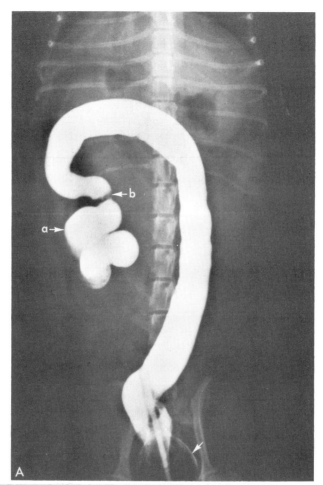

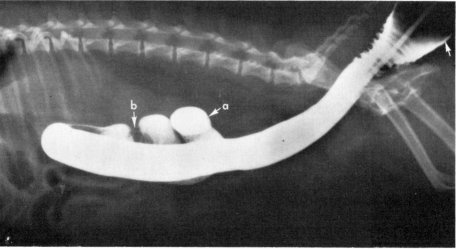

Figure 16–27. Opacification of the colon. *A,* Positive contrast study. The wall is smooth in outline and the lumen is uniform in width. The colon assumes a "shepherd's crook" or "question mark" configuration in the VD view. In this study, the cecum (a) and cecocolic valve (b) are seen. Cecal opacification during radiography of the colon is not always satisfactory. Note the air-filled cuff of the Bardex catheter (arrows). *B,* Post-evacuation study. After as much of the contrast medium as possible is removed from the colon, the lower bowel is found to be collapsed. It should not have changed in general location however. *C,* Double contrast study. A volume of air equal to the amount of contrast medium recovered prior to the post-evacuation study adequately distends the barium coated large bowel. The wall is well visualized and is normally smooth and of uniform thickness. The cecum (*a*) and cecocolic valve (*b*) are seen.

(Illustration continued on opposite page)

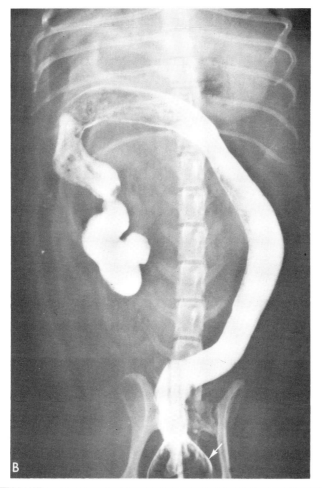

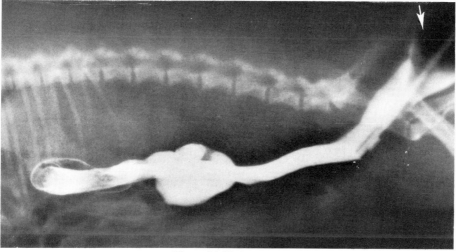

Figure 16–27 *Continued*

(Illustration continued on the following page)

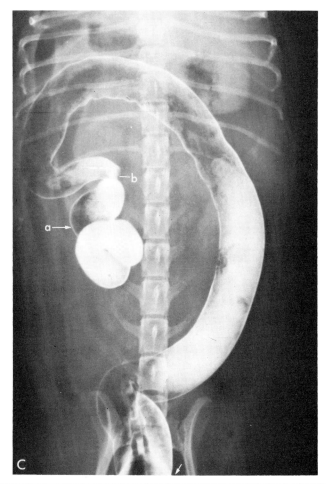

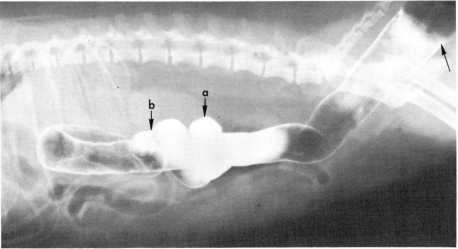

Figure 16–27 *Continued*

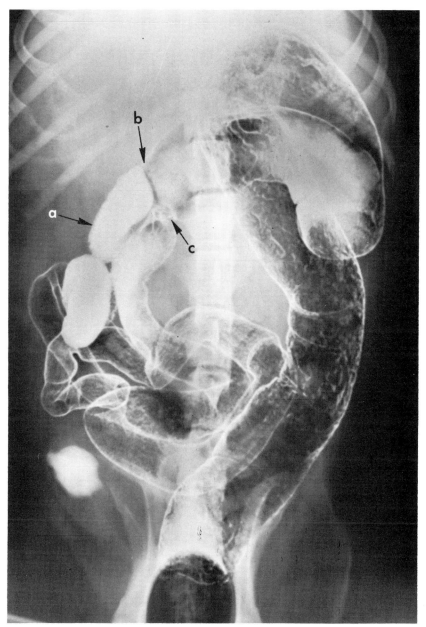

Figure 16–28. Normal variant canine colon. VD projection of double contrast study of a redundant canine colon. Retrograde filling of the ileum and terminal jejunum has occurred. This is not unusual and may be due merely to overfilling of the colon. It is otherwise unremarkable, and is considered a variation of normal. The smooth "shepherd's crook" configuration seen in Figure 16–27 is not present. The cecum (a), cecocolic valve (b) and ileocolic valve (c) are seen. Because of the presence of the multiple convolutions, it is sometimes difficult to remove enough contrast material to perform satisfactory post-evacuation and double contrast studies in patients with this type of colon.

when using one of the water-soluble agents, because no appreciable coating of viable colonic mucosa occurs.

REFERENCES

Allan, G. S., Rendano, V. T., Quick, C. B., and Meunier, P. C.: Gastrografin as a contrast medium in the cat. Vet. Radiol., 20:110, 1979.

Allan, G. S., Wentworth, R. A., Rendano, V. T., Meunier, P. C., and Marmor, P.: The renal excretion of iodine following oral administration of gastrografin to domestic cats. Invest. Radiol., 15:47, 1980.

Bargai, U.: The effect of xylazine hydrochloride on the radiographic appearance of the stomach and intestine in the dog. Vet. Radiol., 23:60, 1982.

Barrett, R. B.: Radiology of the small bowel and colon. Scientific Program, American Veterinary Radiology Society, Boston, 1968.

Crago, W. R.: Use of contrast media in radiological diagnosis. J. Amer. Vet. Rad. Soc., 1:6, 1960.

Douglas, S. W., and Williamson, H. D.: Veterinary Radiological Interpretation. Philadelphia, Lea & Febiger, 1970.

Douglas, S. W., and Williamson, H. D.: Principles of Veterinary Radiography. 2nd ed. Baltimore, Williams & Wilkins Co. 1972.

Dunbar, J. S.: An investigation of effects of opaque media on the lungs with comparison of barium sulfate, lipiodol, and dionosil. Amer. J. Roentgenol., 82:902, 1959.

Evans, S. M., and Laufer, I.: Double contrast gastrography in the normal dog. Vet. Radiol., 22:2, 1981.

Farrow, C. S., and Back, R. T.: Gastrointestinal contrast examination in the cat. Feline Pract., 10:20, 1980.

Ferrucci, J. T., and Benedict, K. T.: Anticholinergic-aided study of the gastrointestinal tract using effervescent substances. Radiol. Clin. N. Amer., 9:25, 1971.

Freeny, P. C.: Double-contrast gastrography of the fundus and cardia: normal landmarks and their pathologic changes. Am. J. Radiol., 133:481, 1979.

Gelfund, D. W.: High density, low viscosity barium for fine mucosal detail on double-contrast upper gastrointestinal examinations. Am. J. Roentgenol., 130:831, 1978.

Gelfund, D. W., and Hachiya, J.: The double contrast examination of the stomach using gas-producing granules and tablets. Radiology, 93:1381, 1969.

Gillette, E. L., Thrall, D. E., and Lebel, J. L.: Carlson's Veterinary Radiology. 3rd ed. Philadelphia, Lea & Febiger, 1977.

Gomez, J. A.: The gastrointestinal contrast study; Methods and interpretation. Vet. Clin. N. Amer., 4:805, 1974.

Grandage, J.: The radiological appearance of stomach gas in the dog. Aust. Vet. J., 50:529, 1974.

Grossman, R. I., Miller, W. T., and Dunn, R. W.: Oral barium sulfate in partial large-bowel obstruction. Radiology, 136:321, 1980.

Kealy, J. K.: Diagnostic Radiology of the Dog and Cat. Philadelphia, W. B. Saunders Co., 1979.

Kelly, M. L.: Silicone-foam molding of the canine ileocolonic junctional zone. Amer. J. Dig. Dis., 12:813, 1967.

Kinsell, R., and Swick, C. R.: Formulary of the Purdue University School of Veterinary Medicine Pharmacy, 1981.

Kneller, S. K., and Lewis, R. E.: Contrast radiography of the normal cat esophagus. J. Amer. Anim. Hosp. Assoc., 9:50, 1973.

Laufer, I.: A simple method for routine double-contrast study of the upper gastrointestinal tract. Radiology, 117:513, 1975.

McAlister, W. H., and Margulis, A. R.: Small bowel transit time of barium sulfate preparations and iodine contrast media in dogs. Am. J. Roentgenol., 91:814, 1964.

Morgan, J. P.: Normal radiographic anatomy of the gastrointestinal tract of the dog. Scientific Proceeding, American Veterinary Medical Association, 101st Annual Meeting. Vol. 155, 1964.

Morgan, J. P.: The upper gastrointestinal tract in the cat: A protocol for contrast radiography. J. Am. Vet. Radiol. Soc., 18:134, 1977.

Morgan, J. P.: The upper gastrointestinal tract in the cat: Normal radiographic appearance using positive contrast medium. Vet. Radiol., 22:159, 1981.

Nelson, S. W., Christoforidis, A. J., and Pratt, P.: Further experience with barium sulfate as a bronchographic contrast medium. Amer. J. Roentgenol., 92:595, 1964.

Nelson, S. W., Christoforidis, A. J., and Roenigk, W. J.: Dangers and fallibilities of iodinated radiopaque media in obstruction of the small bowel. Am. J. Surg., 109:546, 1965.

Nice, C. M.: Bronchography in infants and children: Barium sulfate as a contrast agent. Amer. J. Roentgenol., 91:564, 1964.

O'Brien, T. R.: Radiographic Diagnosis of Abdominal Disorders in the Dog and Cat: Radiographic Interpretation, Clinical Signs, Pathophysiology. Philadelphia, W. B. Saunders Co., 1978.

O'Brien, T. R., Morgan, J. P., and Lebel, J. L.: Pseudo-ulcers in the duodenum of the dog. J. Amer. Vet. Med. Assoc., 155:713, 1969.

Pearson, H., Darke, P. G. G., Gibbs, C., Kelly, D. F., and Orr, C. M.: Reflux esophagitis and stricture formation after anesthesia: A review of seven cases in dogs and cats. J. Small Anim. Pract., 19:507, 1978a.

Pearson, H., Gibbs, C., and Kelly, D. F.: Oesophageal diverticulum formation in the dog. J. Small Anim. Pract., 19:341, 1978b.

Ridgway, R. L., and Suter, P. F.: Clinical and radiographic signs in primary and metastatic esophageal neoplasms of the dog. J. Amer. Vet. Med. Assoc., 174:700, 1979.

Root, C. R., and Lord, P. F.: Linear radiolucent gastrointestinal foreign bodies in cats and dogs: Their radiographic appearance. J. Am. Vet. Radiol. Soc., 12:45, 1971.

Root, C. R., and Morgan, J. P.: Contrast radiology of the upper gastrointestinal tract in the dog—a comparison of micropulverized barium sulfate and U.S.P. barium sulfate suspensions in clinically normal dogs. J. Small Anim. Pract., 10:279, 1969.

Schnelle, G. B.: Radiology in Small Animal Practice. 2nd ed. Evanston, IL, The North American Veterinarian, Inc., 1950.

Seward, C. O.: The use of barium in studying the digestive tract of the dog. J. Amer. Vet. Med. Assoc., 119:125, 1951.

Shook, C. D., and Felson, B.: Inhalation bronchography. Chest, *58*:333, 1970.

Strombeck, D. R.: Small Animal Gastroenterology. Davis, CA, Stonegate Publishing, 1979.

VanStee, E. W., Ward, C. L., and Duffy, M. L.: Recurrent esophageal hairballs in a cat. Vet. Med./ Sm. Anim. Clinician, *75*:1873, 1980.

Vessal, K.: Evaluation of barium and gastrografin as contrast media for suspected esophageal perforation and rupture. 59th Scientific Assembly and Annual Meeting of the Radiological Society of North America, Scientific Program, Vol. 70, 1973.

Watrous, B. J., and Suter, P. F.: Normal swallowing in the dog: A cineradiographic study. J. Amer. Vet. Radiol. Soc., *20*:99, 1979.

Watters, J. W.: Radiography of the canine colon using different contrast agents. J. Amer. Vet. Med. Assoc., *156*:423, 1970.

Woods, C. B., Rawlings, C., Barber, D., and Walker, M.: Esophageal deviation in four English Bulldogs. J. Amer. Vet. Med. Assoc., *172*.934, 1978.

Zezulin, W.: Effective 24-hour preparations for the radiologic examination of the colon. Surg. Clin. N. Amer., *51*:799, 1971.

Zontine, W. J.: Effect of chemical restraint drugs on the passage of barium sulfate through the stomach and duodenum in dogs. J. Amer. Vet. Med. Assoc., *162*:878, 1973.

Contrast Radiography of the Urinary System

In small animal practice, the urinary system is easier to evaluate radiographically than is the gastrointestinal tract. None of the techniques requires general anesthesia, and most of them are less time-consuming than those used for the G.I. tract. Special or expensive equipment is not needed. Contrast radiography can be used to outline the urinary system and can yield valuable information about form, location and (in excretory urography) qualitative function (Kneller, 1974; Feeney et al., 1982; Owens, 1982; Osborne et al., 1969; Ackerman, 1974). Although nephrographic, renal diverticular, pyelographic and ureteral densities have been variously correlated to serum urea nitrogen values and plasma osmolality (Feeney et al., 1980b), quantitative renal function is poorly assessed by contrast radiography, since up to 50 per cent loss of renal function is not detectable by excretory urography (Dure-Smith et al., 1972). All of the contrast radiographic examinations described below may be used by the practitioner and are limited only by the capability to produce good radiographs of the abdomen.

EXCRETORY UROGRAPHY (INTRAVENOUS PYELOGRAPHY, I.V.P., INTRAVENOUS UROGRAPHY)

Indications

Abnormal renal size or shape (determined by palpation or survey radiography) is a common indication for contrast radiography of the kidneys (Gillette et al., 1977; Owens, 1982; Morgan and Silverman, 1982; Biery, 1978; Douglas and Williamson, 1970; Goldman and Freedman, 1971; Lord et al., 1974; McEwan, 1971; Osborne et al., 1969; Watters, 1980b). Contrast radiography of the kidneys, ureters and urinary bladder is also justified when there are suspected renal masses, sublumbar masses, prostatic masses or other intrapelvic masses, or when there is persistent hematuria (Ackerman, 1974; Watters, 1980b) and other forms of abnormal urine (Morgan and Silverman, 1982). This study can be used to verify the presence of renal or ureteral calculi (Finco et al., 1970; Walker and Douglas, 1970). Other conditions that can be demonstrated by excretory urography include hydronephrosis (either congenital or acquired), ureteral ectopia (Pearson and Gibbs, 1971; Walker and Douglas, 1970; Johnston et al., 1977; Osborne et al., 1975; Owen, 1973), ureterocele (Pearson and Gibbs, 1971; Scott et al., 1974), exstrophy of the bladder (Hobson and Ader, 1979), multiple congenital urinary tract abnormalities (Schwartz et al., 1974; Bargai and Bark, 1982), renal ectopia (Johnson, 1979), and renal and ureteral duplication (O'Handley et al., 1979). Traumatic rupture of ureters may be visualized and characterized (Burt and Root, 1971; Lord et al., 1974; Pechman, 1982; Selcer, 1982). When catheterization is impossible or difficult, excretory urography can be used to evaluate the urinary bladder (Borthwick and Robbie, 1971).

Contraindications

In humans, excretory urography is contraindicated in severely debilitated patients, especially in the presence of marked dehydration (Talner, 1972). Presumably, the same is true in animals. High arterial concentrations of certain older types of intravascular contrast materials have been shown to be contraindicated because of renal damage (Andrew et al., 1964; Dean et al., 1964; Killen et al., 1962; Luttwak et al., 1961; Stokes and Bernard, 1961), but there is little,

374

if any, danger of renal toxicity with today's contrast media even if given in high doses (Lord et al., 1974; Stokes and Bernard, 1961) or to an uremic patient, unless that patient is severely dehydrated (Talner, 1972). In fact, diagnostic excretory urography in man is possible and safe even in the presence of markedly elevated creatinine or blood urea nitrogen (B.U.N.) levels using dosages in excess of 650 mg/kg of body weight (Bosniak and Schweizer, 1972).

Preparation of Patient

Standard clinical pathologic tests should be completed if they have not been done as part of the animal's medical work-up. Recent survey radiographs of the abdomen are necessary. The animal should be fasted for 24 hours and should have a thorough enema. Warm, soapy enema solution should not be used, as enemas given in this manner generally result in persistence of considerable luminal gas. Rather, the colon should be flushed repeatedly with isotonic salt solution (8 tsp table salt/gallon tap water or 45 g table salt/5 L tap water) at slightly less than body temperature. Using this procedure, evacuation will be more complete and there will be less residual gas than after using warm soapy enema solution. Water may be withheld for 12 hours if the patient is not severely dehydrated and if short-term water deprivation can be tolerated by the animal, since mild dehydration facilitates opacification of the collecting system (McClennan and Becker, 1971; McClennan et al., 1971; Talner, 1972) in spite of the fact that nephrographic density is not affected by patient hydration (Biery, 1978). Sedation or tranquilization should be avoided unless absolutely necessary, and the urinary bladder should be empty, since this induces diuresis (Morgan and Silverman, 1982).

Materials

Many different types of intravenous infusion devices are satisfactory for delivery of the contrast material. One of the longer indwelling devices (Angiocath Intravenous Placement Unit, Deseret Pharmaceutical Co.; I. V. Intrafusor, Sorenson Research Co.) should be used, since perivascular injection of urographic contrast materials results in severe tissue damage and probable slough.

The type of contrast material used is a matter of personal preference, although the tri-iodinated preparations seem to be the most popular agents at the present time (Biery, 1978). Of these, mixtures of sodium and meglumine diatrizoates are recommended (Renovist II, Sodium and Meglumine Diatrizoate Injection, Squibb and Sons; Hypaque-M, 75%, Sodium and Meglumine Diatrizoates, Sterile Aqueous Injection, Winthrop Laboratories), since they seem to provide an acceptable combination of radiopacity and patient tolerance. Normally, the tri-iodinated contrast agents are nearly exclusively excreted by glomerular filtration, over 99 per cent being eliminated renally and less than 1 per cent being eliminated by alimentary and hepatic routes (Talner, 1972). Although certain types of intravascular contrast materials have been found to be nephrotoxic if injected into the aorta or renal arteries (Andrew et al., 1964; Dean et al., 1964; Luttwak et al., 1961; Stokes and Bernard, 1961), the diatrizoate salts are safe even in uremia, provided the patient is not severely dehydrated (Talner, 1972). It has been found that satisfactory opacification of the urinary system of an uremic patient often can be accomplished by increasing the dose of contrast material (Voltz et al., 1971), since renal opacification is directly related to the amount of contrast material in the blood (Dure-Smith et al., 1972; McEwan, 1971). Nephrographic density is a function of plasma concentration of contrast material, renal tubular osmolality and glomerular filtration rate (Bosniak and Schweizer, 1972). Sodium diatrizoate alone may cause the patient to vomit, but (possibly because of its lower molecular weight) it produces a higher renal concentration of iodine than the meglumine salt alone (Dacie and Fry, 1971). The method used will determine whether or not a 5 per cent glucose solution will be needed. If a procedure requiring abdominal compression is used, a compression device must be available. A simple compression device can be made by grooving a sponge or foam pad on one side (to accommodate the penis in male dogs). The grooved pad is placed securely on the ventral abdomen just cranial to the brim of the pelvis and is held in that position by a tight encircling elastic bandage or similar wrapping material placed around the caudal

Table 16–5. IODINE CONCENTRATIONS OF VARIOUS EXCRETORY UROGRAPHIC MEDIA

Product	mgI/ml
Hypaque, 50% (Winthrop Laboratories)	300
Hypaque-M, 75% (Winthrop Laboratories)	385
Renovist II (Squibb and Sons)	310
Renografin-60 (Squibb and Sons)	288
Renografin-76 (Squibb and Sons)	370

abdomen, just caudal to the wings of the ilia and just cranial to the pubis. Alternatively, conventional compression bands, which are provided as accessories to some x-ray tables, may be used. These require that the patient be held in dorsal recumbency during the compression phase of the procedure, with the compression band passing across the ventral abdomen, immediately cranial to the pubis (Douglas and Williamson, 1972; Suter, 1973).

Dosage of Contrast Material. The dosage of contrast material depends upon several factors—the concentration of iodine in the contrast medium (Table 16–5), the type of excretory urography to be done (Table 16–6), and the renal function of the patient (as evaluated by determination of B.U.N. and/or creatinine levels). If the contrast material is delivered rapidly or as a bolus, the dose should be 425 to 850 mgI/kg of body weight. If the high volume, prolonged or drip infusion technique is used, 1200 mgI/kg of body weight should be administered. Maximum dose probably should not exceed 35 g.

In uremic animals, the recommended dose may be safely doubled (up to 35 g). Arbitrarily, this should be done if the B.U.N. is in excess of 40 mg/100 ml. In the author's experience, satisfactory concentration of contrast material in the presence of markedly elevated B.U.N. and/or creatinine levels may be considerably delayed; excretory urography, in these instances, is usually not rewarding.

Procedure (Table 16–6)

Low Volume, Rapid Infusion Technique With Abdominal Compression. The intravenous catheter is placed in a convenient peripheral vein, and the compression device is applied. The total dose of contrast material (425 mgI/kg) is administered rapidly. Ventrodorsal and lateral radiographs of the abdomen are made immediately and at 1, 3, 5, 10

and 15 minutes. Abdominal compression should be released just prior to the 10 minute film. The purpose of the compression device is to press the urinary bladder against the spine and occlude the terminal ureters, causing stasis and accumulation of opacified urine in the renal pelves and proximal ureters. Some feel that abdominal compression is not physiologic and introduces artifacts (Lord et al., 1974; Owens, 1982), such as tortuosity, dilation and distention of the obstructed ureters and distortion of the renal pelvis. However, in radiographs made after the compression band is released, relatively normal ureteral course and diameter should be appreciated. Patient discomfort during compression is usually well tolerated and, contrary to one opinion (Owens, 1982), does not require anesthesia or other forms of chemical restraint. VD oblique radiographs are necessary to visualize the terminal ureters.

Low Volume, Rapid Infusion Technique, Without Abdominal Compression. Using this method (Lord et al., 1974), the contrast material (850 mgI/kg) is delivered as rapidly as possible through a large intravenous catheter after the patient has been positioned in VD recumbency over the cassette. Ten seconds after injection commences, the first exposure (VD only) is made. After the first radiograph, VD and lateral radiographs are made as soon as possible, and at 1 minute, at 3 to 5 minutes and at 15 minutes after the contrast medium was injected. VD oblique radiographs are necessary to visualize the terminal ureters. Often an arteriographic phase is seen on the radiograph made 10 seconds after beginning injection of contrast material; at the same time, the vascular nephrogram phase is appreciated. Abdominal compression is not done, therefore avoiding ureteral distention and tortuosity. Ureteral opacification is usually much less pronounced with this technique than with one of the techniques employing abdominal compression.

Low Volume, Slow Infusion Technique, Without Abdominal Compression. Using this technique, the contrast material (425 mgI/kg) is infused over a 2 to 3 minute period. Lateral and VD radiographs are made immediately and at 3, 5, 10 and 15 minutes after the injection is complete. VD oblique radiographs are necessary to visualize the terminal ureters. No ureteral artifacts are seen, but visualization of the collecting systems may be poor even if renal clearance and ureteral function are normal.

High Volume, Prolonged or Drip Infusion Technique, With Abdominal Compression. Contrary to one opinion (Thrall, 1980), this method is felt to produce the best visualization of the urinary system (Borthwick and Robbie, 1969; Suter, 1973; Walker and Douglas, 1970). It has the advantage of requiring fewer radiographs than the other procedures, allowing simultaneous visualization of the kidneys, ureters and urinary bladder.

This procedure is normally less expensive and less time-consuming than any of the rapid infusion techniques employing both lateral and ventrodorsal projections, since only six radiographs are usually required to complete the study and very little time is required to apply the compression bandage. Additionally, the animal need not be restrained on its back while contrast material is being administered. The calculated dose of contrast ma-

---

Table 16–6. SUMMARY OF EXCRETORY UROGRAPHY PROCEDURES

1. Fast the animal for 24 hours and give a thorough enema.
2. Obtain current survey radiographs of the abdomen.
3. *Low volume, rapid infusion technique with abdominal compression:*
   a. Place an indwelling catheter in a convenient peripheral vein.
   b. Apply a compression band just cranial to the pubis.
   c. Rapidly administer 425 mgI/kg of one of the mixtures of sodium and meglumine diatrizoates intravenously.
   d. Make lateral and VD radiographs of the abdomen immediately and at 1, 3 and 5 minutes.
   e. Remove the compression band immediately prior to the 10 minute radiographs and make lateral and VD abdominal radiographs at 10 and 15 minutes.
   f. VD oblique radiographs of the pelvis made immediately after removal of the compression band are necessary for visualization of the terminal ureters.
4. *Low volume, rapid infusion technique without abdominal compression:*
   a. Place an indwelling catheter in a convenient peripheral vein.
   b. Position the animal over the cassette in dorsal recumbency.
   c. Inject 850 mgI/kg of one of the mixtures of sodium and meglumine diatrizoate intravenously as rapidly as possible.
   d. The first radiograph (VD only) is made 10 seconds after injection is commenced.
   e. Make VD and lateral abdominal radiographs as soon as possible and at 1 minute, at 3 to 5 minutes and at 15 minutes following injection.
   f. VD oblique views of the pelvis may be made if terminal ureters are of special interest.
5. *Low volume, slow infusion technique without abdominal compression:*
   a. Place an indwelling catheter in a convenient peripheral vein.
   b. Over a 2 to 3 minute period of time,
   infuse 425 mgI/kg of one of the mixtures of sodium and meglumine diatrizoates intravenously.
   c. When the contrast material has been injected, make lateral and VD radiographs of the abdomen immediately and at 3, 5, 10 and 15 minutes after completion of injection of the contrast material.
   d. VD oblique views of the pelvis may be made if terminal ureters are of special interest.
6. *High volume, drip infusion technique with abdominal compression:*
   a. Place an indwelling catheter in a convenient peripheral vein.
   b. Mix 1200 mgI/kg body weight of one of the mixtures of sodium and meglumine diatrizoates (maximum dose, 35 g) with an equal volume of 5% dextrose and water.
   c. By drip infusion, administer the mixture over a 10 minute period of time, accelerating the rate of infusion near the end of this period if necessary to insure injection of all the contrast material within the specified time. Alternatively, administer the contrast material with a large syringe, injecting 1/40 of the total volume every 15 seconds.
   d. At the end of the infusion, make radiographs of the abdomen in both projections.
   e. Immediately apply a compression band to the caudal abdomen.
   f. If renal function was determined to be normal, repeat radiographs in both projections 10 minutes later.
   g. If renal function was abnormal, make radiographs of the abdomen 20 minutes later.
   h. Remove the compression band.
   i. Additional radiographs after removal of the compression band are optional. VD oblique films of the trigone should be made at this time if the terminal ureters are of special interest.

terial (1200 mgI/kg, not to exceed 35 g) is mixed with an equal volume of 5 per cent glucose solution, and is administered over a 10 minute period through a suitable intravenous catheter. The total volume of contrast-containing solution can be administered with one or more large syringes, injecting 1/40 of the total volume each 15 seconds. This insures a relatively uniform delivery rate. Alternatively, the contrast preparation may be administered by drip infusion. The duration of infusion should be approximately 10 minutes in order to allow the entire urinary system to be satisfactorily opacified. Contrast material remaining approximately 8 minutes after the beginning of infusion may be administered within the last 2 minutes. Lateral and VD radiographs are made of the abdomen at the completion of administration of the contrast material, and a compression device is applied. Placement of the compression device is critical if consistent ureteral compression is to be obtained. It must encircle the abdomen caudal to the iliac crests and cranial to the pubis. If renal opacification is determined to be normal, radiographs of the abdomen are repeated 10 minutes later, and the compression band is removed. If renal clearance is radiographically suboptimal, the compression band remains in place and radiographs are made 20 minutes later. When renal and proximal ureteral opacification has been determined to be acceptable, the compression device is removed and the radiographs are repeated, allowing visualization of the caudal ureters. If the vesicoureteral junctions are to be visualized, VD oblique radiographs of the pelvic region must be made immediately after removal of the compression device.

Complications

If the contrast material is injected too rapidly, vomiting may be induced, especially when a contrast medium containing only the sodium salt of the diatrizoate molecule is used. Vomiting is less common when a combination of the sodium and meglumine diatrizoates is used, but it can occur. Emesis should not effect the outcome of the study, but it may cause a slight delay in the filming sequence.

Because perivascular deposition or significant extravasation of the contrast material

will cause a severe slough (McAlister and Palmer, 1971), an indwelling type of venous catheter is strongly recommended. If perivascular deposition of media occurs, immediate local infiltration of the perivascular swelling with sterile saline, lidocaine HCl and a corticosteroid is helpful in reducing the severity of the reaction.

Anaphylactoid reactions to the contrast agent are rare in animals and man. In human studies, most radiologists no longer administer a preliminary "test dose" of the contrast material because reactions are uncommon and often delayed. Reactions to the "test dose" are often as severe as reactions to the entire dose. In man, the incidence of severe reactions may be lessened by giving atropine sulfate prior to injection of contrast material (Svendsen and Wilson, 1971).

Pancytopenia is reported to have resulted from the administration of diatrizoates in man (Stemerman et al., 1971). This has not been reported in dogs or cats.

It has been suggested that abdominal compression is potentially hazardous in the presence of an abdominal mass (Thrall, 1980). However, such an abdominal mass, especially if large enough to complicate abdominal compression, would be detected by survey radiography. Its presence probably should suggest employment of a non-compressive excretory urographic procedure, even though intraperitoneal pressure is only slightly increased during compression of the caudal abdomen (Olin and Rees, 1973). Further, although the diagnostic accuracy of excretory urography with abdominal compression has not been objectively shown to be superior to that without abdominal compression, as has been pointed out (Thrall, 1980), the reverse is also true. The anatomic structures are unequivocally better visualized, however, when using abdominal compression than when abdominal compression is omitted during excretory urography; therefore, the author is confident that diagnostic accuracy can be proved to be superior when using caudal abdominal compression during excretory urography.

Compression of the caudal abdomen produces a transient rise in renal blood flow and decreases the glomerular filtration rate within 15 minutes (Olin and Rees, 1973). Therefore, in spite of the fact that ureteral compression causes stasis and dilation of the diverticulae, the renal pelves and the proximal ureters, prolonged ureteral compression appears to be counterproductive.

Results of urinalysis, particularly specific gravity, obtained after excretory urography should be considered inaccurate (Feeney et al., 1980); normal results probably cannot be obtained for at least 8 hours, even if the urinary bladder is completely emptied after excretory urography.

Normal Findings (Figs. 16–29 and 16–30)

Both kidneys should be visualized. The left kidney in the dog is normally located caudomedial to the spleen, adjacent to the second, third, fourth and fifth lumbar vertebrae (Osborne et al., 1969; Kealy, 1979), while the right kidney normally is located approximately half its length further craniad, at the level of T13 to L3. Renal position is much more variable in the cat. Normal kidney length is approximately 2½ adjacent vertebral bodies in the dog (Douglas and Williamson, 1970; Root and Scott, 1971) and approximately 2 adjacent vertebral bodies in the cat (Lord et al., 1974). In both species, this measurement includes the widths of the interposed intervertebral disc spaces. The radiographic ratio of kidney length to the length of L2 has been determined to be approximately 2.5:1 to 3.5:1 in the dog (Finco et al., 1971) and 2.4:1 to 3.0:1 in the cat (Barrett and Kneller, 1972). This method eliminates the widths of the intervertebral spaces but apparently has not been objectively compared to previously used guidelines for assessment of kidney size. The kidneys should be smooth in outline (Kealy, 1979). Feline kidneys normally are more rounded than those of the dog. The renal cortical shadows should be diffusely opaque, indicating uniform function of all areas.

Both pelves and both ureters should be visualized. If compression is not used, these structures may be difficult to see; because of long peristaltic waves, only portions of each ureter may be visualized. The ureters should be straight in the absence of obstruction or abdominal compression. The pelves and collecting systems will be faint densities, often incomplete in outline. However, if a compression device is applied, the collecting systems, renal pelves and proximal ureters are well delineated and slightly dilated; the

ureters may be slightly tortuous, owing to their increased length from overdistention.

Whether or not abdominal compression is used, visualization of the terminal ureters is usually poor, unless supplemental oblique projections of the pelvic region are made. The urinary bladder should become progressively opaque and should contain no filling defects. The bladder wall should be smooth in outline and uniform in thickness. Urinary bladder shape may reflect extrinsic pressures of adjacent structures unless fully distended.

CONTRAST RADIOGRAPHY OF THE URINARY BLADDER (CYSTOGRAPHY, PNEUMOCYSTOGRAPHY, CYSTOGRAM-PNEUMOCYSTOGRAM)

Indications

The most common indication for contrast radiography of the urinary bladder is hematuria (Park, 1974), especially if it is accompanied by vesical tenesmus. However, straining to urinate without hematuria is also a valid indication for this study. Pneumocystography (Rhodes and Biery, 1967) or cystography may be the only methods by which radiolucent urinary calculi can be demonstrated. Contrast radiography is important for definitive localization of the urinary bladder in instances of perineal or other herniae (Gillette et al., 1977; Park, 1974), caudal abdominal or pelvic masses (Douglas and Williamson, 1972), prostatic enlargement (Douglas and Williamson, 1972; Leav and Ling, 1968; Pearson and Gibbs, 1971) or suspected rupture of the bladder (Gillette et al., 1977; Owens, 1982). Suspected patent urachus also may be evaluated by opacification of the urinary bladder (Greene and Bohning, 1971; Pearson and Gibbs, 1971).

Contraindications

Contrast radiography of the urinary bladder is unrewarding and possibly contraindicated in the presence of massive bladder enlargement resulting from atony, since true atony is most often due to neurologic dysfunction rather than obstructive disease. Although contrast radiography is not truly con-

Text continued on page 386.

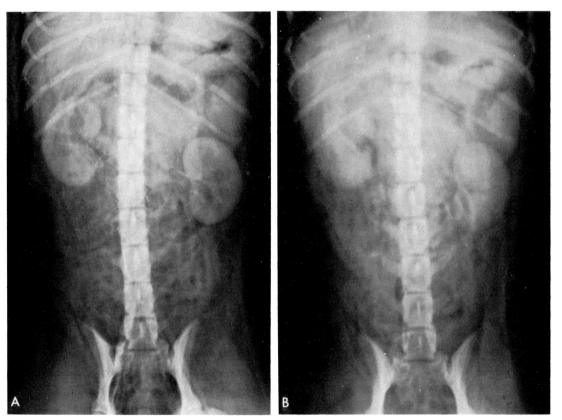

Figure 16–29. Normal excretory urogram, low volume, rapid injection without compression. Radiographs of the abdomen of a normal dog made 8 seconds (*A*), 15 seconds (*B*), 3 minutes (*C*), 10 minutes (*D*), and 15 minutes (*E*) after rapid intravenous injection of organic iodide solution containing 450 mg of organic iodine per kg of body weight (using a mixture of sodium and meglumine diatrizoates). At 8 seconds (A) and at 15 seconds (B), the renal outlines (nephrogram phase) are well visualized. At 3 minutes, faint opacification of the renal collecting systems and ureters (pyelogram-ureterogram phase) is seen. At 10 (D) and 15 minutes (E), there is progressive opacification of the urinary bladder.

(Illustration continued on opposite page)

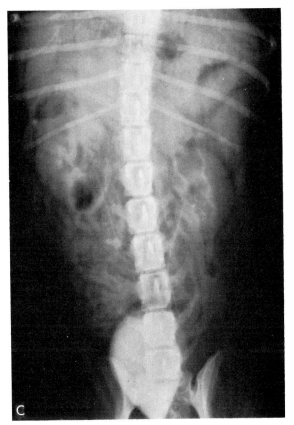

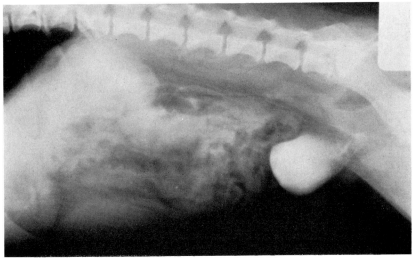

Figure 16–29 *Continued*

(Illustration continued on the following page)

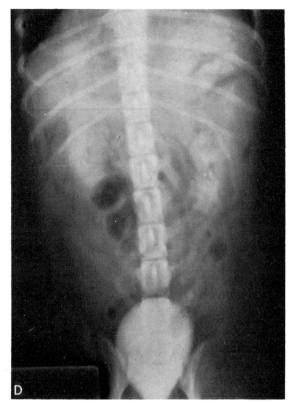

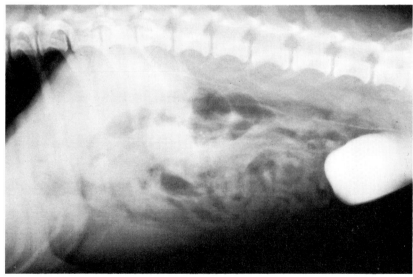

Figure 16–29 *Continued*

(Illustration continued on opposite page)

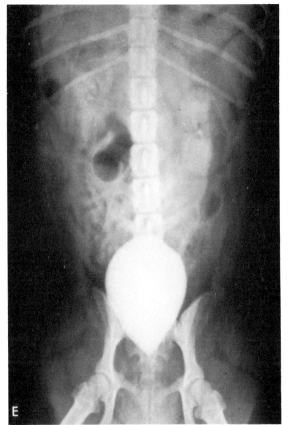

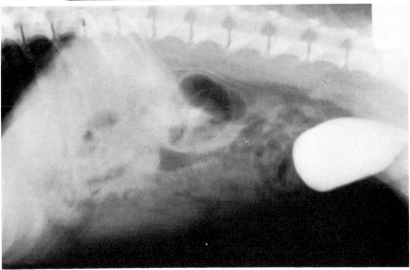

Figure 16–29 *Continued*

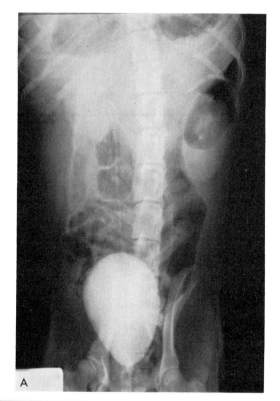

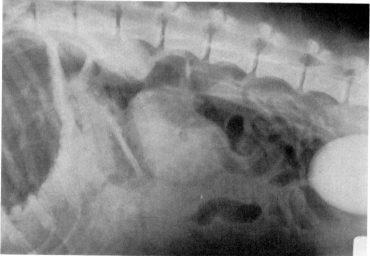

Figure 16–30. Normal excretory urogram — high volume drip infusion with compression. *A,* VD and lateral abdominal radiographs of a normal dog at the completion of slow intravenous injection of organic iodide containing 850 mg of iodine per kg of body weight (using a mixture of sodium and meglumine diatrizoates). The kidneys, ureters and urinary bladder are faintly opacified. *B,* VD and lateral abdominal radiographs of the same dog 20 minutes after commencement of injection (10 minutes after cessation of infusion and application of a tight compression bandage around the caudal abdomen). The renal collecting systems, ureters, and urinary bladder are distended and well visualized.

(Illustration continued on opposite page)

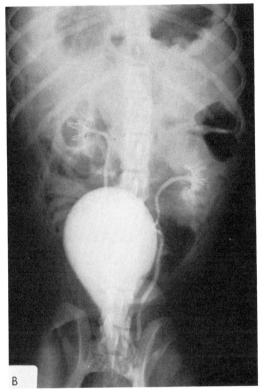

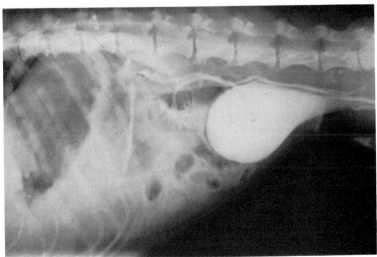

Figure 16–30 *Continued*

traindicated in the presence of radiopaque cystic calculi, it is usually not necessary, since the wall of the urinary bladder may be viewed directly during subsequent cystotomy, or since prescription dietary therapy alone may be effective in controlling clinical signs.

Pneumocystography in which luminal pressure may have been increased much above normal physiologic levels to accomplish distention of the urinary bladder appears to have been associated with fatal air embolism (Zontine and Andrews, 1978; Thayer et al., 1980; Ackerman et al., 1972). This seems particularly true in the presence of damaged urinary mucosal surfaces. Under no circumstances should manual urethral occlusion be used to forcibly distend a thickened, inflamed urinary bladder.

Preparation of Patient

The patient should be fasted for 12 to 24 hours (Gillette et al., 1977; Park, 1974) and a cleansing enema should be given (Gillette et al., 1977; Park, 1974; Rhodes and Biery, 1967). As in most other contrast procedures involving abdominal viscera, commercial hypertonic enema solutions usually are not thorough enough, and warm soapy enemas leave too much gas in the bowel. Therefore, isotonic saline solution (8 tsp table salt per gallon tap water or 45 g table salt per 5 L tap water), slightly less than body temperature, should be used for cleansing of the colon. A current urinalysis is recommended before opacification of the urinary bladder, since it will provide information useful in differential diagnosis. Survey radiographs of the abdomen are required (Gillette et al., 1977).

Materials

A three-way stopcock, a catheter adapter (Rubber Catheter Adapter, Rusch, Inc.), a male catheter (Ureteral Catheters, 3–10 French, Rusch, Inc.) and a large syringe are necessary for performing contrast radiography of the urinary bladder. Rigid female catheters are not needed because females may be easily and safely catheterized with large male catheters, with reduced risk of puncturing the urinary bladder or lacerating the urethra. Flexible male catheters also appear to be more comfortable and therefore may be allowed to remain in place during the study.

Any of the diatrizoate media (Hypaque-M, 75%, Winthrop Laboratories; Renovist II, Squibb and Sons) may be used for cystography, but must be diluted to 5 to 10 per cent iodine (W/V). Sodium iodide solution (Park, 1974) probably should not be used because it causes irritation of the bladder mucosa (Breton et al., 1978). Further, it will produce a transient but severe peritonitis if it gains access to the peritoneal cavity (Park, 1978). Room air is used for pneumocystography.

Dosage of Contrast Material. The urinary bladder must be moderately distended with contrast medium. This usually requires 6 to 12 ml of medium per kg of body weight. The desired concentration of iodine in the urinary bladder may be accomplished in several ways. The easiest and most accurate method is to empty the bladder completely before instilling a known concentration (5 to 10% iodine, W/V) of contrast material.

Procedure (Table 16–7)

In veterinary medicine, often either positive contrast cystography or negative contrast cystography (pneumocystography) is performed (Kealy, 1979; Morgan and Silverman, 1982). Unfortunately, this often results in obtaining less than maximal information about the character of the wall of the urinary bladder. It is recommended, therefore, that pneumocystography routinely follow positive contrast cystography, since the mucosal surface of the urinary bladder is best appreciated when the bladder is opacified and the thickness of its wall is best seen when contrasted with air. Cystography alone is indicated only

Table 16–7. SUMMARY OF CYSTOGRAPHY–PNEUMOCYSTOGRAPHY PROCEDURE

1. Fast the patient for 12 to 24 hours.
2. Give a cleansing enema (see text).
3. Obtain current survey radiographs of the abdomen.
4. Catheterize and empty urinary bladder.
5. Instill 6 to 12 ml/kg of body weight of 5 to 10% organic iodide solution. PALPATE THE URINARY BLADDER WHILE FILLING TO AVOID OVERDISTENTION OR RUPTURE.
6. Make lateral and VD radiographs of the caudal abdomen, leaving the catheter in place.
7. Remove the iodide solution and replace it with an equal volume of air.
8. Make lateral and VD radiographs of the caudal abdomen.

if rupture of the urinary bladder is suspected. Either cystography or pneumocystography will verify suspected rupture of the urinary bladder. Cystography, however, sometimes clearly delineates the site of disruption of the bladder wall.

A catheter is introduced, as aseptically as possible (Park, 1974, 1978), and as much of the urine as possible is removed. Several authors recommend instilling 5 to 10 ml of 2 per cent lidocaine solution to minimize pain and spasm during filling of the urinary bladder with contrast material (Park, 1978; Morgan and Silverman, 1982). The urinary bladder is then filled with 6 to 12 ml/kg of body weight of a 5 to 10 per cent solution (W/V) of one of the mixtures of sodium and meglumine diatrizoate. Filling of the urinary bladder must be monitored by abdominal palpation, since luminal masses, mural masses and severely thickened urinary bladders will not permit instillation of the entire calculated volume of contrast medium (Morgan and Silverman, 1982; Park, 1978). After the urinary bladder is filled with an appropriate volume of contrast material, radiographs of the caudal abdomen are made in the lateral and VD projections. The contrast material is then replaced with an equal volume of air, and the radiographs of the caudal abdomen are repeated.

Complications

Overdistention of the urinary bladder will lead to rupture. This is not a common sequelum to contrast radiography of the urinary bladder if normal precautions are used and recommended volumes of contrast media are not exceeded. However, if there are large masses within the urinary bladder, 6 to 12 ml/kg may cause overdistention and may lead to rupture. Palpation of the urinary bladder during filling is therefore strongly advised. Careless catheterization can lead to urethral trauma (Owens, 1982; Park, 1978) or cystitis, but these problems can be minimized by using caution and antiseptic technique.

Fatal air embolism has been reported after pneumocystography in cats (Zontine and Andrews, 1978; Thayer et al., 1980) and in a dog (Ackerman et al., 1972). Care must be taken not to increase the luminal tension significantly above physiological pressures, especially if the urinary mucosa is thought to be inflamed and/or the urinary bladder is difficult to distend.

Normal Findings (Fig. 16–31)

The pitfalls of cystographic interpretation and the common radiographic signs of disease have been described (Park, 1974, 1978). If normal, the urinary bladder should be uniformly distended. Its wall should be intact and should be thin and regular in width. There should be no mural or luminal filling defects. Contrast material should be present only in the lumen of the urinary system and should not fill the prostatic ducts in the male. In the female, the apex of the urinary bladder is more pointed than in the male. The distended urinary bladder displaces the small bowel cranially and dorsally. Ventrally, the urinary bladder is usually in contact with the ventral body wall. The colon is usually displaced to the left, but in some animals it may be displaced to the right if the bladder is markedly distended, if the colon is redundant, or if the animal had been placed in left lateral recumbency for several minutes immediately before ventrodorsal radiography. Retrograde opacification of one or both ureters may be a normal finding (Christie, 1971, 1973a, b; Newman et al., 1973). This finding is most common in young dogs (Christie, 1971, 1973a, b) and in patients positioned in lateral recumbency during distention of the urinary bladder with contrast material (Newman et al., 1973).

URETHROGRAPHY (RETROGRADE URETHROGRAPHY, PROSTATIC URETHROGRAPHY)

Indications

Clinical signs commonly associated with urethrographically demonstrable lesions include dysuria, tenesmus and/or hematuria (Ticer et al., 1980a; Morgan and Silverman, 1982).

Retrograde urethrography is indicated when there is suspicion of penile or extrapelvic urethral disease, when urethral catheterization is difficult or impossible, or when there may have been trauma to the prostatic, pelvic, or peripheral portions of the urethra (Kleine and Thornton, 1971; Park, 1974; Zontine, 1975; Johnston et al., 1977; Acker-

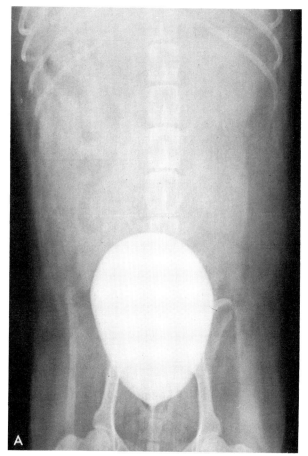

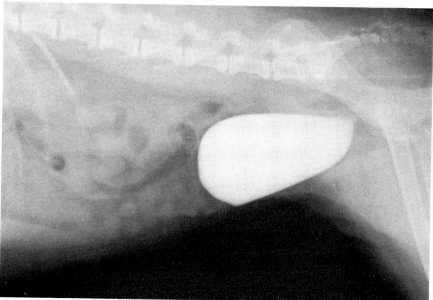

Figure 16–31. Normal cystogram-pneumocystogram. *A,* VD and lateral radiographs of the abdomen of a normal female dog after distention of the urinary bladder with 9 ml of 7.5% organic iodide solution per kg of body weight. *B,* VD and lateral radiographs of the same dog after replacement of the iodine solution with an equal volume of room air. The wall of the urinary bladder is smooth and uniform in width. No mural or luminal filling defects are seen. The tip of the catheter (arrow) is seen in the apex of the urinary bladder during the pneumocystogram.

(Illustration continued on opposite page)

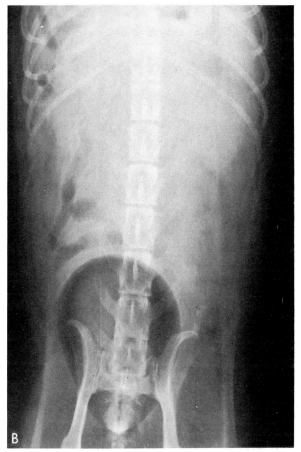

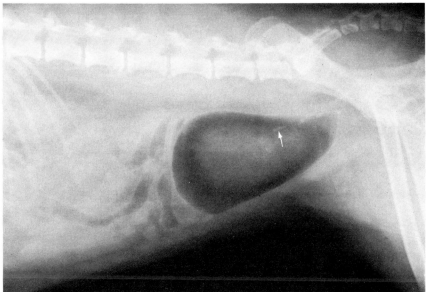

Figure 16–31 *Continued*

man, 1980; Ticer et al., 1980a; Watters, 1980a; Pechman, 1982; Selcer, 1982). Severe pelvic trauma, in which one or both of the pubes are fractured and displaced, is a strong indication for retrograde urethrography (Kleine and Thornton, 1971; Ticer et al., 1980a), especially if the patient has hematuria. In rare fractures of the *os penis,* retrograde opacification of the urethra can determine whether or not the damage includes disruption of the urethral mucosal lining or extrinsic compression of the urethra.

Prostatic urethrography, on the other hand, should be reserved for those instances in which prostatic disease is considered likely. This study, although sometimes done as an independent procedure in male dogs, is usually part of the standard cystogram-pneumocystogram described above.

Contraindications

There are few contraindications for urethrography. Retrograde urethral filling requiring high pressure should be avoided, particularly if loss of urethral mucosal integrity is suspected (Park, 1978). In such cases, surgical exploration of the obstructed portion of the urethra is indicated. In the presence of severe urethral hemorrhage, hemostasis should be accomplished before contrast radiography of the urethra is performed. Urethrography can be performed in female dogs (Johnston et al., 1977; Ticer et al., 1980b) but is difficult because the urethra is relatively short in length and wide in diameter.

Preparation of Patient

Cleansing of only the terminal colon and rectum usually is satisfactory, and the commercial hypertonic enema solutions are adequate for this purpose, if properly administered. Fasting is not necessary unless studies of the kidneys and urinary bladder are also needed (Johnston et al., 1977). Survey radiography of the pelvis and perineum in the lateral and VD projections is required.

Materials

An organic iodide solution is recommended, and the diatrizoates (Renovist II,

Squibb and Sons; Hypaque-M 75%, Winthrop Laboratories) are the agents of choice. Depending upon the portion of the urethra to be studied, either an 8 to 12 French gauge pediatric Foley catheter (Pediatric Gilbert Foley Catheters, 8 to 12 French, Bard Hospital Division, C.R. Bard, Inc.) or a male urethral catheter (Ureteral Catheters, 3 to 10 French, Rusch, Inc.) is needed. If the Foley catheter is chosen, 2 per cent lidocaine HCl solution and gel (Xylocaine HCl Injection or Gel, 2%, Ayerst Laboratories) are also required. With either catheter, an appropriate catheter adapter (Rubber Catheter Adapters, Rusch, Inc.) and a three-way stopcock are necessary.

Dosage of Contrast Material. The amount of contrast material is not critical, but the urethra must be distended at the time the films are made. This usually requires 5 to 10 ml of contrast material.

Procedure (Table 16–8)

Retrograde Urethrography

The Foley catheter is used to administer the medium to the extrapelvic or penile portion of the urethra. Its introduction may be facilitated through the use of a stylet to produce rigidity (Johnston et al., 1977), but this is usually unnecessary and should not be used unless catheterization is impossible without it, since air bubbles are usually introduced into the lumen when the stylet is withdrawn. The catheter lumen is filled with 2 per cent lidocaine HCl solution (for males) or with contrast medium (for females) prior to catheterization in order to eliminate air bubbles (Ticer et al., 1980a, b). The syringe should remain on the catheter. Using a small amount of the lidocaine gel for lubrication and topical anesthesia, the catheter is inserted so that its cuff is within that portion of the urethra contained by the os penis. In the female, catheterization should be visualized by using a speculum, and the catheter tip is inserted an additional centimeter after the retention bulb enters the urethra (Ticer et al., 1980a, b). The stylet (if used) is removed, 2 to 3 ml of 2 per cent lidocaine HCl solution or gel are slowly injected, and the cuff is gently inflated. Several more milliliters of lidocaine HCl are injected slowly to topically anesthetize the proximal urethral mucosa. Topical anesthesia is not necessary

Table 16–8. SUMMARY OF
URETHROGRAPHY PROCEDURES

1. Fasting is not necessary, but cleansing the colon is advised.
2. *Retrograde Urethrography:*
   a. Introduce an appropriate Foley catheter into the penile urethra, using lidocaine HCl gel and a stylet if necessary.
   b. Instill several milliliters of lidocaine HCl solution or gel into the penile urethra through the Foley catheter. Inflate the cuff.
   c. Slowly inject 2 to 5 ml of lidocaine HCl solution into the urethra.
   d. Slowly inject 5 to 10 ml of the contrast material with the animal positioned for lateral radiography.
   e. As the injection is terminated, while the urethra is pressurized by the injection, make an exposure, centering on the perineum.
   f. Repeat the injection with the patient in a slightly oblique VD position if desired.
3. *Prostatic Urethrography:*
   a. During positive contrast cystography, deliver 5 to 10 ml of 5 to 10% organic iodide solution or opacified urine into the prostatic urethra (the location of which is 1 to 3 cm distal to the point at which aspiration is not possible during slow withdrawal of the catheter from the urinary bladder).
   b. Radiograph the prostatic urethra in the lateral projection as the injection is completed, while the urethra is still under pressure.

in the female (Ticer et al., 1980a, b). Gentle traction on the catheter will verify whether or not it is satisfactorily seated after the prepuce is allowed to slip back over the glans. Male dogs should be positioned in lateral recumbency and the rear limbs pulled forward, with the x-ray beam centered on the perineum. Cats and female dogs should be positioned in a slight lateral oblique position, with the upper leg elevated out of the x-ray beam, preventing superimposition of the pubis and femurs over the intrapelvic urethra (Ticer et al., 1980a, b). Five to 10 ml of contrast medium are slowly injected and the film is exposed as the last of the contrast medium is infused. The urethra must be distended at the time of exposure. In the female dog, distension will not be accomplished, owing to a lack of injection resistance (Ticer et al., 1982a, b). Additional injections may be made with the animal in VD oblique

view, if desired; however, the lateral projection is the most valuable in the male dog.

Prostatic Urethrography

If the prostatic urethra is to be specifically studied, a standard male catheter is used. This study should be a part of the standard positive contrast cystogram in the male dog. After the required volume of 5 to 10 per cent iodide solution has been instilled into the urinary bladder, the catheter is slowly withdrawn into the prostatic urethra while some of the opaque medium from the urinary bladder is aspirated until backflow into the syringe ceases. The catheter is then withdrawn 1 to 3 cm further to ensure that the delivery holes in the catheter are within the prostatic urethra. Then the contrast material is slowly reinjected. As the last of the contrast material is injected, a lateral radiograph of the caudal abdomen and perineum is made. A slightly oblique VD projection also may be worthwhile. If the contrast medium is re-injected too rapidly or too far distally, reflex micturition may be stimulated.

Complications

Theoretically, overdistention of the cuff of the Foley catheter can traumatize the urethra (Johnston, 1980), but this potential complication has not been observed by the author and does not appear to have been documented in the literature. Suffice it to say that only enough pressure to distend the cuff and retain it in place is required.

Air bubbles may be difficult to differentiate from calculi (Zontine, 1975); they may be prevented by injecting enough contrast medium to flush them retrograde into the urinary bladder. If the catheter lumen is filled with either contrast medium (in females) or lidocaine (in males) prior to inserting the catheter into the urethra, this artifact rarely occurs (Ticer et al., 1980a, b). If, during prostatic urethrography, the tip of the standard male catheter is too distally located, the animal may be stimulated to urinate. If this occurs, and one is not quick enough to obtain a voiding urethrogram, the study may have to be repeated. If topical anesthesia is inadequate or omitted during the Foley catheter technique in males, a long spasm of the pelvic urethra (particularly proximal to the ischial arch) may be seen.

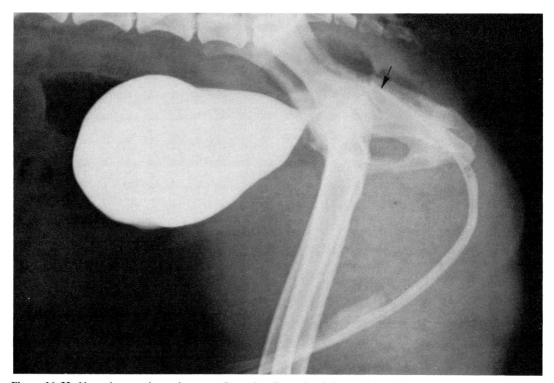

Figure 16–32. Normal prostatic urethrogram. Lateral radiograph of the caudal pelvis of a male dog, made during routine cystography after injection of 10 ml of 7.5% organic iodide solution into the prostatic portion of the urethra. Not only is the prostate gland totally within the pelvic canal, but no contrast material has entered the prostatic ducts. Some of the contrast material also opacifies the penile portion of the urethra. The catheter tip (arrow) is seen in the caudal prostatic urethra.

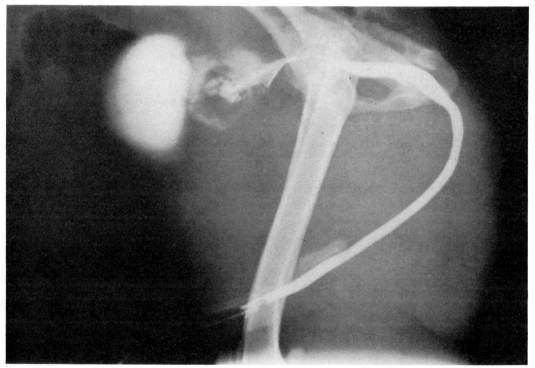

Figure 16–33. Normal retrograde urethrogram. Lateral radiograph of the caudal abdomen and perineum of a male dog at the conclusion of retrograde opacification of the urethra with 15 ml of 75% organic iodide solution injected through a Foley catheter. The urethral mucosa had been topically anesthetized by retrograde flushing of lidocaine HCI solution before instillation of contrast agent. The prostatic urethra in this animal is narrowed by spasm but may be dilated in other normal patients. The entire penile urethra is smooth in outline and uniform in width. No filling defects are present.

Normal Findings (Figs. 16–32 and 16–33)

The male dog urethra should be smooth in outline throughout its entire course, but in the presence of spasm of its pelvic portion it may not be uniform in width. A common site for spastic luminal narrowing is at the ischial arch. This narrowing may be differentiated from stricture by repeating the examination. Nonpathological narrowing usually has tapered margins that are unlike the abrupt change in diameter that occurs with most strictures (Ticer et al., 1980a). The prostatic urethra usually is slightly wider than the extrapelvic urethra. No filling defects are seen in the urethral lumen, and no contrast material normally enters the prostatic ducts or glandular tissue.

In the female dog, the luminal outline is smooth and has longitudinal striations due to mucosal folding (Ticer et al., 1980a).

REFERENCES

Ackerman, N.: Intravenous pyelography. J. Am. Anim. Hosp. Assoc., *10*:227, 1974.

Ackerman, N.: Use of the pediatric foley catheter for positive-contrast retrograde urethrography. Mod. Vet. Pract., *61*:684, 1980.

Ackerman, N., Wingfield, W. E., and Corley, E. A.: Fatal air embolism associated with pneumourethrography and pneumocystography in a dog. J. Am. Vet. Med. Assoc., *160*:1616, 1972.

Andrew, J. H., et al.: Renal damage from angiographic media. Arch. Surg., *88*:812, 1964.

Bargai, U., and Bark, H.: Multiple congenital urinary tract abnormalities in a bitch: A case history report. Vet. Radiol., *23*:10, 1982.

Barrett, R. B., and Kneller, S. K.: Feline kidney mensuration. Acta Radiol. Suppl., *319*:279, 1972.

Biery, D. N.: Upper urinary tract. *In* O'Brien, T. R.: Radiographic Diagnosis of Abdominal Disorders in the Dog and Cat. Philadelphia, W. B. Saunders Co., 1978.

Borthwick, R., and Robbie, B.: Urography in the dog by an intravenous infusion technique. J. Small Anim. Pract., *10*:465, 1969.

Borthwick, R., and Robbie, B.: Large volume urography in the cat. J. Small Anim. Pract., *12*:579, 1971.

Bosniak, M. A., and Schweizer, R. D.: Urographic findings in patients with renal failure. Radiol. Clin. N. Amer., *10*:433, 1972.

Breton, L., Pennock, P. W., and Valli, V. E.: The effects of hypaque 25% and sodium iodide 10% in the canine urinary bladder. J. Am. Vet. Radiol. Soc., *19*:116, 1978.

Burt, J. K., and Root, C. R.: Radiographic manifestations of abdominal trauma. J. Amer. Anim. Hosp. Assoc., *7*:328, 1971.

Christie, B. A.: Incidence and etiology of vesicoureteral reflux in apparently normal dogs. Invest. Urol., *9*:184, 1971.

Christie, B. A.: The occurrence of vesicoureteral reflux and pyelonephritis in apparently normal dogs. Invest. Urol., *10*:359, 1973a.

Christie, B. A.: Vesicoureteral reflux in dogs. J. Amer. Vet. Med. Assoc., *169*:772, 1973b.

Dacie, J. E., and Fry, I. K.: A comparison of sodium and methylglucamine diatrizoate in clinical urography. Brit. J. Radiol., *44*:51, 1971.

Dean, R. E., Andrew, J. H., and Read, R. C.: Renal damage from angiographic media. J.A.M.A., *187*:27, 1964.

Douglas, S. W., and Williamson, H. D.: Veterinary Radiological Interpretation. Philadelphia, Lea & Febiger, 1970.

Douglas, S. W., and Williamson, H. D.: Principles of Veterinary Radiography, 2nd ed. Baltimore, Williams and Wilkins, 1972.

Dure-Smith, P., Simenhoff, M., Brodsky, S., and Zimskind, P. D.: Opacification of the urinary tract during excretory urography: Concentration vs. amount of contrast medium. Invest. Radiol., *7*:407, 1972.

Feeney, D. A., Barber, D. L., and Osborne, C. A.: The fundamental aspects of the nephrogram in excretory urography: A review. Vet. Radiol., *23*:42, 1982.

Feeney, D. A., Osborne, C. A., and Jessen, C. R.: Effects of radiographic contrast media on results of urinalysis with emphasis on alteration in specific gravity. J. Amer. Vet. Med. Assoc., *176*:1378, 1980.

Feeney, D. A., Barber, D. L., Culver, D. H., Prasse, K. W., Thrall, D. E., and Lewis, R. E.: Canine excretory urogram: Correlation with base-line measurements. Am. J. Vet. Res., *41*:279, 1980.

Finco, D. R., Kurtz, H. J., and Porter, T. E.: Renal and ureteral urolithiasis in a dog. J. Amer. Vet. Med. Assoc., *157*:837, 1970.

Finco, D. R., Stiles, N. S., Kneller, S. K., Lewis, R. E., and Barrett, R. B.: Radiologic estimation of kidney size of the dog. J. Amer. Vet. Med. Assoc., *159*:995, 1971.

Gillette, E. L., Thrall, D. E., and Lebel, J. L.: Carlson's Veterinary Radiology. 3rd ed. Philadelphia, Lea & Febiger, 1977.

Goldman, H. S., and Freeman, L. M.: Radiographic and radioisotopic methods of evaluation of the kidneys and urinary tract. Pediatr. Clin. N. Amer., *18*:409, 1971.

Greene, R. W., and Bohning, R. H.: Patent persistent urachus associated with urolithiasis in a cat. J. Amer. Vet. Med. Assoc., *158*:489, 1971.

Hobson, H. P., and Ader, P. L.: Exstrophy of the bladder in a dog. J. Am. Anim. Hosp. Assoc., *15*:103, 1979.

Johnson, C. A.: Renal ectopia in a cat: A case report and literature review. J. Amer. Anim. Hosp. Assoc., *15*:599, 1979.

Johnston, D. E.: Editor's note. *In* Watters, J. W.: Urinary tract radiography—bladder and urethra. Comp. Cont. Ed., *2*:124, 1980.

Johnston, G. R., Jessen, C. R., and Osborne, C. A.: Retrograde contrast urethrography. *In* Kirk, R. W.: Current Veterinary Therapy VI. Philadelphia, W. B. Saunders Co., 1977.

Johnston, G. R., Osborne, C. A., Wilson, J. W., and Yano, B. L.: Familial ureteral ectopia in the dog. J. Amer. Anim. Hosp. Assoc., *13*:168, 1977.

Kealy, J. K.: Diagnostic Radiology of the Dog and Cat. Philadelphia, W. B. Saunders Co., 1979.

Killen, D. A., Foster, J. H., and Scott, H. W.: Toxic reactions incident to urokon aortography. Ann. Surg., 155:472, 1962.

Kleine, L. J., and Thornton, G. W.: Radiographic diagnosis of urinary tract trauma. J. Amer. Anim. Hosp. Assoc., 7:318, 1971.

Kneller, S. K.: Role of the excretory urogram in the diagnosis of renal and ureteral disease. Vet. Clin. N. Amer., 4:843, 1974.

Leav, I., and Ling, G. V.: Adenocarcinoma of the canine prostate. Cancer, 22:1329, 1968.

Lord, P. F., Scott, R. C., and Chan, K. F.: Intravenous urography for evaluation of renal diseases in small animals. J. Amer. Anim. Hosp. Assoc., 10:139, 1974.

Luttwak, E. M., Reed, G. E., and Breed, E. S.: Effect of aortography on renal function. Ann. Surg., 154:190, 1961.

McAlister, W. H., and Palmer, K.: The histologic effects of four commonly used media for excretory urography and an attempt to modify the responses. Radiology, 99:511, 1971.

McClennan, B. L., and Becker, J. A.: Excretory urography: Choice of contrast material—clinical. Radiology, 100:591, 1971.

McClennan, B. L., Becker, J. A., and Berdon, W. E.: Excretory urography: Choice of contrast material—experimental. Radiology, 100:585, 1971.

McEwan, A. D.: The clinical diagnosis of renal disease in the dog. J. Small Anim. Pract., 12:543, 1971.

Morgan, J. P., and Silverman, S.: Techniques of Veterinary Radiography. 3rd ed. Davis, CA, Veterinary Radiology Associates, 1982.

Newman, L., Bucy, J. G., and McAlister, W. H.: Incidence of naturally occurring vesicoureteral reflux in mongrel dogs. Invest. Radiol., 8:354, 1973.

O'Handley, P., Carrig, C. B., and Walshaw, R.: Renal and ureteral duplication in a dog. J. Amer. Vet. Med. Assoc., 174:484, 1979.

Olin, T. R., and Rees, D. O.: Renal function at urography with compression—an experimental investigation in the rabbit. Acta Radiol., 14:613, 1973.

Osborne, C. A., Dieterich, H. F., Hanlon, G. F., and Anderson, L. D.: Urinary incontinence due to ectopic ureter in a male dog. J. Amer. Vet. Med. Assoc., 166:911, 1975.

Osborne, C. A., Yoho, B. C., Low, D. G., and Wall, B. E.: Radiographic evaluation of the canine urinary system. J. Amer. Anim. Hosp. Assoc., 5:136, 1969.

Owen, R.: Three case reports of ectopic ureters in bitches. Vet. Rec., 93:2, 1973.

Owens, J. M.: Radiographic Interpretation for the Small Animal Clinician. St. Louis, MO, Ralston Purina Co., 1982.

Park, R. D.: Radiographic contrast studies of the lower urinary tract. Vet. Clin. N. Amer., 4:863, 1974.

Park, R. D.: Radiology of the urinary bladder and urethra. In O'Brien, T. R.: Radiographic Diagnosis of Abdominal Disorders in the Dog and Cat. Philadelphia, W. B. Saunders Co., 1978.

Pearson, H., and Gibbs, C.: Urinary tract abnormalities in the dog. J. Small Anim. Pract., 12:67, 1971.

Pechman, R. D.: Urinary trauma in dogs and cats: A review. J. Amer. Anim. Hosp. Assoc., 18:33, 1982.

Rhodes, W. H., and Biery, D. N.: Pneumocystography in the dog. J. Amer. Vet. Radiol. Soc., 8:45, 1967.

Root, C. R., and Scott, R. C.: Emphysematous cystitis and other radiographic manifestations of diabetes mellitus in dogs and cats. J. Amer. Vet. Med. Assoc., 158:279, 1971.

Schwartz, A., Lipowitz, A. J., and Burt, J.: Urinary incontinence due to multiple urogenital anomalies in a mature dog. J. Amer. Vet. Med. Assoc., 164:1021, 1974.

Scott, R. C., Greene, R. W., and Patnaik, A. K.: Unilateral ureterocele associated with hydronephrosis in a dog. J. Amer. Anim. Hosp. Assoc., 10:126, 1974.

Selcer, B. A.: Urinary tract trauma associated with pelvic trauma. J. Amer. Anim. Hosp. Assoc., 18:785, 1982.

Stemerman, M., Goldstein, M. L., and Schulman, P. L.: Pancytopenia associated with diatrizoate. N. Y. State J. Med., 71:1220, 1971.

Stokes, J. M., and Bernard, H. R.: Nephrotoxicity of iodinated contrast media. Ann. Surg., 153:299, 1973.

Suter, P. F.: Personal communication. January, 1973.

Svendsen, P., and Wilson, J.: Adverse reactions during urography and modification by atropine. Acta Radiol., 11:427, 1971.

Talner, L. B.: Urographic contrast media in uremia: Physiology and pharmacology. Radiol. Clin. N. Amer., 10:421, 1972.

Thayer, G. W., Carrig, C. B., and Evans, A. T.: Fatal air embolism associated with pneumocystography in a cat. J. Amer. Vet. Med. Assoc., 176:643, 1980.

Thrall, D. E.: Reviewer's note. In Watters, J. W.: Urinary tract radiography—kidneys and ureters. Comp. Cont. Ed., 2:224, 1980.

Ticer, J. W., Spencer, C. P., and Ackerman, N.: Positive contrast retrograde urethrography: A useful procedure for evaluating urethral disorders in the dog. Vet. Radiol., 21:2, 1980a.

Ticer, J. W., Spencer, C. P., and Ackerman, N.: Transitional cell carcinoma of the urethra in four female dogs: Its urethrographic appearance. Vet. Radiol., 21:2, 1980b.

Voltz, P. W., Logan, B., and Wolff, H. L.: Adequate dose excretory urography: Experience with 25,000 cases. South. Med. J., 64:903, 1971.

Walker, R. G., and Douglas, S. W.: The use of contrast media in the diagnosis of urinary tract abnormalities in the dog, with particular reference to infusion urography: A report of two cases. Vet. Rec., 87:287, 1970.

Watters, J. W.: Urinary tract radiography—bladder and urethra. Comp. Cont. Ed., 2:124, 1980a.

Watters, J. W.: Urinary tract radiography—kidneys and ureters. Comp. Cont. Ed., 2:224, 1980b.

Zontine, W. J.: Radiographic interpretation—the urethra. Mod. Vet. Pract., 56:411, 1975.

Zontine, W. J., and Andrews, L. K.: Fatal air embolism as a complication of pneumocystography in two cats. J. Amer. Vet. Rad. Soc., 19:8, 1978.

17

SAM SILVERMAN

Avian Radiographic Technique

Radiographic examination of the avian patient is a practical procedure applicable to the diagnosis of skeletal, abdominal, and thoracic diseases, some of which are manifested in similar nonspecific clinical signs. When treating avian patients, it is not uncommon to base a diagnosis on specific radiographic changes and nonspecific clinical signs. The relative inability to rely on clinical pathological tests when treating the avian patient increases the diagnostic and prognostic importance of the radiographic examination (Altman, 1973; Lafeber, 1966, 1968). Over 50 per cent of the avian patients examined at the Veterinary Medical Teaching Hospital at the University of California at Davis are radiographed.

INDICATIONS

Skeletal Conditions

All suspected skeletal diseases or injuries are radiographed in order to obtain the maximum information concerning their extent, chronicity, and possible etiology. The frequency of metabolic bone disease due to dietary imbalance is high. The evaluation of dietary therapy and orthopedic procedures is almost totally dependent on repeated radiographic examinations.

Inflammatory and infectious processes of soft tissue that may extend to skeletal structures such as bumblefoot should also be evaluated radiographically.

Abdominal Diseases

Clinical signs produced by abdominal diseases are often non-organ specific, such as ruffled feathers, general depression, or abdominal distention. The additional information provided by abdominal radiography can supplement physical findings and help to formulate a diagnosis. Identification of altered size, shape, or position of organs (such as hepatomegaly due to fatty infiltration, free abdominal fluid due to peritonitis, and inflammatory processes such as air sacculitis) can be made radiographically.

Respiratory Diseases

Dyspnea is one of the most common clinical signs detected on physical examination of the avian patient. Its etiology often cannot be defined with physical diagnostic techniques, but radiographic examination will usually indicate the site and sometimes the nature of the pathologic condition, and help to differentiate inflammatory, neoplastic, and traumatic etiology. The following are some of the radiographically detectable conditions that may cause dyspnea: tracheitis, tracheal collapse, infraorbital sinusitis, pneumonia, pulmonary hemorrhage, pulmonary gout, air sacculitis, air sac mites, and compression of air sacs and/or lungs by abdominal mass lesions or fluid.

CONTRAINDICATIONS

Radiographic examination of the avian patient is contraindicated when the physical and psychological stresses produced in positioning and restraining the patient are judged to be in excess of what the patient can tolerate. In these cases, radiography is frequently postponed until the patient's general condition is improved by supportive therapy.

ANATOMY

Normal avian abdominal and thoracic structures are easily delineated radiographically—often more completely than is possible in the mammalian species. This phenomenon is due primarily to the presence of the intra-abdominal and intrathoracic gas-filled air sacs, which reproduce the equivalent of a negative contrast study. Figures 17–1 and 17–2 illustrate the normal avian radiographic anatomy (Petrak, 1969).

Alteration in the size, shape, or position of abdominal and thoracic structures can result in the opacification of the air sacs, or in the displacement of other organs. The ventriculus (usually identifiable by its radiodense contents) can be displaced characteristically in a number of abdominal diseases. Hepatomegaly displaces the ventriculus caudally and dorsally; caudal abdominal masses displace the ventriculus cranially; and dorsal abdominal masses (e.g., renal tumors) produce ventral displacement of the ventriculus. The proventriculus may be relatively large in raptors and some sea birds in which it serves as a storage organ.

Pneumatization and the cortical thickness of the long bones is species-dependent. Increased endosteal and intramedullary bone densities are often noted in egg-producing females. This is a normal finding but can be quite bizarre in appearance.

MATERIALS

X-Ray Machine

The small size of the patient and the rapid respiratory movements necessitate that x-ray exposure times of 1/60 sec or less be used. Increased radiographic detail can be obtained from an x-ray unit that has a small focal spot (0.3 mm). If possible, the aluminum filter should be removed, in order to utilize lower kv x-rays.

X-Ray Film and Cassette

Non-screen medical film (Kodak NS 5 4T, Eastman Kodak Co.) or screen film (Cronex 6, E. I. DuPont De Nemours and Co.) with ultra detail intensifying screens (Radelin Ultra Detail Aluminized Maximum Radiation Screens, United States Radium Corporation) may be used. The choice of film depends largely on the detail required in the radiograph and the nature of the examination. The increased detail obtained from nonscreen film must be balanced against the additional exposure required for this film. The longer exposure time required for the nonscreen film often produces radiographs that are less diagnostic than screen film when patient motion is a problem (as in the case of dyspneic patients). The use of detail or fine rare earth phosphor intensifying screen will allow exposure times that are about the same as those used with par speed calcium tungstate screen. The radiographic detail can be increased markedly without requiring increased exposure times. The radiographic contrast is also improved by using intensifying screens.

Restraint Apparatus

Positioning the patient on a clear, acrylic material board, utilizing masking tape for restraint, is the method of choice for avian radiography. The masking tape is easy to work with, relatively atraumatic to the patient, and radiolucent compared with other types of adhesive tape. Pipe cleaners attached to Velcor strips may also be used for leg and neck restraint. The acrylic sheet provides a movable restraint surface, which allows the examiner to change film for multiple exposures without having to reposition the patient on a new cassette or film envelope (Figs. 17–3 and 17–4). The acrylic board should not be more than ¼ inch thick so that the attenuation of the lower kv x-rays is minimized.

TECHNIQUE

Anesthesia

Ketamine hydrochloride (Ketamine Hydrochloride, Ketalar 100 mg/ml, Parke Davis & Co.) administered intramuscularly at a dosage of 10 to 30 mg/lb of body weight, is used routinely when radiographing fractious or excited avian patients. This technique has proven successful in over 200 avian patients, with no adverse reactions attributed to the anesthetic technique. Full recovery usually

Text continued on page 403.

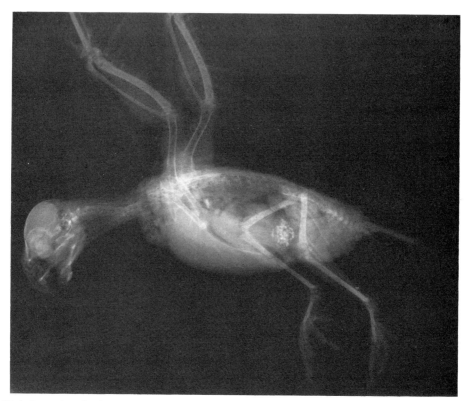

Figure 17–1. Lateral projection of a normal cockatoo. Note that the medullary cavities of most of the long bones show mottled radiodensities that are commonly seen in female birds during egg production.

(Illustration continued on the opposite page.)

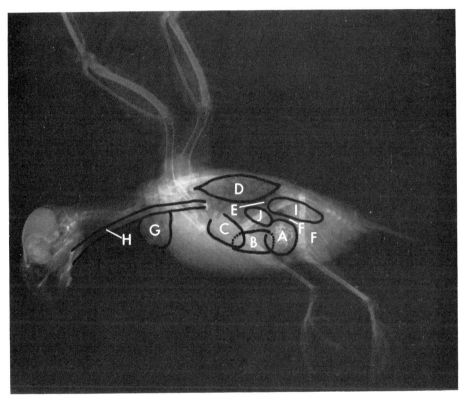

Figure 17–1. *Continued.* Lateral projection of a normal cockatoo. *A,* Ventriculus; *B,* liver; *C,* heart; *D,* lungs; *E,* air sacs; *F,* small intestines; *G,* crop; *H,* trachea; *I,* kidney; *J,* proventriculus.

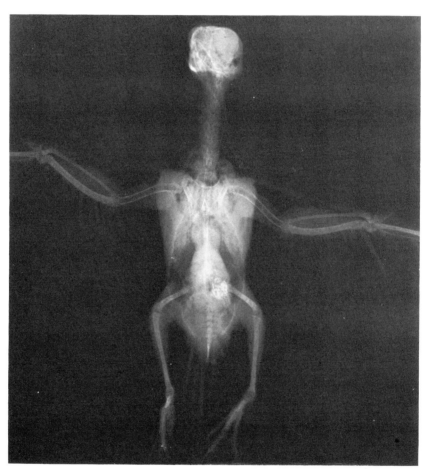

Figure 17–2. Ventrodorsal projection of a normal cockatoo (same patient as in Figure 17–1).
(Illustration continued on the opposite page.)

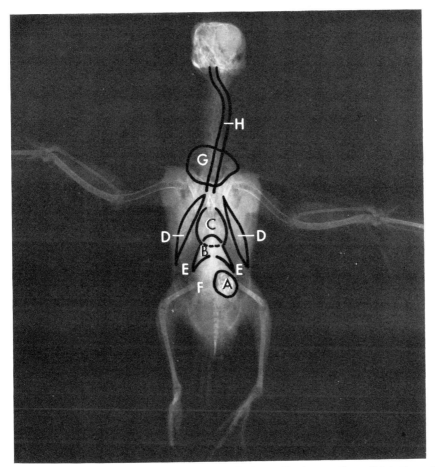

Figure 17–2. *Continued. A,* Ventriculus; *B,* liver; *C,* heart; *D,* lungs; *E,* air sacs; *F,* small intestines; *G,* crop; *H,* trachea.

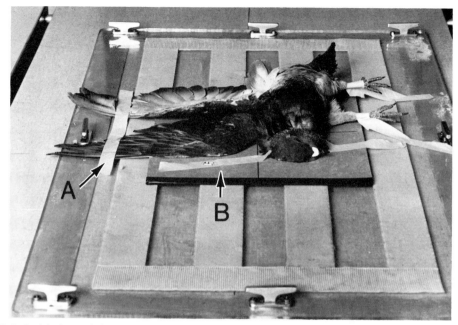

Figure 17–3. Positioning technique for lateral radiograph of an unanesthetized pigeon. The patient is restrained with masking tape (*A*) and is in direct contact with a nonscreen x-ray cassette (*B*). The method shown in Figure 17–4 may also be used if desired.

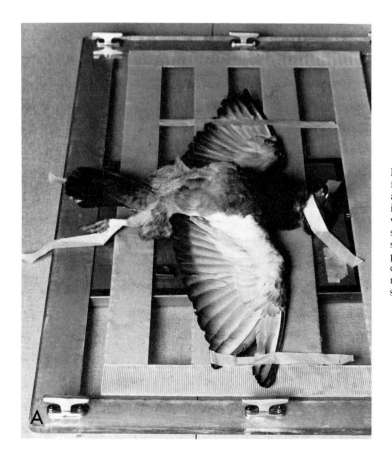

Figure 17–4. Positioning technique for ventrodorsal body radiograph of an unanesthetized pigeon. The bird is attached to a plastic sheet (*A*) with masking tape. The x-ray cassette is placed under the plastic sheet. This method allows for repeated exposures with a minimum of patient movement. The patient may be taped directly to the cassette.

Table 17–1. AVIAN RADIOGRAPHIC TECHNIQUES

Subject	Film Type	F.F.D. (Inches)	ma	sec	kv
Canary	NS 54 T	30	100	1/60	70
Parakeet	NS 54 T	27	100	1/60	72
Parrot	NS 54 T	21	100	1/60	72
Red Tail Hawk	Cronex 6*	40	100	1/60	65
Pigeon	Cronex 6*	40	100	1/60	60
Macaw	Cronex 6*	40	100	1/60	72

*Cronex 6 used with ultra-detail intensifying screens.

occurs in 30 to 45 minutes after administration of the anesthesia, thus allowing adequate time to perform the radiographic examination.

Positioning

Abdominal and Thoracic Studies. The entire body cavity of the avian patient is usually radiographed simultaneously, which allows evaluation of abdominal, thoracic, and a portion of the skeletal structures on a single study.

Patients manifesting marked dyspnea should not be positioned in such a way that the respiratory excursions of their abdominal and thoracic cavities are compromised. Oxygen therapy and the maintenance of body temperature with heat lamps may be used to support the patient during the radiographic examination. On completion of the examination, the patient should be placed in an incubator where temperature, humidity, and oxygen can be regulated.

Lateral body radiographs are produced with the dependent side marked with an appropriate right or left marker, and the dependent extremities positioned cranial to the contralateral extremity (Fig. 17–3). Full extension of the wings and legs will preclude their superimposition on the abdominal or thoracic structures. This projection will also provide a lateral radiograph of the wings or legs. The x-ray beam is centered at the middle of the body.

Ventrodorsal body radiographs require full and symmetrical extension and abduction of the limbs to preclude their superimposition on other organs of interest (Fig. 17–4). The x-ray beam is centered on the midline, slightly cranial to the caudal tip of the sternum. Craniocaudal projections of the legs will be obtained on the ventrodorsal body projections.

Extremity Examinations. Craniocaudal projections of the wings are best obtained with manual positioning of the patient. The remainder of the extremity examination can be obtained with positioning techniques described for abdominal and thoracic radiography. The x-ray beam should be appropriately centered on the area of interest.

Exposure

Exposure factors for some representative avian species are given in Table 17–1. These techniques may require slight modification for use with other x-ray units. Minimization of exposure time and utilization of a small focal spot are desired. Although decreasing the focal film distance from the standard 40 inches will produce some geometric distortion of the image (primarily magnification), it will produce quality diagnostic radiographs because the patient-film distance is small for most avian species (see Chap. 2).

Radiographic Interpretation

Basic radiographic changes in the avian species are similar to those detected in the mammalian species. Familiarization with avian anatomy and establishment of a "normal" file of radiographs, arranged according to species, will enhance interpretative ability.

REFERENCES

Altman, R. J.: Cage Birds: Radiography. Vet. Clin. N. Amer., 3:165–173, 1973.

Lafeber, T. J.: Bird clinic cage bird practice today. Animal Hospital, 2:48–55, 1966.

Lafeber, T. J.: Radiography in the caged bird clinic. Animal Hospital, 4:41–48, 1968.

Petrak, M. L.: Diseases of Caged and Aviary Birds. Philadelphia, Lea & Febiger, 1969.

SECTION III

*An Atlas of
Radiographic
Positioning and
Technique of
Large Animals*

18

Thoracic Limb

SHOULDER JOINT

Mediolateral (ML) View. The patient is placed with the shoulder to be examined adjacent to a wall-mounted grid cabinet or cassette holder. The limb is pulled forward so that the shoulder and elbow joints are extended. The shoulder is displaced as far as possible cranially so that there is a minimum overlay of the contralateral pectoral musculature (Fig. 18–1). The x-ray beam is directed from medial to lateral in a horizontal plane. In some well-muscled horses, it is necessary to angle the x-ray slightly from a cranial to caudal direction in order to minimize pectoral muscle overlay.

Patients that are uncooperative or in pain may require general anesthesia in order to obtain this view. In such cases, the patient is placed in lateral recumbency with the shoulder being examined placed on the floor. The limb is then extended and the contralateral limb is retracted caudally. A vertical x-ray beam is used to produce the radiograph.

A grid must be used to minimize fog-producing scatter radiation. Alternatively the exposure may be made through the back of the cassette (see p. 69). The caudocranial view cannot be obtained unless the patient is anesthetized.

Figure 18–2 illustrates the radiographic anatomy of the equine shoulder joint in ML view.

ELBOW JOINT

Craniocaudal (CrCd) View. (Formerly anteroposterior [AP] view.) The limb is lifted and pulled cranially as far as possible and a

cassette holder is placed on the caudal surface (Fig. 18–3). The x-ray beam is directed at the humeroradial joint space so that it is as near perpendicular to the cassette surface as possible. A grid must be used to minimize fog-producing scatter radiation. The grid lines must be oriented parallel to the longitudinal axis of the limb in order to minimize grid cut if the x-ray beam angle varies slightly from the perpendicular. Alternatively, the exposure may be made through the back of the cassette (see p. 69).

General anesthesia may be required to produce this view in uncooperative patients. In these cases the patient is placed in lateral recumbency with the affected limb up, abducted slightly and extended. The x-ray beam is directed in a horizontal plane (parallel to the floor).

Figure 18–4 illustrates the radiographic anatomy of an equine elbow joint in CrCd view.

Mediolateral (ML) View. The patient is placed with the elbow to be examined adjacent to a wall-mounted grid cabinet or cassette holder. The limb is pulled forward so that the elbow and shoulder joints are extended. The elbow is displaced cranially as far as possible so that there is minimal overlay of the pectoral musculature (Fig. 18–5). The x-ray beam is directed at the humeroradial joint from medial to lateral in a horizontal plane. In some well-muscled horses it is necessary to angle the x-ray beam slightly from a cranial to caudal direction in order to minimize pectoral muscle overlay. Care must be taken, therefore, to assure that the cassette surface remains perpendicular to the x-ray beam in order to avoid grid cut.

A grid is usually necessary to reduce fog-

404

producing scatter radiation. Alternatively, the exposure may be made through the back of the cassette (see p. 69). If olecranon pathology is suspected, a second, reduced exposure is usually required.

In uncooperative patients, general anesthesia may be required, in which case the patient is placed in lateral recumbency with the affected elbow placed on the floor. The limb is then extended and cranially displaced and the contralateral limb is retracted caudally. A vertical x-ray beam is used to produce the radiograph.

Figure 18–6 illustrates the radiographic anatomy of an equine elbow joint in ML view.

CARPAL JOINT

Dorsopalmar (DPa) View. (Formerly anteroposterior [AP] view.) The patient is allowed to stand normally and the cassette holder is placed against the palmar surface of the carpus (Fig. 18–7). The x-ray beam is directed parallel to the floor and centered at the midportion of the carpus along the midsagittal line of the dorsal surface. A grid is usually not necessary. In uncooperative patients, the contralateral limb may be lifted to help reduce motion.

Figure 18–8 illustrates the radiographic anatomy of a mature equine carpus in DPa view. Figure 18–9 shows the anatomy of an immature equine carpus in DPa view to illustrate the normal appearance of the distal radial physis (b) and the ossification center for the distal ulnar epiphysis (c). This center fuses to the radial epiphysis at between 2 and 9 months of age and becomes the lateral styloid process.

Lateromedial (LM) View. The patient is allowed to stand normally and the cassette holder is placed against the medial surface of the carpus (Fig. 18–10). The x-ray beam is directed parallel to the floor and centered at the midportion of the carpus on the lateral surface. A grid is usually not used.

In uncooperative patients, the contralateral limb may be lifted to help reduce motion. The person lifting the limb should stand clear of the primary x-ray beam.

Figure 18–11 illustrates the radiographic anatomy of an equine carpus in LM view.

Flexed Lateromedial (LM [flexed]) View. The limb being examined is lifted, the carpus is flexed and the cassette holder is placed against the medial surface of the carpus (Fig. 18–12). The x-ray beam is directed parallel to the floor and centered at the midportion of the carpus on the lateral surface. A grid is usually not used.

Care must be taken to avoid exposure of the person lifting the limb to the primary x-ray beam.

Figure 18–13 illustrates the radiographic anatomy of an equine carpus in LM (flexed) view.

Dorsolateral-Palmaromedial Oblique (D60°L-PaMO) View. (Formerly dorsopalmar medial oblique or anteroposterior medial oblique [APMO] view.) The patient is allowed to stand normally and the cassette holder is placed on the palmaromedial surface of the carpus. The x-ray beam is directed parallel to the floor and centered at the midportion of the carpus on the dorsolateral surface 60 degrees lateral to the dorsal surface (Fig. 18–14). The exact angle may vary slightly with the specific anatomical region to be examined. A grid is usually not used. The contralateral limb should not be lifted in an effort to control motion, since the person performing this task would be in the primary x-ray beam.

Figure 18–15 illustrates the radiographic anatomy of an equine carpus in D60°L-PaMO view.

Dorsomedial-Palmarolateral Oblique (D60°M-PaLO) View. (Formerly dorsopalmar lateral oblique or anteroposterior lateral oblique [APLO] view.) The patient is allowed to stand normally and the cassette holder is placed on the palmarolateral surface of the carpus. The x-ray beam is directed parallel to the floor and centered at the midportion of the carpus on the dorsomedial surface 60 degrees medial to the dorsal surface (Fig. 18–16). The exact angle may vary slightly with the specific anatomical region to be examined. A grid is usually not used. The contralateral limb may be lifted to help control motion in an uncooperative patient.

Figure 18–17 illustrates the normal radiographic anatomy of an equine carpus in D60°M-PaLO view.

Proximodistal (PrDi) View of the Proximal Row of Carpal Bones. (Formerly the skyline or proximodistal tangential view.) The limb to be examined is lifted, the carpus is flexed and the cassette holder is placed against the dorsal surface of the proximal

Text continued on page 422.

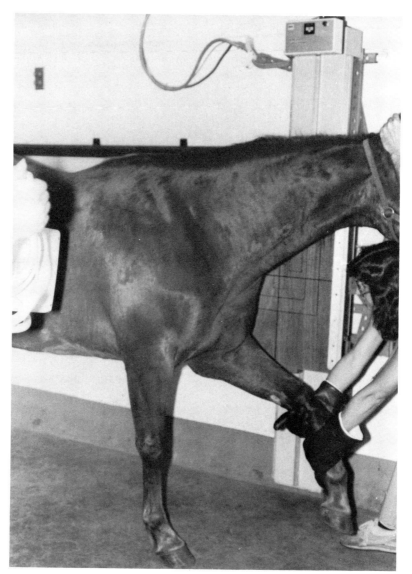

Figure 18–1. Position for mediolateral (ML) view of the equine shoulder.

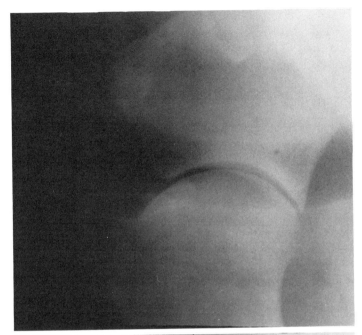

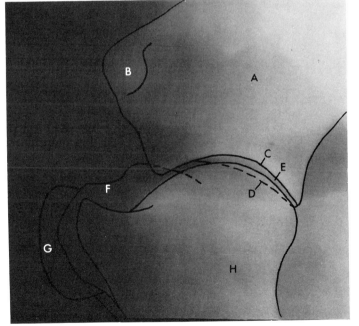

Figure 18–2. Mediolateral (ML) view of an equine shoulder.
A. Scapula
B. Supraglenoid tubercle
C. Rim of the glenoid cavity
D. Opposite rim of the glenoid cavity
E. Scapulohumeral articulation
F. Lesser tubercle of the humerus
G. Greater tubercle of the humerus.

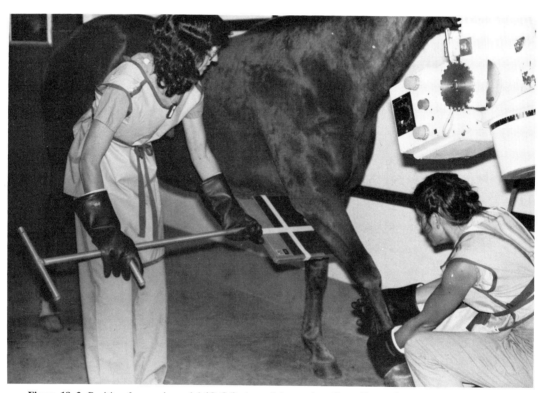

Figure 18–3. Position for craniocaudal (CrCd) view of the equine elbow (formerly anteroposterior [AP]).

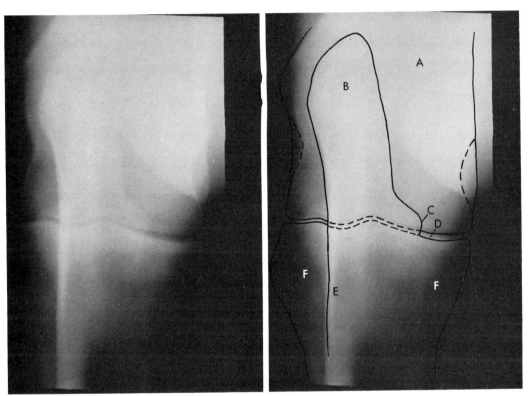

Figure 18–4. Craniocaudal (CrCd) view of an equine elbow.
    A. Humerus
    B. Olecranon of the ulna
    C. Coronoid process of the ulna
    D. Humeroradial articulation
    E. Ulna
    F. Radius

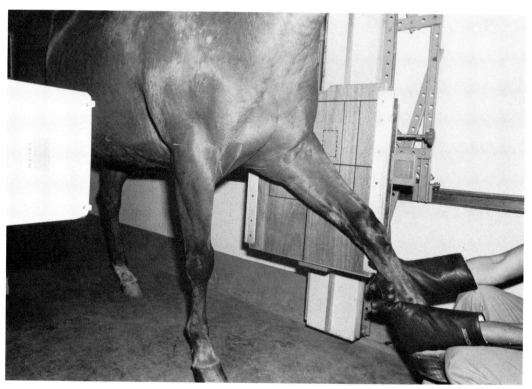

Figure 18–5. Position for mediolateral (ML) view of the equine elbow.

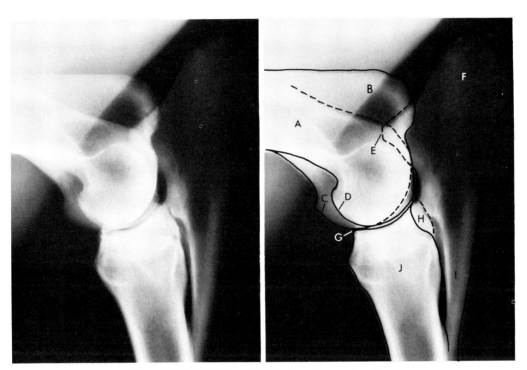

Figure 18–6. Mediolateral (ML) view of an equine elbow.
- A. Humerus
- B. Medial epicondyle of the humerus
- C. Lateral condyle of the humerus
- D. Medial condyle of the humerus
- E. Anconeal process of the ulna
- F. Olecranon of the ulna
- G. Humeroradial articulation
- H. Coronoid process of the ulna
- I. Ulna
- J. Radius

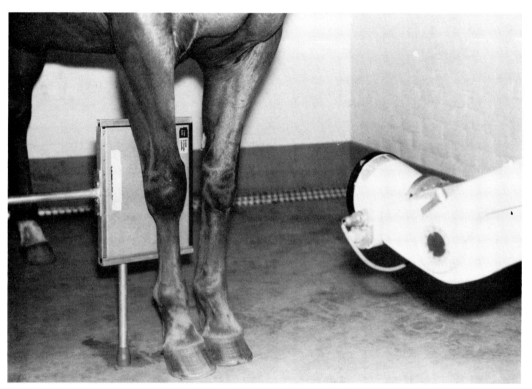

Figure 18–7. Position for dorsopalmar (DPa) view of the equine carpus (formerly anteroposterior [AP]).

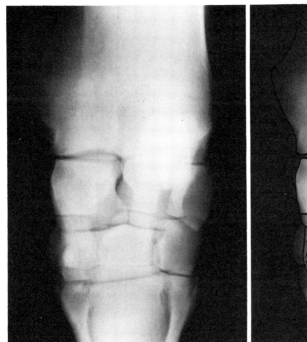

Figure 18–8. Dorsopalmar view of an equine carpus.

A. Radius
B. Accessory carpal bone
C. Antibrachiocarpal joint
D. Radial carpal bone
E. Intermediate carpal bone
F. Ulnar carpal bone
G. First carpal bone
H. Second carpal bone
I. Third carpal bone
J. Fourth carpal bone
K. Second metacarpal bone
L. Third metacarpal bone
M. Fourth metacarpal bone

Figure 18–9. Dorsopalmar (DPa) view of a two-week-old equine carpus showing open distal radial physis and ossification center for the distal ulnar epiphysis.

A. Radial metaphysis
B. Radial physis
C. Ossification center for the distal ulnar epiphysis
D. Radial epiphysis
E. Antibrachiocarpal joint

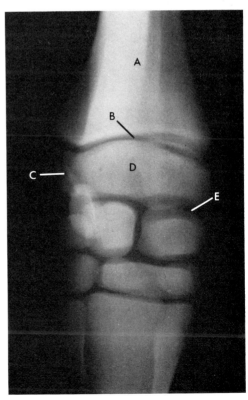

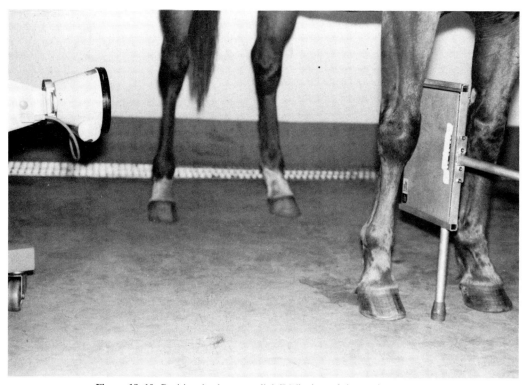

Figure 18–10. Position for lateromedial (LM) view of the equine carpus.

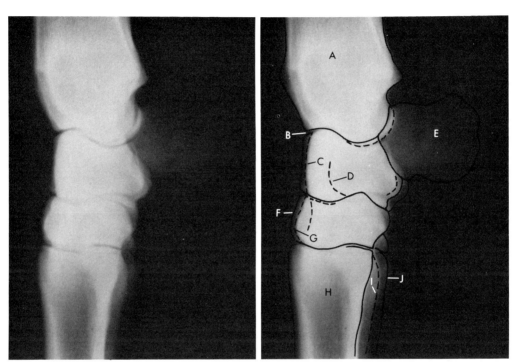

Figure 18–11. Lateromedial (LM) view of an equine carpus.
  A. Radius
  B. Intermediate carpal bone
  C. Radial carpal bone
  D. Ulnar carpal bone
  E. Accessory carpal bone
  F. Third carpal bone
  G. Second carpal bone
  H. Third metacarpal bone
  I. Second metacarpal bone
  J. Fourth metacarpal bone

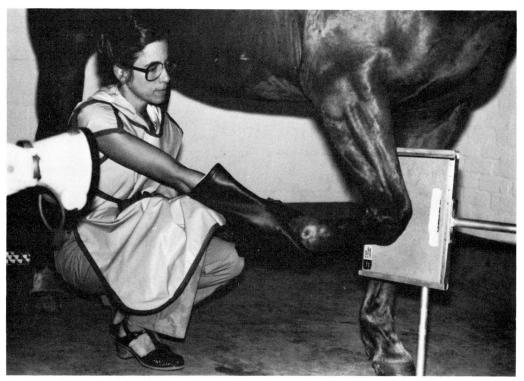

Figure 18–12. Position for flexed lateromedial (LM [flexed]) view of the equine carpus.

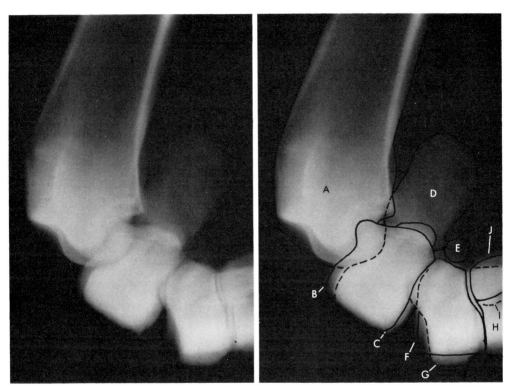

Figure 18–13. Flexed lateromedial (LM [flexed]) view of an equine carpus

A. Radius
B. Intermediate carpal bone
C. Radial carpal bone
D. Accessory carpal bone
E. First carpal bone
F. Fourth carpal bone
G. Third carpal bone
H. Third metacarpal bone
I. Second metacarpal bone
J. Fourth metacarpal bone

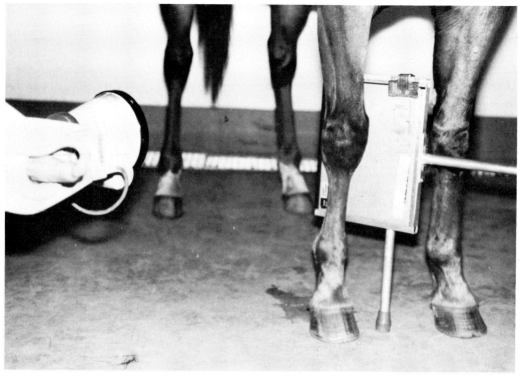

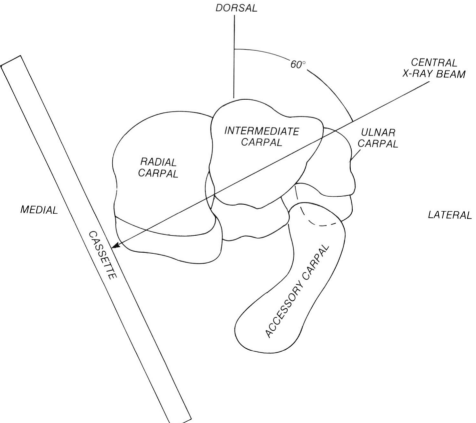

Figure 18–14. Position for dorsolateral-palmaromedial oblique (D60°L-PaMO) view of the equine carpus (formerly dorsopalmar medial oblique or anteroposterior medial oblique [APMO]).

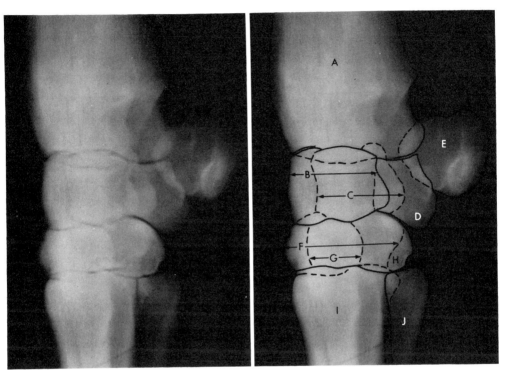

Figure 18–15. Dorsolateral-palmaromedial oblique (D60°L-PaMO) view of an equine carpus.

A. Radius
B. Radial carpal bone
C. Intermediate carpal bone
D. Ulnar carpal bone
E. Accessory carpal bone
F. Third carpal bone
G. Second carpal bone
H. Fourth carpal bone
I. Third metacarpal bone
J. Fourth metacarpal bone

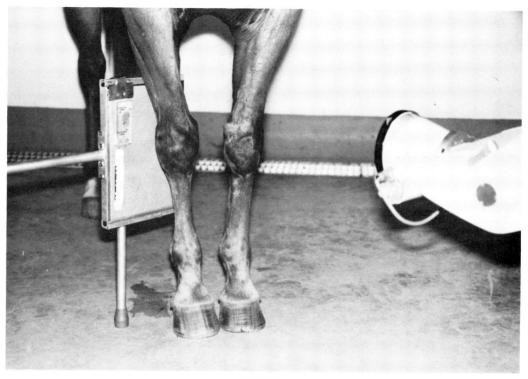

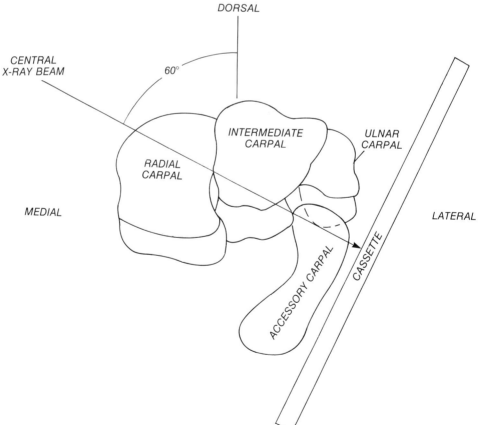

Figure 18–16. Position for dorsomedial-palmarolateral oblique (D60°M-PaLO) view of the equine carpus (formerly dorsopalmar lateral oblique or anteroposterior lateral oblique [APLO]).

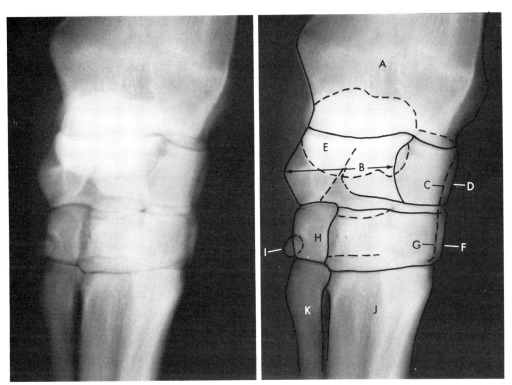

Figure 18–17. Dorsomedial-palmarolateral oblique (D60°M-PaLO) view of an equine carpus.

A. Radius
B. Ulnar carpal bone
C. Intermediate carpal bone
D. Radial carpal bone
E. Accessory carpal bone
F. Fourth carpal bone
G. Third carpal bone
H. Second carpal bone
I. First carpal bone
J. Third metacarpal bone
K. Second metacarpal bone

metacarpal region and parallel to the floor. The x-ray beam is directed perpendicular to the cassette surface from the proximal direction in such a manner as to profile the dorsal surface of the proximal row of carpal bones (Fig. 18–18). The cranial surface of the distal end of the radius may also be examined with similar positioning if the carpus is retracted caudally a short distance. This will result in an angularity between the cassette and the x-ray beam and thus cause some distortion of the radiographic appearance of the distal radius.

Figure 18–19 illustrates the radiographic anatomy of an equine carpus in PrDi view.

Proximodistal (PrDi) View of the Distal Row of Carpal Bones. (Formerly skyline or proximodistal tangential view.) The limb to be examined is lifted, the carpus is flexed and the cassette holder is placed against the dorsal surface of the proximal metacarpal region and parallel to the floor. The x-ray beam is directed 30 degrees proximal to the cassette surface in such a manner as to profile the dorsal surface of the distal row of carpal bones (Fig. 18–20).

Figure 18–21 illustrates the radiographic anatomy of the distal row of equine carpal bones in PrDi view. Note that the distortion of the anatomical appearance caused by the lack of a perpendicular relationship of the x-ray beam and the cassette surface does not prevent the detection of a fracture (c) of the third carpal bone (b) dorsal surface.

METACARPUS (METATARSUS)

Dorsopalmar (DPa) View. (Formerly anteroposterior [AP] view.) The patient is allowed to stand normally and the cassette holder is placed against the palmar surface of the metacarpus (Fig. 18–22). A 7 × 17 inch cassette allows the study of the entire metacarpal region, including the proximal and distal articulations. The x-ray beam is directed parallel to the floor and centered at the midmetacarpal region along the midsagittal line of the dorsal surface. A grid is not necessary.

In uncooperative patients, the contralateral limb may be lifted to help reduce motion.

Figure 18–23 illustrates the radiographic anatomy of an equine metacarpal region in DPa view.

Lateromedial (LM) View. The patient is allowed to stand normally and the cassette holder is placed against the medial surface of the metacarpus (Fig. 18–24). A 7 × 17 inch cassette allows the study of the entire metacarpal region, including the proximal and distal articulations. The x-ray beam is directed parallel to the floor and centered at the midmetacarpal region on the lateral surface. A grid is not necessary.

In uncooperative patients, the contralateral limb may be lifted to help reduce motion. The person lifting the limb should stand clear of the primary x-ray beam.

Figure 18–25 illustrates the radiographic anatomy of an equine metacarpal region in LM view.

Dorsolateral-Palmaromedial Oblique (D40°L-PaMO) View. (Formerly dorsopalmar medial oblique or anteroposterior medial oblique [APMO] view.) This view is especially useful for examining the fourth metacarpal bone. The patient is allowed to stand normally and the cassette holder is placed on the palmaromedial surface of the metacarpal region. The x-ray beam is directed parallel to the floor and centered at the midportion of the metacarpus on the dorsolateral surface 40 degrees lateral to the dorsal surface (Fig. 18–26). The exact angle may vary slightly with the conformation of the horse and can be best determined by palpation. A grid is not necessary.

The contralateral limb should not be lifted in an effort to control motion, since the person performing this task would be in the primary x-ray beam.

Figure 18–27 illustrates the radiographic anatomy of an equine metacarpus in D40°L-PaMO view.

Dorsomedial-Palmarolateral Oblique (D40°M-PaLO) View. (Formerly dorsopalmar lateral oblique or anteroposterior lateral oblique [APLO] view.) This view is especially useful for examining the second metacarpal bone. The patient is allowed to stand normally and the cassette holder is placed on the palmarolateral surface of the metacarpal region. The x-ray beam is directed parallel to the floor and centered at the midportion of the metacarpus on the dorsomedial surface 40 degrees medial to the dorsal surface (Fig. 18–28). The exact angle may vary slightly with the conformation of the horse and can best be determined by palpation. A grid is not necessary. In uncooperative patients, the contralateral limb may be lifted to help control motion.

Figure 18–29 illustrates the radiographic anatomy of a equine metacarpus in D40°M-PaLO view.

METACARPOPHALANGEAL (FETLOCK) JOINT AND PROXIMAL SESAMOID BONES (METATARSOPHALANGEAL JOINT)

Dorsopalmar (DPa) View. (Formerly anteroposterior [AP] view.) The patient is allowed to stand normally and the cassette holder is placed against the palmar surface of the proximal phalanx and allowed to extend proximally at least as far as the proximal aspect of the proximal sesamoid bones (Fig. 18–30). The angle of the cassette to the floor will vary with the angle of the joint. The x-ray beam is directed perpendicular to the cassette surface and centered at the joint space along the midsagittal line of the dorsal surface. A grid is not necessary. In uncooperative patients, the contralateral limb may be lifted to help reduce motion.

Figure 18–31 illustrates the radiographic anatomy of the metacarpophalangeal (fetlock) joint and proximal sesamoid bones in DPa view.

Lateromedial (LM) View. The patient is allowed to stand normally and the cassette holder is placed against the medial surface of the joint (Fig. 18–32). The x-ray beam is directed parallel to the floor and centered at the joint space on the lateral surface. A grid is not necessary.

In uncooperative patients, the contralateral limb may be lifted to help reduce motion. The person lifting the leg should stand clear of the primary x-ray beam.

Figure 18–33 illustrates the radiographic anatomy of an equine metacarpophalangeal (fetlock) joint in LM view.

Flexed Lateromedial (LM [flexed]) View. The limb being examined is lifted, the joint is flexed and the cassette holder is placed against the medial surface of the joint (Fig. 18–34). The x-ray beam is directed parallel to the floor and centered at the joint space on the lateral surface. A grid is not necessary. Care must be taken to avoid exposure of the person lifting the leg to the primary x-ray beam.

Figure 18–35 illustrates the radiographic anatomy of an equine metacarpophalangeal joint in LM (flexed) view.

Dorsolateral-Palmaromedial Oblique (D35°L-PaMO) View. (Formerly dorsopalmar medial oblique or anteroposterior medial oblique [APMO] view.) This view is especially useful for examining the lateral proximal sesamoid bone. The patient is allowed to stand normally, and the cassette holder is placed on the palmaromedial surface of the proximal phalanx and allowed to extend proximally at least as far as the proximal aspect of the sesamoid bones. The angle of the cassette to the floor will vary with the angle of the joint. The x-ray beam is directed perpendicular to the cassette surface and centered at the joint space on the dorsolateral surface 35 degrees lateral to the dorsal surface (Fig. 18–36). The exact angle from the dorsal surface toward the lateral surface will vary depending upon the specific region to be examined; however, 35 degrees is usually sufficient for examining the lateral proximal sesamoid bone. A grid is not necessary.

The contralateral limb should not be lifted in an effort to reduce motion, since the person performing the task would be in the primary x-ray beam.

Figure 18–37 illustrates the radiographic anatomy of an equine metacarpophalangeal (fetlock) joint in D35°L-PaMO view.

Dorsomedial-Palmarolateral Oblique (D35°M-PaLO) View. (Formerly dorsopalmar lateral oblique or anteroposterior lateral oblique [APLO] view.) This view is especially useful for examining the medial proximal sesamoid bone. The patient is allowed to stand normally, and the cassette holder is placed on the palmarolateral surface of the proximal phalanx and allowed to extend proximally at least as far as the proximal aspect of the sesamoid bones. The angle of the cassette to the floor will vary with the angle of the joint. The x-ray beam is directed perpendicular to the cassette surface and centered at the joint space on the dorsomedial surface 35 degrees medial to the dorsal surface (Fig. 18–38). The exact angle from the dorsal surface will vary depending upon the specific region to be examined; however, 35 degrees is usually sufficient for examining the medial proximal sesamoid bone. A grid is not necessary. In uncooperative patients, the contralateral limb may be lifted to help control motion.

Figure 18–39 illustrates the radiographic anatomy of an equine metacarpophalangeal (fetlock) joint in D35°M-PaLO view.

Text continued on page 446

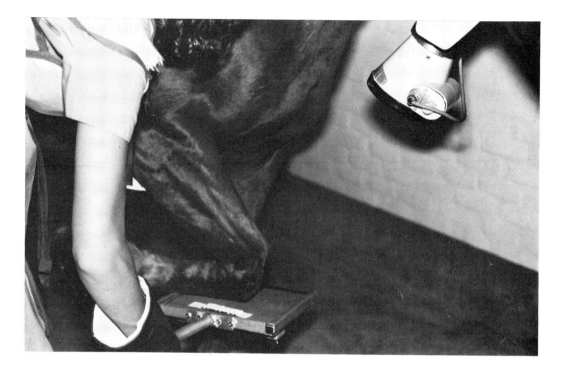

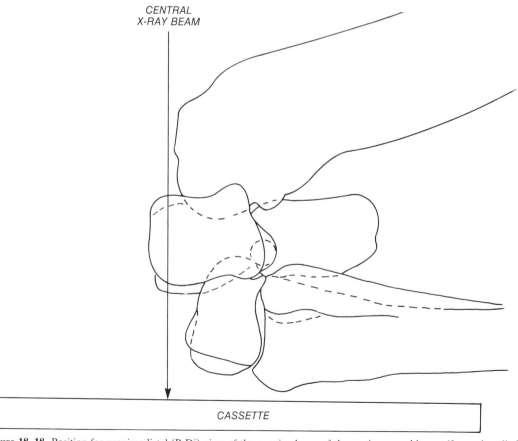

CENTRAL
X-RAY BEAM

CASSETTE

Figure 18–18. Position for proximodistal (PrDi) view of the proximal row of the equine carpal bones (formerly called the skyline or proximodistal tangential view).

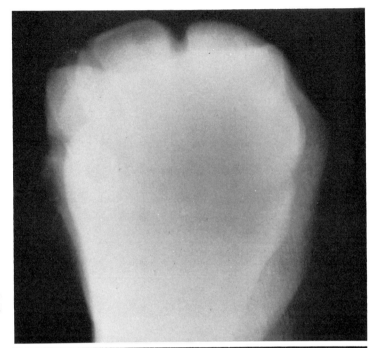

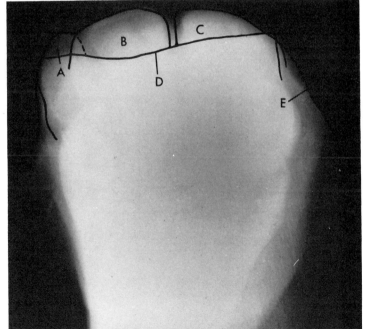

Figure 18–19. Proximodistal (PrDi) view of the proximal row of carpal bones of an equine.
  A. Ulnar carpal bone
  B. Intermediate carpal bone
  C. Radial carpal bone
  D. Articular surface of the distal radius
  E. Radius

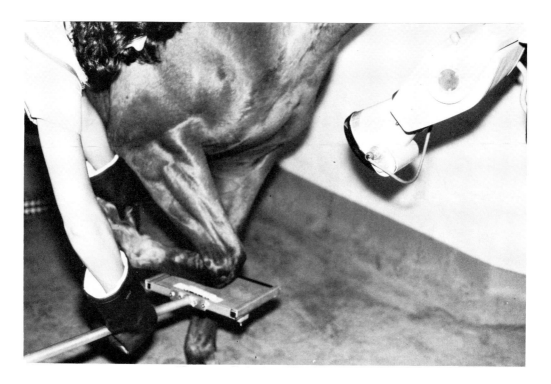

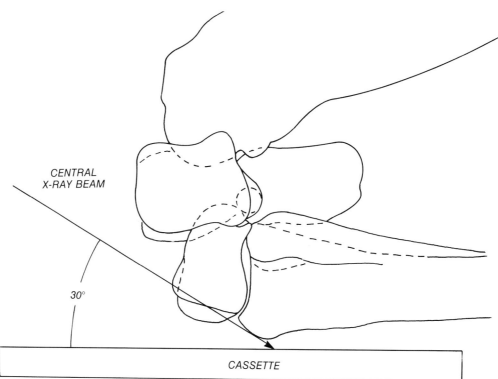

Figure 18–20. Position for proximodistal (PrDi) view of the distal row of the equine carpal bones (formerly called the skyline or proximodistal tangential view).

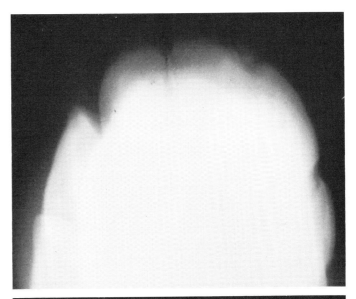

Figure 18–21. Proximodistal (PrDi) view of the distal row of carpal bones of an equine. Note the fracture (C) of the dorsal surface of the third carpal bone (B).

A. Fourth carpal bone
B. Third carpal bone
C. Fracture fragment from the dorsal surface of the third carpal bone
D. Second carpal bone
E. Ulnar carpal bone
F. Accessory carpal bone
G. Intermediate carpal bone
H. Radial carpal bone

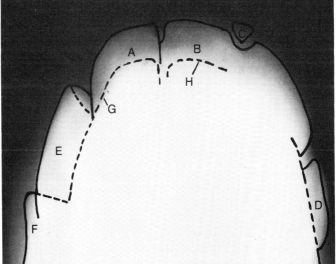

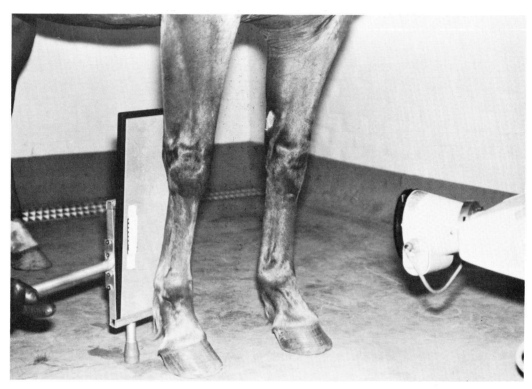

Figure 18–22. Position for dorsopalmar (DPa) view of the equine metacarpus (formerly anteroposterior [AP]).

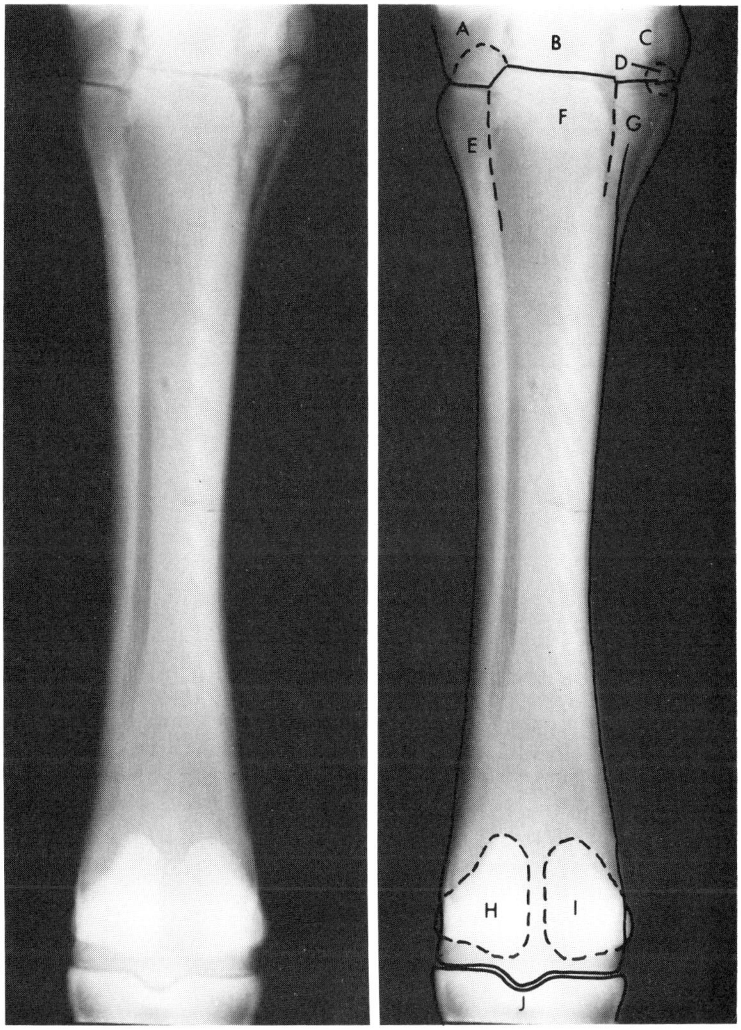

Figure 18–23. Dorsopalmar (DPa) view of an equine metacarpus.
  A. Fourth carpal bone
  B. Third carpal bone
  C. Second carpal bone
  D. First carpal bone
  E. Fourth metacarpal bone
  F. Third metacarpal bone
  G. Second metacarpal bone
  H. Lateral proximal sesamoid bone
  I. Medial proximal sesamoid bone
  J. Proximal phalanx

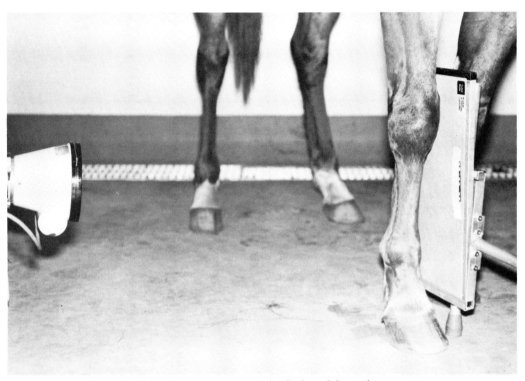

Figure 18–24. Position for lateromedial (LM) view of the equine metacarpus.

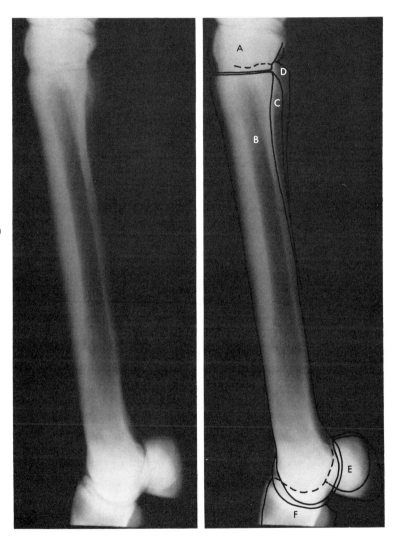

Figure 18–25. Lateromedial (LM) view of an equine metacarpus.
  A. Distal row of carpal bones
  B. Third metacarpal bone
  C. Second metacarpal bone
  D. Fourth metacarpal bone
  E. Proximal sesamoid bones
  F. Proximal phalanx

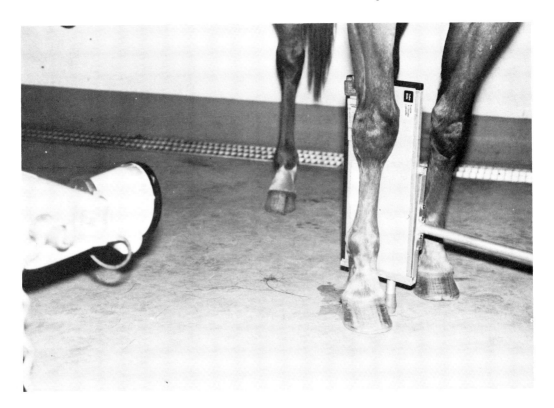

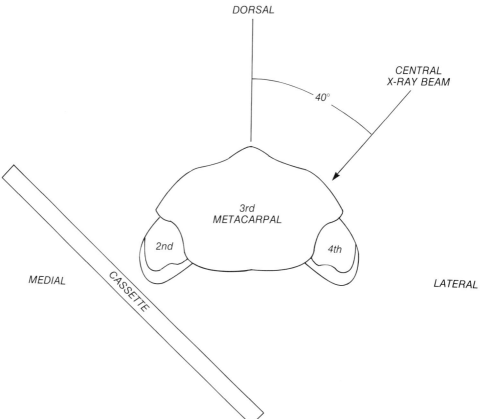

Figure 18–26. Position for dorsolateral-palmaromedial oblique (D40°L-PaMO) view of the equine metacarpus (formerly dorsopalmar medial oblique or anteroposterior medial oblique [APMO]).

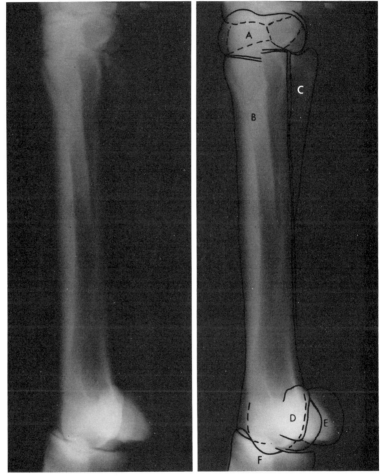

Figure 18–27. Dorsolateral-palmaromedial oblique (D40°L-PaMO) view of an equine metacarpus.
A. Distal row of carpal bones
B. Third metacarpal bone
C. Fourth metacarpal bone
D. Medial proximal sesamoid bones
E. Lateral proximal sesamoid bone
F. Proximal phalanx

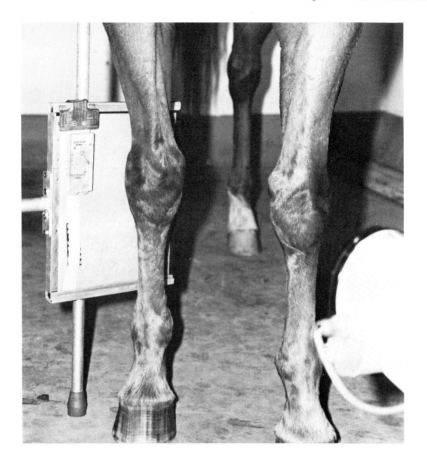

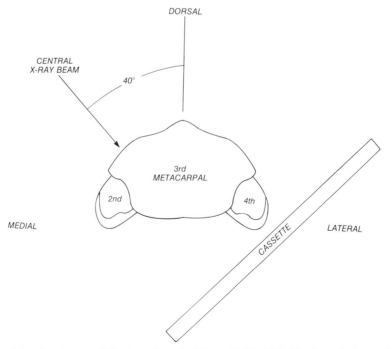

Figure 18–28. Position for dorsomedial-palmarolateral oblique (D40°M-PaLO) view of the equine metacarpus (formerly dorsopalmar lateral oblique or anteroposterior lateral oblique [APLO]).

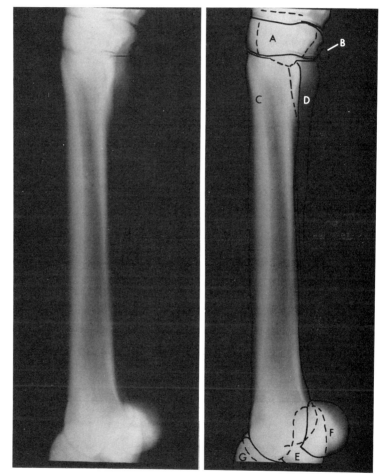

Figure 18–29. Dorsomedial-palmarolateral oblique (D40°M-PaLO) view of an equine metacarpus.
A. Distal row of carpal bones
B. First carpal bone
C. Third metacarpal bone
D. Second metacarpal bone
E. Lateral proximal sesamoid bone
F. Medial proximal sesamoid bone
G. Proximal phalanx

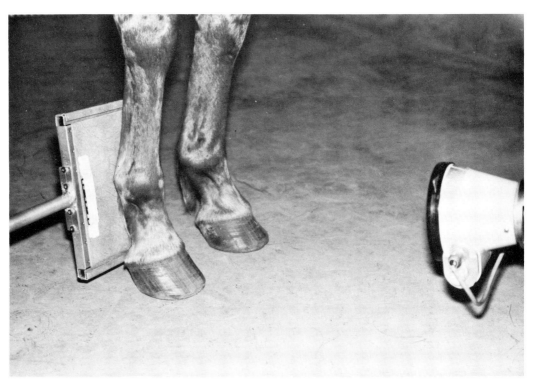

Figure 18–30. Position for dorsopalmar (DPa) view of the metacarpophalangeal (fetlock) joint and the proximal sesamoid bone in the equine (formerly anteroposterior [AP]).

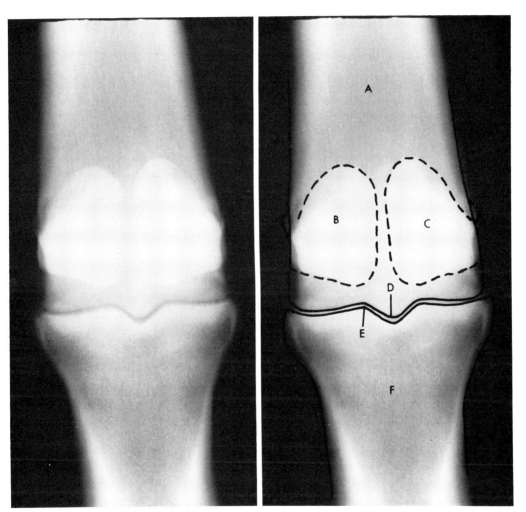

Figure 18–31. Dorsopalmar (DPa) view of the metacarpophalangeal (fetlock) joint and the proximal sesamoid bones in an equine.

A. Distal end of the third metacarpal bone
B. Medial proximal sesamoid bone
C. Lateral proximal sesamoid bone
D. Sagittal ridge of the third metacarpal bone
E. Metacarpophalangeal joint
F. Proximal phalanx

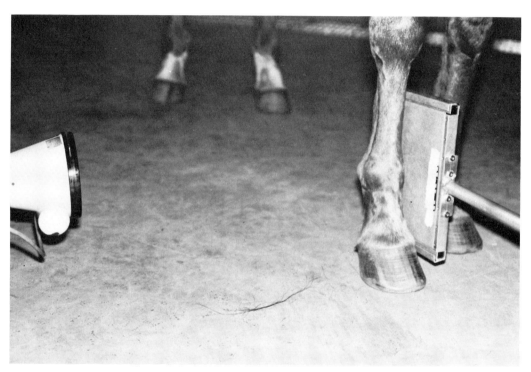

Figure 18–32. Position for lateromedial (LM) view of the metacarpophalangeal (fetlock) joint and the proximal sesamoid bones in the equine.

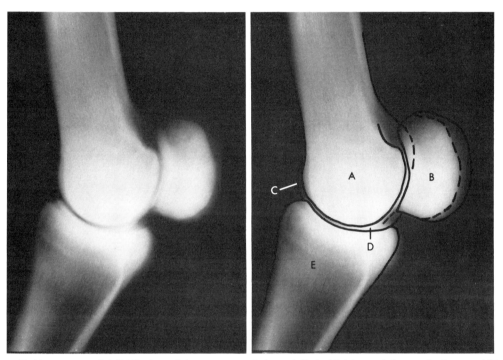

Figure 18–33. Lateromedial (LM) view of the metacarpophalangeal (fetlock) joint and the proximal sesamoid bone in an equine.

A. Distal end of the third metacarpal bone
B. Proximal sesamoid bones
C. Sagittal ridge of the third metacarpal bone
D. Metacarpophalangeal joint
E. Proximal phalanx

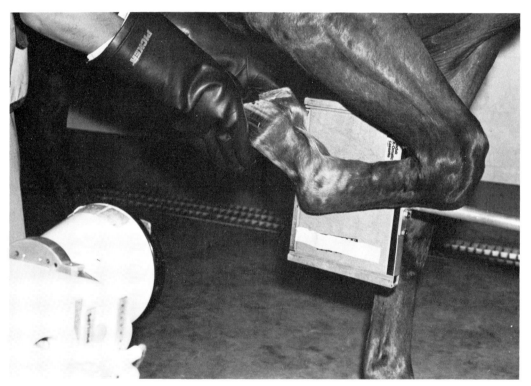

Figure 18–34. Position for the flexed lateromedial (LM-flexed) view of the metacarpophalangeal (fetlock) joint and proximal sesamoid bones in the equine.

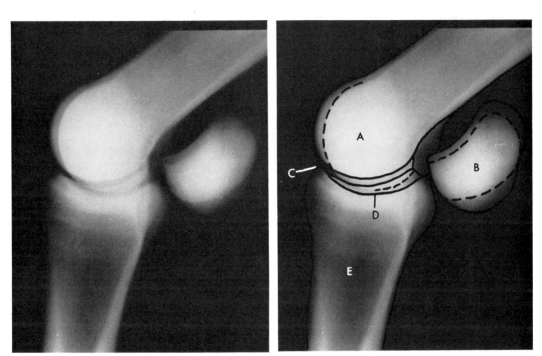

Figure 18–35. Flexed lateromedial (LM-flexed) view of the metacarpophalangeal (fetlock) joint and proximal sesamoid bones in an equine.

A. Distal end of the third metacarpal bone
B. Proximal sesamoid bones
C. Sagittal ridge of the third metacarpal bone
D. Metacarpophalangeal joint
E. Proximal phalanx

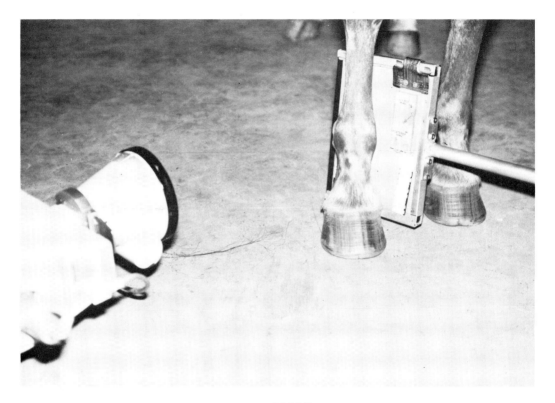

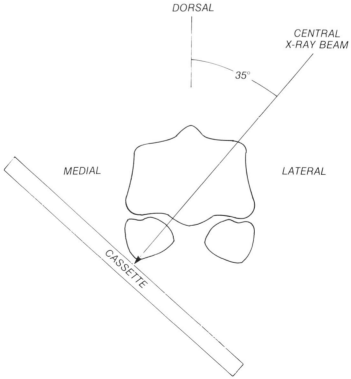

Figure 18–36. Position for the dorsolateral-palmaromedial oblique (D35°L-PaMO) view of the equine lateral proximal sesamoid bone (formerly dorsopalmar medial oblique or anteroposterior medial oblique [APMO]).

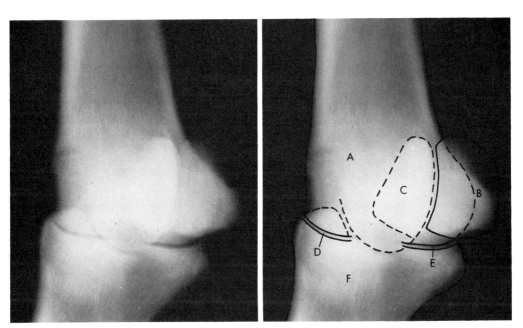

Figure 18–37. Dorsolateral-palmaromedial oblique (D35°L-PaMO) view of an equine lateral proximal sesamoid bone.

    A. Distal end of the third metacarpal bone
    B. Lateral proximal sesamoid bone
    C. Medial proximal sesamoid bone superimposed upon the metacarpal bone
    D. Dorsomedial aspect of the metacarpophalangeal joint
    E. Palmarolateral aspect of the metacarpophalangeal joint
    F. Proximal phalanx

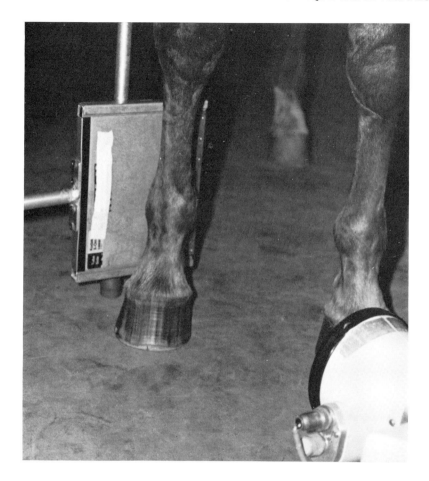

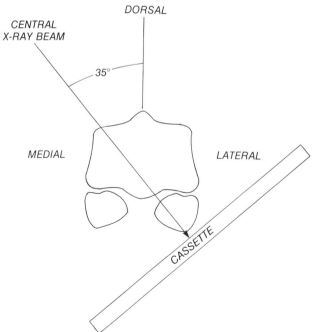

Figure 18–38. Position for the dorsomedial-palmarolateral oblique (D35°M-PaLO) view of the equine medial proximal sesamoid bone (formerly dorsopalmar lateral oblique or anteroposterior lateral oblique [APLO]).

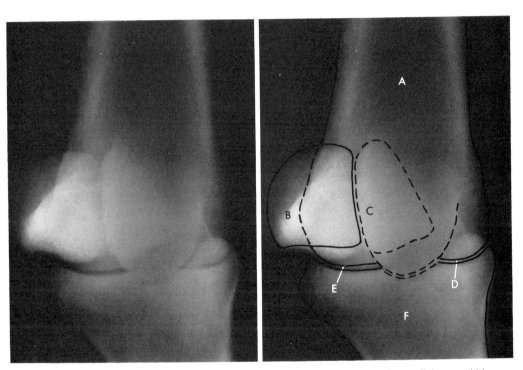

Figure 18–39. Dorsomedial-palmarolateral oblique (D35°M-PaLO) view of an equine medial sesamoid bone.
- A. Distal end of the third metacarpal bone
- B. Medial proximal sesamoid bone
- C. Lateral proximal sesamoid bone
- D. Dorsolateral aspect of the metacarpophalangeal joint
- E. Palmaromedial aspect of the metacarpophalangeal joint
- F. Proximal phalanx

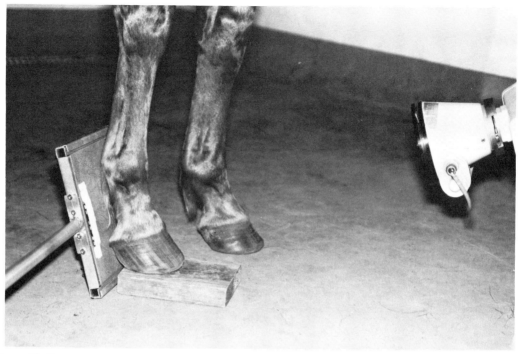

Figure 18–40. Position for dorsopalmar (DPa) view of the equine proximal and middle phalanges (formerly anteroposterior [AP]).

DIGIT

Dorsopalmar (DPa) View. (Formerly anteroposterior [AP] view.) The patient is allowed to stand normally and the cassette holder is placed against the palmar surface of the phalanges (Fig. 18–40). If the distal interphalangeal (coffin) joint is of particular interest, the foot should be placed on a wooden block so that the cassette may extend distal to the distal phalanx. The x-ray beam is directed perpendicular to the cassette surface and centered at the region of specific interest along the midsagittal line of the dorsal surface. Survey examination of the digit may be done by centering the x-ray beam at the proximal interphalangeal (pastern) joint. A grid is not necessary. In uncooperative patients, the contralateral limb may be lifted to help reduce motion.

Figure 18–41 illustrates the radiographic anatomy of an equine digit in DPa view.

Lateromedial (LM) View. The patient is allowed to stand normally and the cassette holder is placed against the medial surface of the digit (Fig. 18–42). The x-ray beam is directed parallel to the floor and centered at the region of specific interest on the lateral surface. Survey examination of the digit may be done by centering the x-ray beam at the proximal interphalangeal (pastern) joint. A grid is not necessary.

In uncooperative patients, the contralateral limb may be lifted to help reduce motion. The person lifting the leg should stand clear of the primary x-ray beam.

Figure 18–43 illustrates the radiographic anatomy of an equine digit in LM view.

DISTAL PHALANX AND DISTAL SESAMOID (NAVICULAR) BONE

Dorsoproximal-Palmarodistal Oblique (D65°Pr-PaDiO) View. (Formerly dorsopalmar or anteroposterior [AP] view.) This view is especially designed to examine the distal phalanx and distal sesamoid (navicular) bone in dorsopalmar projection. The foot is placed on a cassette tunnel and the patient is allowed to stand normally. The x-ray beam

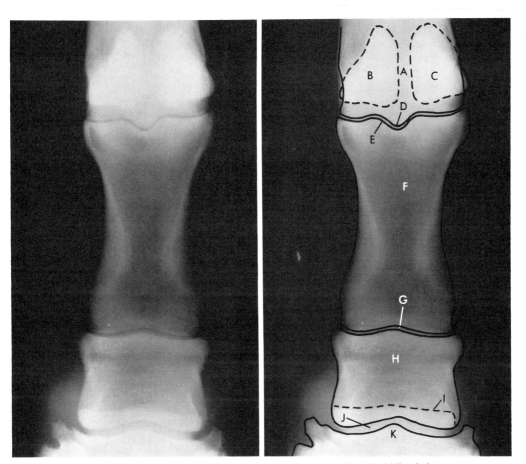

Figure 18–41. Dorsopalmar (DPa) view of the equine proximal and middle phalanges.

A. Third metacarpal bone
B. Lateral proximal sesamoid bone
C. Medial proximal sesamoid bone
D. Sagittal ridge of the third metacarpal bone
E. Metacarpophalangeal (fetlock) joint
F. Proximal phalanx
G. Proximal interphalangeal (pastern) joint
H. Middle phalanx
 I. Proximal border of the distal sesamoid bone (navicular)
J. Distal interphalangeal (coffin) joint
K. Distal phalanx

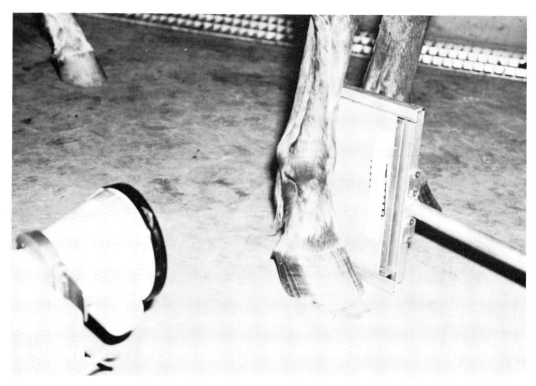

Figure 18–42. Position for lateromedial (LM) view of the equine proximal and middle phalanges.

is directed 65 degrees proximal to the floor[1] and centered at the coronary border of the hoof along the midsagittal line of the dorsal surface (Fig. 18–44). The angle of the x-ray beam to the floor will vary with patient conformation, but 65 degrees will usually produce a satisfactory examination of the distal sesamoid (navicular) bone. The angle may be reduced to as little as 45 degrees if the distal phalanx is of primary interest.

The exposure should be reduced if the body and solar borders of the distal phalanx are of primary interest. If the distal interphalangeal joint or distal sesamoid (navicular) bone is of interest, a normal grid expo-

sure for the thickness of the part should be used.

If the patient has pain in the flexor apparatus, such as in severe navicular disease, a normal standing position may not be possible. In these cases the foot can be placed in a wooden supporting device (Hickman block) in such a manner that the toe is pointed downward and the interphalangeal joints are allowed to flex, thereby removing the pain-producing pressure. The x-ray beam is directed parallel to the floor and centered at the coronary border of the hoof on the midsagittal line of the dorsal surface (Fig. 18–45).

When the distal phalanx and distal sesamoid (navicular) bone are examined, the shoe should be removed and the sole and frog of the hoof should be cleaned and packed with a substance that will eliminate air from the sole of the hoof. Play-Doh[2] works well for this purpose.

Figure 18–46 illustrates the radiographic anatomy of an equine distal phalanx in D65°Pr-PaDiO view.

---

[1]The nomenclature committee of the American College of Veterinary Radiology (Shively et al., 1982) concedes that the supporting surface is not equivalent to the transverse plane through this body part. In an effort to avoid the complexities of angles in the distal limb, the nomenclature is based on a simplified schematic perspective in which the animal is considered to have vertically oriented limbs; therefore, the supporting surface is used rather than the true transverse plane of the limb in naming the positions. Additional justification for this recommendation includes the fact that the angle indicators on most x-ray tube heads are based on horizontal and vertical axes.

---

[2]Rainbow Crafts, Cincinnati, Ohio.

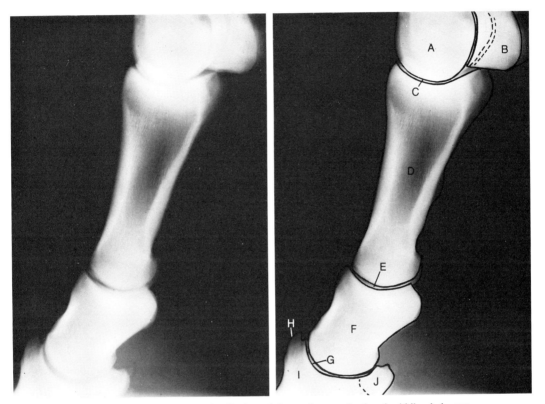

Figure 18–43. Lateromedial (LM) view of the equine proximal and middle phalanges.

    A. Third metacarpal bone
    B. Proximal sesamoid bones
    C. Metacarpophalangeal (fetlock) joint
    D. Proximal phalanx
    E. Proximal interphalangeal (pastern) joint
    F. Middle phalanx
    G. Distal interphalangeal (coffin) joint
    H. Extensor process distal phalanx
    I. Distal phalanx
    J. Distal sesamoid (navicular) bone

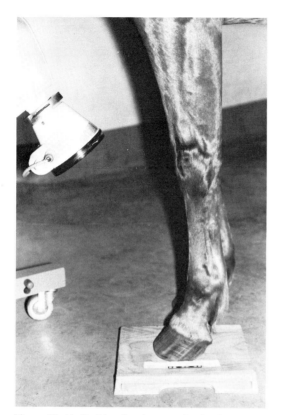
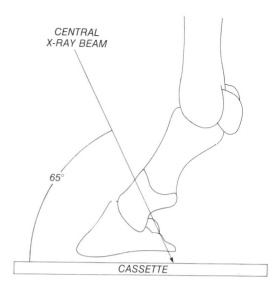

Figure 18–44. Position for dorsoproximal-palmarodistal oblique (D65°Pr-PaDiO) view of the equine distal phalanx and distal sesamoid (navicular) bone (formerly dorsopalmar or anteroposterior [AP]) view).

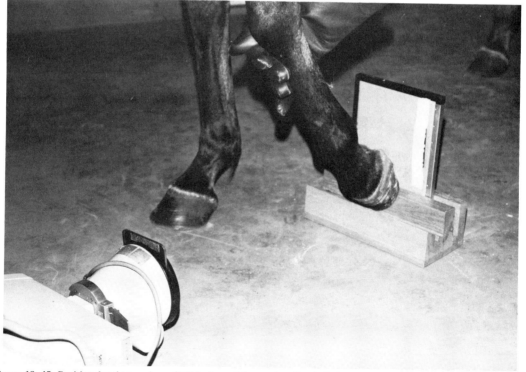

Figure 18–45. Position for dorsopalmar (DPa) view of the equine distal phalanx and distal sesamoid (navicular) bone using a wooden positioning block.

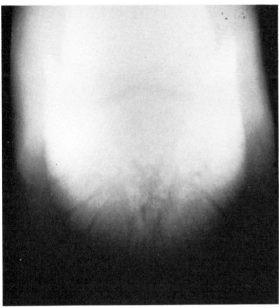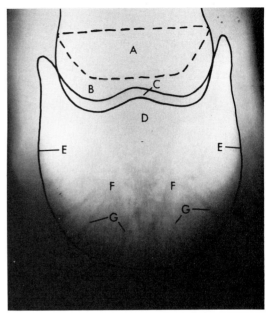

Figure 18–46. Dorsoproximal-palmarodistal oblique (D65°Pr-PaDiO) view of an equine distal phalanx.

  A. Distal sesamoid (navicular) bone
  B. Middle phalanx
  C. Distal interphalangeal joint
  D. Distal phalanx
  E. Volar borders
  F. Volar canal
  G. Vascular channels

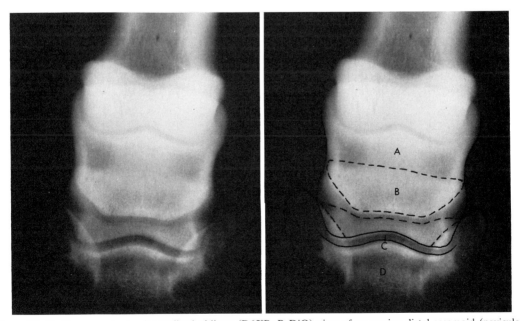

Figure 18–47. Dorsoproximal-palmarodistal oblique (D65°Pr-PaDiO) view of an equine distal sesamoid (navicular) bone.

  A. Middle phalanx
  B. Distal sesamoid (navicular) bone
  C. Distal interphalangeal joint
  D. Distal phalanx

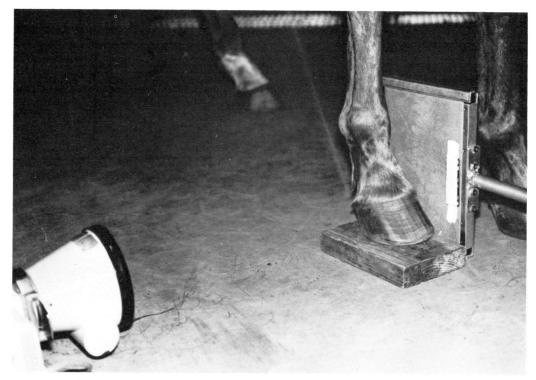

Figure 18–48. Position for lateromedial (LM) view of the equine distal extremity.

Figure 18–47 illustrates the radiographic anatomy of an equine distal sesamoid (navicular) bone in D65°Pr-PaDiO view.

Lateromedial (LM) View. The foot is placed on a wooden block so that the x-ray beam may be centered at the coronary border of the hoof with the tube head lowered to the floor. The cassette holder is placed on the medial surface, and the x-ray beam is directed parallel to the floor and centered on the lateral surface at the level of the coronary border of the hoof (Fig. 18–48). A grid is not needed.

In uncooperative patients the contralateral limb may be lifted to help reduce motion. The person lifting the leg should stand clear of the primary x-ray beam.

Figure 18–49 illustrates the radiographic anatomy of an equine distal extremity in ML view.

Laterodorsoproximal-Mediopalmarodistal Oblique (L45°D50°Pr-MPaDiO) View. (Formerly oblique view of the distal phalanx.) The foot is placed on a cassette tunnel and the patient is allowed to stand normally. The x-ray beam is directed 45 degrees dorsal to the lateral surface and 50 degrees proximal to the floor and centered at the coronary border of the hoof (Fig. 18–50). The exposure should be reduced if the volar borders of the distal phalanx are of primary interest.

In uncooperative patients, the contralateral limb may be lifted to help control motion.

Figure 18–51 illustrates the radiographic anatomy of an equine distal extremity in L45°D50°Pr-MPaDiO view.

Palmaroproximal-Dorsodistal Oblique (Pa75°Pr-DDiO) View. (Formerly flexor view of the distal sesamoid [navicular] bone.) This view is especially designed to examine the palmar cortex (flexor surface) of the distal sesamoid (navicular) bone. The foot is placed on a cassette tunnel as far caudally as possible so that the metacarpophalangeal (fetlock) joint is maximally extended. If the patient is not cooperative owing to discomfort when maximum tension is placed on inflamed flexor tendons or bursa, the heel may be elevated by placing a wooden block or dowel such as a broomhandle between the bulbs of the heel and the cassette tunnel. The patient is then allowed to stand in a normal position with

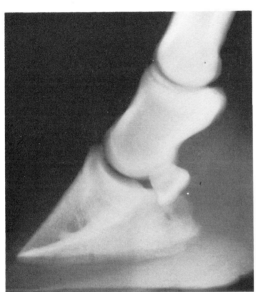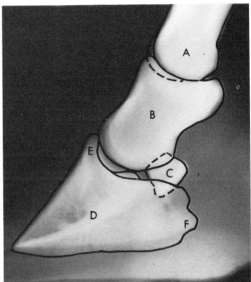

Figure 18–49. Lateromedial (LM) view of an equine distal extremity.
- A. Proximal phalanx
- B. Middle phalanx
- C. Distal sesamoid (navicular) bone
- D. Distal phalanx
- E. Extensor process
- F. Palmar processes

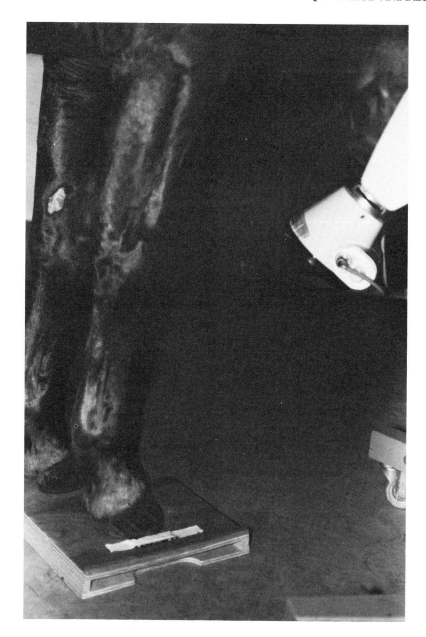

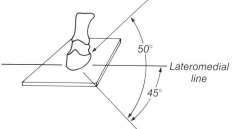

Laterodorsalproximal-mediopalmarodistal
oblique
(L45°D50°Pr-MPaDiO)

50°

Lateromedial
line

45°

Figure 18–50. Position for laterodorsoproximal-mediopalmarodistal oblique (L45°D50°Pr-MPaDiO) view of the equine distal sesamoid (navicular) bone and distal phalanx of the equine (formerly oblique view of the distal phalanx).

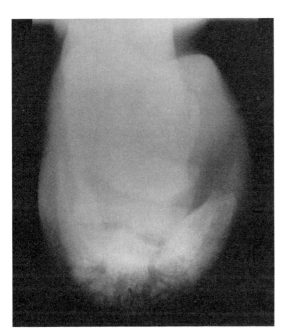 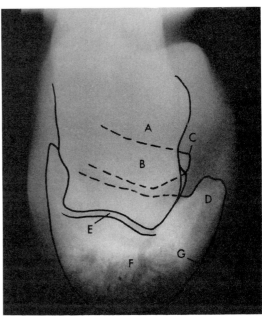

Figure 18–51. Laterodorsoproximal-mediopalmarodistal oblique (L45°D50°Pr-MPaDiO) view of an equine distal sesamoid (navicular) bone and distal phalanx.

        A. Middle phalanx
        B. Distal sesamoid (navicular) bone
        C. Lateral angle of the distal sesamoid (navicular) bone
        D. Lateral palmar process
        E. Distal interphalangeal joint
        F. Distal phalanx
        G. Lateral volar border

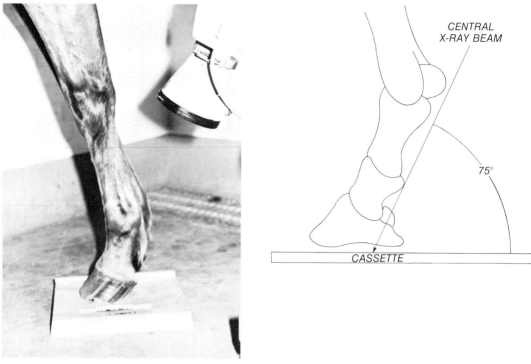

Figure 18–52. Position for palmaroproximal-dorsodistal oblique (Pa75°Pr-DDiO) view of the flexor surface of the equine distal sesamoid (navicular) bone (formerly flexor view).

less tension on the flexor apparatus (Root and Taylor, 1982).

The x-ray beam is directed 75 degrees proximal to the floor and centered on the bulbs of the heel at the midsagittal line of the palmar surface (Fig. 18–52). The FFD must be decreased so that the tube head may be placed under the thoracic wall.

In uncooperative patients, the contralateral limb may be lifted to help control motion. If pain in the flexor apparatus is severe, lifting the contralateral limb may not be beneficial. In these cases, a nerve block may be necessary to control pain.

Figure 18–53 illustrates the radiographic anatomy of an equine distal sesamoid (navicular) bone in Pa75°Pr-DDiO view.

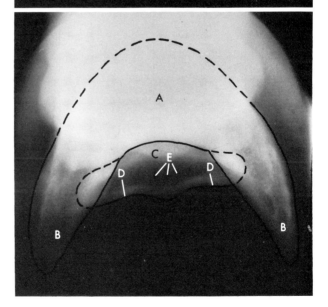

Figure 18–53. Palmaroproximal-dorsodistal oblique (Pa75°Pr-DDiO) view of the flexor surface of an equine distal sesamoid (navicular) bone.
- A. Distal phalanx superimposed over the middle phalanx
- B. Palmar processes
- C. Distal sesamoid (navicular) bone
- D. Palmar cortex
- E. Vascular channels

REFERENCES

Getty, R.: Sisson and Grossman's The Anatomy of the Domestic Animals. 5th ed. Philadelphia, W. B. Saunders Co., 1975.

Morgan, J. P., and Silverman, S.: Techniques in Veterinary Radiography. 3rd ed. Davis, Ca., Veterinary Radiology Associates, 1982.

Rendano, V. T., and Grant, B.: The equine third phalanx: Its radiographic appearance. J. Am. Vet. Radiol. Soc., 19(4):125, 1977.

Root, C. R., and Taylor, S. D.: Louisiana State University, Baton Rouge. Personal Communications. 1982.

Schebitz, H., and Wilkens, H.: Atlas of Radiographic Anatomy of the Horse. Berlin, Paul Parey, 1978.

Shively, M. J., Smallwood, J. E., Habel, R. E., and Rendano, V. T.: A Standardized Nomenclature for Radiographic Views Used in Veterinary Medicine. Unpublished report of the Nomenclature Committee, Am. Coll. Vet. Radiol., 1982.

Smallwood, J. E., and Shively, M. J.: Radiographic and xerographic anatomy of the equine carpus. Equine Practice. 1(1):22, 1979.

19

Pelvic Limb

STIFLE JOINT

Caudocranial (CdCr) View. (Formerly posteroanterior [PA] view.) The patient is allowed to stand normally and the cassette holder is placed adjacent to the cranial surface of the femorotibial (stifle) joint. The cassette will be at an angle that is less than 90 degrees to the floor when the cassette is snugly fitted to the cranial surface (Fig. 19–1). The x-ray beam is directed at a 90 degree angle to the cassette surface (above and directed downward toward the stifle joint) and centered at the joint on the midsagittal plane of the caudal surface. A grid should be used to minimize fog-producing scatter radiation. Alternatively, the exposure may be made through the back of the cassette (see p. 69). In uncooperative patients, a contralateral limb may be lifted to help minimize motion and the danger of kick. Figure 19–2 illustrates the radiographic anatomy of an equine stifle joint in CdCr view.

Lateromedial (LM) View. The patient is allowed to stand normally and the cassette holder is placed on the medial surface of the joint as high in the flank as possible. The x-ray beam is directed parallel to the floor and centered at the joint on the lateral surface (Fig. 19–3). The region of the joint is approximately 10 cm distal to the palpated patella. If the patella or trochleae of the femur are of primary interest, the x-ray beam should be centered at the patella and the exposure reduced.

In some patients the cassette will not be tolerated high in flank region. In these cases, profound sedation or anesthesia may be necessary to perform a satisfactory examination.

Place the affected limb on the table and use a vertical x-ray beam. A grid may be necessary to reduce fog-producing scatter radiation. Alternatively, the exposure may be made through the back of the cassette (see p. 69).

Figure 19–4 illustrates the radiographic anatomy of an equine stifle joint in LM view.

TARSAL (HOCK) JOINT

Dorsoplantar (DPl) View. (Formerly anteroposterior [AP] view.) The patient is allowed to stand normally and the cassette holder is placed on the plantar surface of the tarsal joint (Fig. 19–5). The x-ray beam is directed parallel to the floor and centered at the distal intertarsal joint on the midsagittal plane of the dorsal surface. It is helpful if the patient points the foot laterally so that the dorsal surface is perpendicular to the x-ray beam when the tube head is as close to the thorax as possible. If the patient stands with appreciable flexion of the tarsocrural (tibiotarsal) joint, the cassette will be at an angle less than 90 degrees to the floor. In these cases, the x-ray beam should be directed perpendicular to the cassette surface rather than parallel to the floor. This will assure that the intertarsal and tarsometatarsal joints will be oriented perpendicular to the cassette and parallel to the x-ray beam. In uncooperative patients, a contralateral limb may be lifted to help reduce motion. A grid may be necessary to reduce fog-producing scatter radiation.

Text continued on page 467.

459

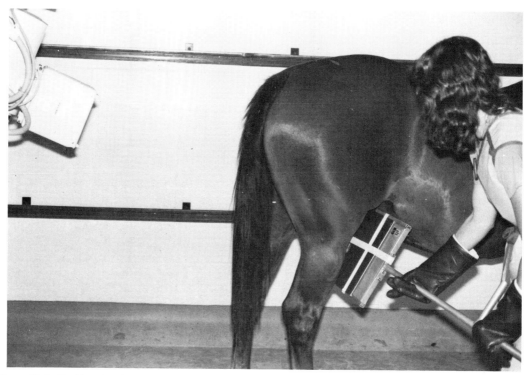

Figure 19–1. Position for the caudocranial (CdCr) view of the equine stifle joint (formerly posteroanterior [PA] view).

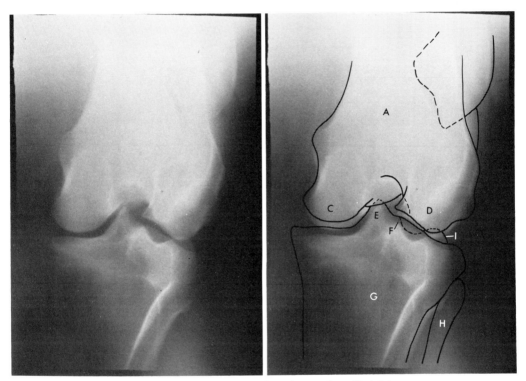

Figure 19–2. Caudocranial view of an equine stifle joint.
- A. Distal femur
- B. Patella
- C. Medial condyle
- D. Lateral condyle
- E. Medial intercondyloid tubercle
- F. Lateral intercondyloid tubercle
- G. Proximal tibia
- H. Fibula
- I. Tibial tuberosity

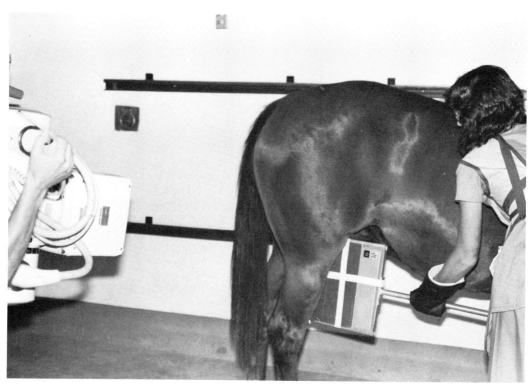

Figure 19–3. Position for the lateromedial (LM) view of the equine stifle joint.

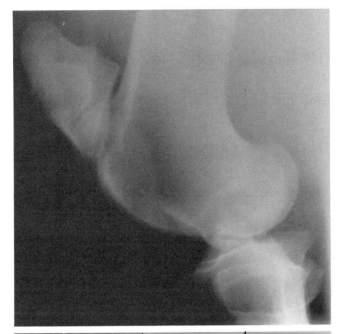

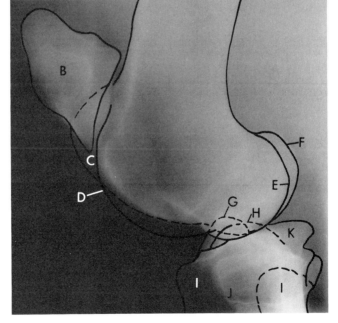

Figure 19–4. Lateromedial (LM) view of an equine stifle joint.

    A. Distal femur
    B. Patella
    C. Medial ridge of the trochlea
    D. Lateral ridge of the trochlea
    E. Lateral condyle
    F. Medial condyle
    G. Medial intercondyloid tubercle
    H. Lateral intercondyloid tubercle
    I. Tibial tuberosity
    J. Proximal tibia
    K. Lateral condyle of the tibia
    L. Fibula

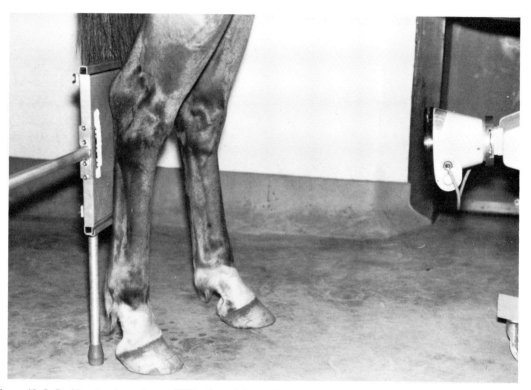

Figure 19–5. Position for dorsoplantar (DPl) view of the equine tarsus (hock joint) (formerly anteroposterior [AP] view).

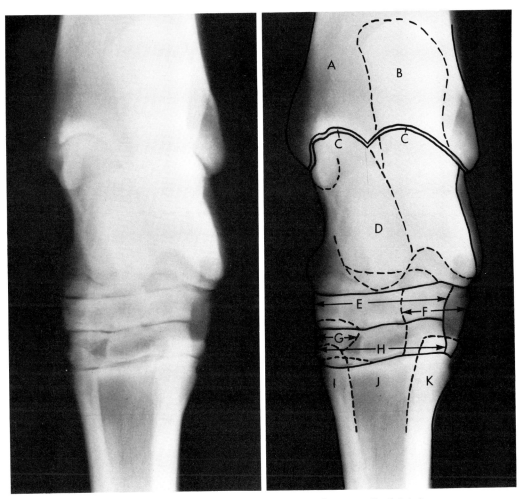

Figure 19–6. Dorsoplantar (DPl) view of an equine tarsus (hock joint).

    A. Distal tibia
    B. Calcaneus (fibular tarsal bone)
    C. Tarso-crural joint (tibiotarsal joint)
    D. Talus (tibial tarsal bone)
    E. Central tarsal bone
    F. Fourth tarsal bone
    G. Fused first and second tarsal bones
    H. Third tarsal bone
    I. Second metatarsal bone
    J. Third metatarsal bone
    K. Fourth metatarsal bone

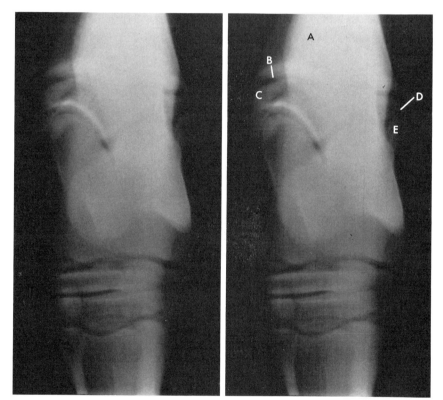

Figure 19–7. Dorsoplantar (DPl) view of a five-week-old equine tarsus (hock joint).
A. Distal tibial metaphysis
B. Distal tibial physis
C. Distal tibial epiphysis
D. Distal fibular physis
E. Distal fibular epiphysis (fuses to the tibial epiphysis to form the lateral malleolus)

Alternatively, the exposure may be made through the back of the cassette (see p. 69).

Figure 19–6 illustrates the radiographic anatomy of a mature equine tarsal joint in DPl view.

Figure 19–7 illustrates the radiographic anatomy of an immature equine tarsal joint in DPl view. Note the ossification center of the distal fibular epiphysis (E) that fuses with the distal tibial epiphysis to form the lateral malleolus at 3 to 24 (most at 12) months of age.

Lateromedial (LM) View. The patient is allowed to stand normally and the cassette holder placed on the medial surface of the tarsus (Fig. 19–8). The x-ray beam is directed parallel to the floor and centered at the distal intertarsal joint on the lateral surface. In large horses or when excessive swelling is present, a grid may be necessary to reduce fog-producing scatter radiation. Alternatively, the exposure may be made through the back of the cassette (see p. 69).

In uncooperative patients, a forelimb may be lifted to reduce motion. The contralateral rear limb should not be lifted because the person lifting the limb will be in the primary x-ray beam.

Figure 19–9 illustrates the radiographic anatomy of an equine tarsus in LM view.

Dorsolateral-Plantaromedial Oblique (D60°L-PlMO) View. (Formerly antero-posterior medial oblique [APMO] or dorso-plantar medial oblique view.) The patient is allowed to stand normally and the cassette holder is placed on the plantaromedial surface of the tarsal joint (Fig. 19–10). The x-ray beam is directed parallel to the floor, 60 degrees lateral to the dorsal surface and centered at the distal intertarsal joint. In large horses or when excessive swelling is present, a grid may be necessary to reduce fog-producing scatter radiation. Alternatively, the exposure may be made through the back of the cassette (see p. 69).

In uncooperative patients, a contralateral limb may be lifted to reduce motion; however, the person lifting the limb should be careful to stand clear of the x-ray beam.

Figure 19–11 illustrates the radiographic anatomy of an equine tarsal joint in D60°L-PlMO view.

Dorsomedial-Plantarolateral Oblique (D60°M-PlLO) View. (Formerly antero-posterior lateral oblique [APLO] or dorso-plantar lateral oblique view). The patient is allowed to stand normally and the cassette holder is placed on the plantarolateral surface of the tarsal joint (Fig. 19–12). The x-ray beam is directed parallel to the floor, 60 degrees medial to the dorsal surface and centered at the distal intertarsal joint. In large horses or when excessive swelling is present, a grid may be necessary to reduce fog-producing scatter radiation. Alternatively, the exposure may be made through the back of the cassette (see p. 69).

In some uncooperative patients, the presence of an x-ray tube under the abdomen may not be tolerated. In these cases a plantarolateral-dorsomedial oblique (Pl60°L-DMO) view may be used to produce similar results. The cassette is placed on the dorsomedial surface of the tarsal joint and the x-ray beam is directed parallel to the floor, 60 degrees lateral from the plantar surface and centered at the distal intertarsal joint. A grid may be necessary to reduce fog-producing scatter radiation. Alternatively, the exposure may be made through the back of the cassette (see p. 69). In uncooperative patients a contralateral limb may be lifted to reduce motion.

Figure 19–13 illustrates the radiographic anatomy of an equine tarsal joint in D60°M-PlLO view.

Pelvic Limb Distal to the Tarsus. The distal pelvic limb may be examined in a manner similar to that for the thoracic limb. The terminology is the same except that the term plantar is substituted for palmar in the position descriptions.

SPECIAL VIEWS OF THE PELVIC LIMB

Ventrodorsal (VD) and Lateral (Le-RtL or Rt-LeL) View of the Pelvis. The pelvis may only be examined in ventrodorsal (VD) recumbent and lateral view while the patient is anesthetized. It is necessary to use an x-ray generator with very high ma (300 to 2000) capacity. Intensifying screens should be of the rare earth phosphor type to reduce exposure requirements. The best detail may be obtained by using a high ratio (12:1) grid to help reduce fog-producing scatter radiation. In very large patients, a pair of 10:1 ratio grids may be placed with the grid lines 90 degrees to each other, thereby producing the so-called cross-hatched arrangement.

The grid and the cassette should be placed under the patient in a protecting tunnel or under a table or cart with a radiolucent top. A lead sheet should be placed under the

Text continued on page 474.

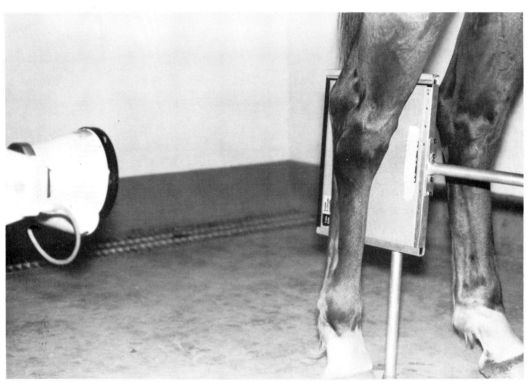

Figure 19–8. Position for the lateromedial (LM) view of the equine tarsus (hock joint).

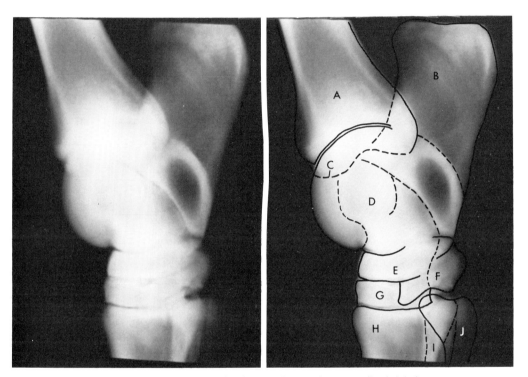

Figure 19–9. Lateromedial (LM) view of an equine tarsus (hock joint).
A. Distal tibia
B. Calcaneus (fibular tarsal bone)
C. Sagittal ridge of the tibial trochlea
D. Talus (tibial tarsal bone)
E. Central tarsal bone
F. Fourth tarsal bone
G. Third tarsal bone
H. Third metatarsal bone
I. Second metatarsal bone
J. Fourth metatarsal bone

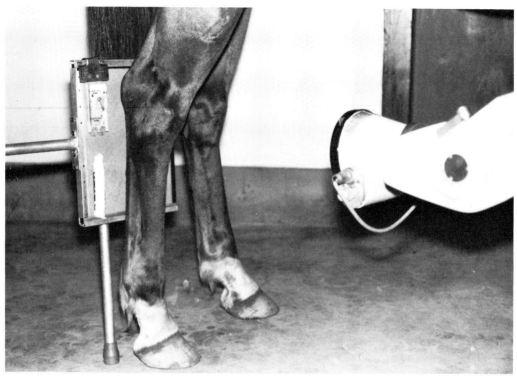

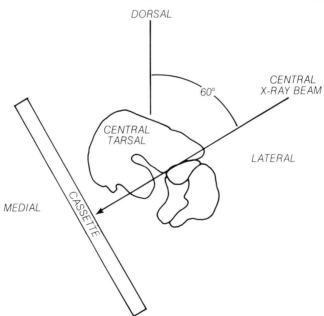

Figure 19–10. Position for dorsolateral-plantaromedial oblique (D60°L-PlMO) view of the equine tarsus (hock joint) (formerly anteroposterior medial oblique [APMO] or dorsoplantar medial oblique).

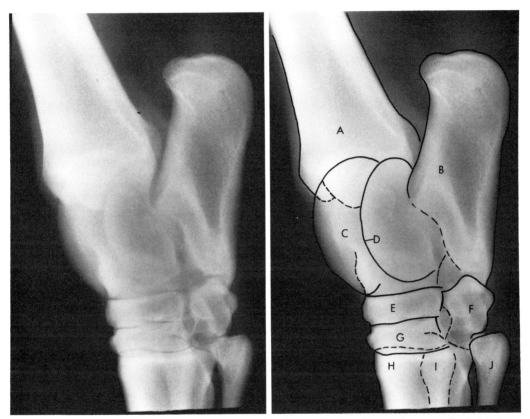

Figure 19–11. Dorsolateral-plantaromedial oblique (D60°L-PlMO) view of an equine tarsus (hock joint).

    A. Distal tibia
    B. Calcaneus (fibular tarsal bone)
    C. Medial ridge of talus trochlea
    D. Lateral ridge of talus trochlea
    E. Central tarsal bone
    F. Fourth tarsal bone
    G. Third tarsal bone
    H. Third metatarsal bone
    I. Second metatarsal bone superimposed over the third
    J. Fourth metatarsal bone

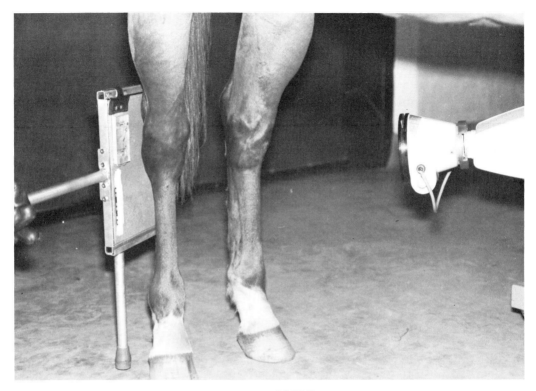

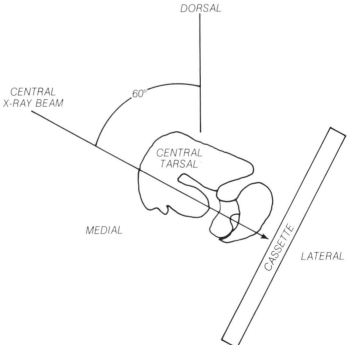

Figure 19–12. Position for dorsomedial-plantarolateral oblique (D60°M-PlLO) view of the equine tarsus (hock joint) (formerly anteroposterior lateral oblique [APLO] or dorsoplantar lateral oblique).

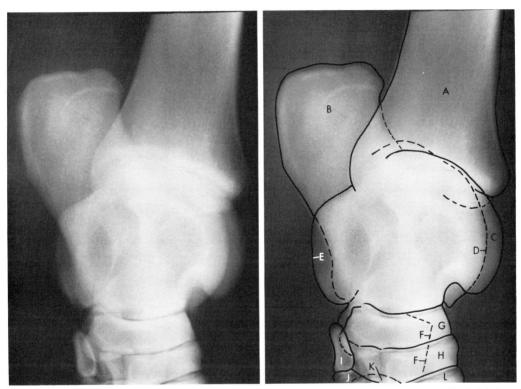

Figure 19–13. Dorsomedial-plantarolateral oblique (D60°M-PlLO) view of an equine tarsus (hock joint).

A. Distal tibia
B. Calcaneus
C. Lateral ridge of talus trochlea
D. Medial ridge of talus trochlea
E. Plantar surface of sustentaculum tali
F. Fourth tarsal bone
G. Central tarsal bone
H. Third tarsal bone
I. Fused first and second tarsal bones
J. Second metatarsal bone
K. Fourth metatarsal bone superimposed
L. Third metatarsal bone

cassette to prevent back scatter from the floor. Exposures of 500-600 mas and 125 kv are typical for these examinations.

Proximodistal (PrDi) View of the Patella and Cranial Surface of the Distal Femur. (Formerly skyline view.) This view requires that the stifle and tarsal joints be flexed and the x-ray beam be directed distally from overhead toward the person flexing the limb when the patient is standing. It is therefore not recommended except in rare instances and then only when the patient is placed in lateral recumbency under general anesthesia.

Dorsoplantar (DPl) View of the Calcaneal Tuber. Occasionally this special view of the calcaneal tuber is required to assess the extent of abnormalities in the region. The stifle and tarsus are flexed and the cassette holder is placed on the plantar surface of the tarsus, parallel to the floor. The x-ray beam is directed vertically from overhead at the dorsal surface of the calcaneal tuber. A grid is not necessary.

REFERENCES

Getty, R.: Sisson and Grossman's The Anatomy of the Domestic Animals. 5th ed. Philadelphia, W. B. Saunders Co., 1975.

Morgan, P., and Silverman, S.: Techniques of Veterinary Radiography. 3rd ed. Davis, Ca., Veterinary Radiology Associates, 1982.

Schebitz, H., and Wilkens, H.: Atlas of Radiographic Anatomy of the Horse. Berlin, Paul Parey, 1978.

20

Vertebral Column

CERVICAL VERTEBRAE

Left-right Lateral (Le-RtL standing/horizontal) or Right-Left Lateral (Rt-LeL standing/horizontal) View. The cervical vertebrae may be examined in lateral view in the standing equine if careful attention is given to positioning and x-ray beam placement. Hyperextension or hyperflexion examinations of the cervical vertebrae in lateral view can be satisfactorily made only with the patient under general anesthesia. VD views require general anesthesia.

The patient is allowed to stand normally against a cassette cabinet (Fig. 20–1) or with a cassette holder placed on the lateral surface in the region to be examined. At least three overlapping radiographs should be made for a routine survey. The x-ray beam is directed horizontal to the floor centered at C2, C4 and at C6 on the lateral surface opposite the cassette. A grid must be used to help reduce fog-producing scatter radiation. Alternatively, the exposure may be made through the back of the cassette (see p. 69).

Figures 20–2, 20–4 and 20–5 illustrate the radiographic anatomy of an equine cervical

region in Le-RtL view. The minimum sagittal diameter of the cranial aspect of each vertebral body from C2 to C7 has been reported (Mayhew, et al., 1978) and is listed in Table 20–1. Patients with minimum sagittal diameters of less than listed values should be considered to have a stenotic vertebral canal.

Figure 20–3 illustrates the radiographic anatomy of an immature equine cervical vertebral column. Note the pair of physeal lines in the cranial aspect of C2 (b and d). These normal structures should not be mistaken for fractures.

REFERENCES

Getty, R.: Sisson and Grossman's The Anatomy of the Domestic Animals. 5th ed. Philadelphia, W. B. Saunders Co. 1975.

Mayhew, I. G., DeLahunta, A., Whitlock, R. H., Krook, L., and Tasker, J. B.: The Cornell Veterinarian. *68*(Suppl. 6):44, 1978.

Morgan, P., and Silverman, S.: Techniques of Veterinary Radiography. 3rd ed. Davis, Ca., Veterinary Radiology Associates, 1982.

Schebitz, H., and Wilkens, H.: Atlas of Radiographic Anatomy of the Horse. Berlin, Paul Parey, 1978.

Illustrations and table follow.

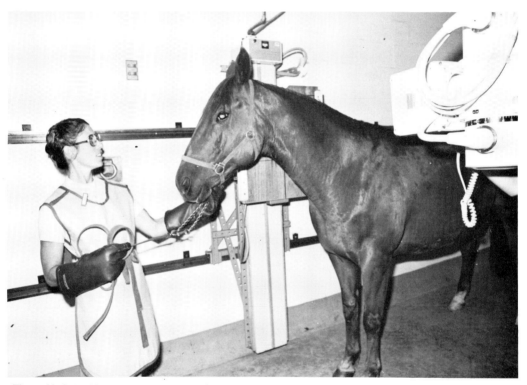

Figure 20–1. Position for left-right lateral (Le-RtL standing/horizontal) view of the equine cervical vertebrae.

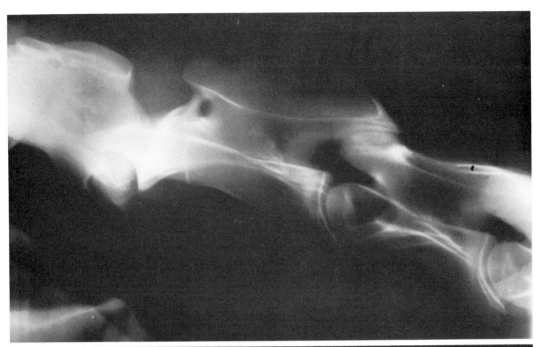

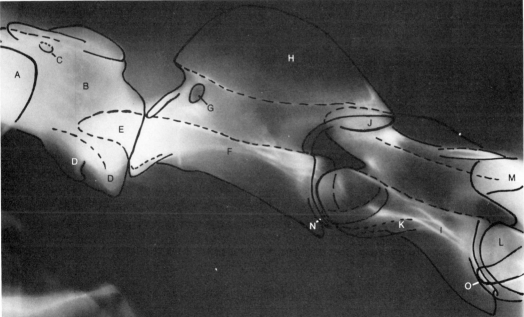

Figure 20–2. Left-right lateral (Le-RtL standing/horizontal) view of the cranial aspect of an equine cervical vertebral column.

A. Occipital condyles
B. C1 (atlas)
C. Transverse foramen
D. Transverse processes of C1
E. Dens
F. Body of C2 (axis)
G. Lateral vertebral foramen
H. Spinous process of C2

I. Body of C3
J. Articular processes of C2 and C3
K. Transverse processes of C3
L. Body of C4
M. Articular processes of C3 and C4
N. Partially closed caudal physis of C2
O. Partially closed caudal physis of C3

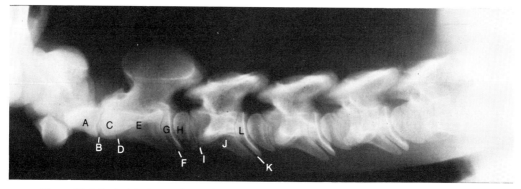

Figure 20–3. Left-right lateral (LèRtL) view of a two-week-old equine cervical vertebral column.

    A. Dens
    B. Physis between dens and the cranial epiphysis of C2 (axis)
    C. Cranial epiphysis of C2
    D. Cranial physis of C2
    E. Body of C2
    F. Caudal physis of C2
    G. Caudal epiphysis of C2
    H. Cranial epiphysis of C3
    I. Cranial physis of C3
    J. Body of C3
    K. Caudal physis of C3
    L. Caudal epiphysis of C3

Table 20–1. MINIMUM SAGITTAL DIAMETER OF THE EQUINE CERVICAL VERTEBRAL CANAL

	Minimum Sagittal Diameter (MM)					
Body Size	*C2*	*C3*	*C4*	*C5*	*C6*	*C7*
Less than 320 kg	20.8	18.1	16.7	17.3	18.3	19.8
Greater than 320 kg	22.1	18.5	17.7	18.7	19.0	22.2

After Mayhew et al., 1978

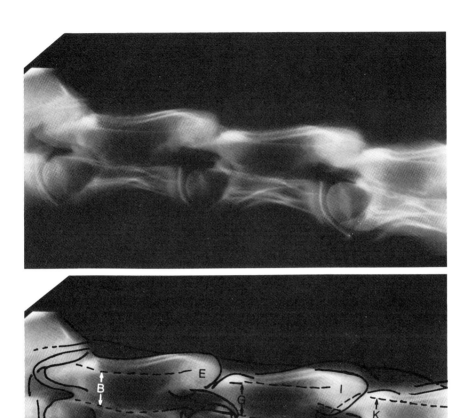

Figure 20–4. Left-right lateral (LeRtL standing/horizontal) view of the midcervical vertebral column in an equine.

A. Body of C3
B. Midsagittal diameter of C3 neural canal
C. Transverse processes of C3
D. Partially closed caudal physis of C3
E. Articular processes of C3 and C4
F. Body of C4
G. Midsagittal diameter of C4
H. Transverse processes of C4
I. Articular processes of C4 and C5
J. Body of C5
K. Midsagittal diameter of C5
L. Transverse processes of C5

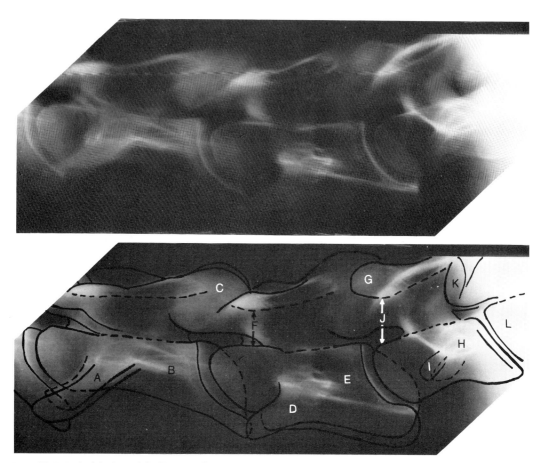

Figure 20–5. Left-right lateral (LeRtL standing/horizontal) view of the caudal cervical vertebral column in an equine.

   A. Transverse processes of C5
   B. Body of C5
   C. Articular processes of C5 and C6
   D. Transverse processes of C6
   E. Body of C6
   F. Midsagittal diameter of C6
   G. Articular processes of C6 and C7
   H. Body of C7
    I. Transverse processes of C7
   J. Midsagittal diameter of C7
   K. Articular processes of C7 and T1
   L. Body of T1

21

Head

SURVEY EXAMINATIONS

Right-Left Lateral (Rt-LeL standing/horizontal) or Left-Right Lateral (Le-RtL standing/horizontal) View. This view is used for survey examinations of the skull or for specific views of the cranial vault, nasal and paranasal sinuses, teeth, mandible, or the pharyngeal, guttural pouch and laryngeal region in lateral view. The halter is replaced by gauze bandage material or radiolucent cord or rope. The patient is allowed to stand normally, and the side of the head where the suspected lesion is located is placed against a cassette cabinet or cassette holder (Fig. 21–1). The x-ray beam is directed parallel to the floor and centered at the region of specific interest. Exposure factors should be reduced for examinations of the nasal and paranasal sinuses and for the pharyngeal, guttural pouch and laryngeal region.

Oblique views of the dental arches may be made by directing the x-ray beam from above (approximately 20 degrees dorsal to the lateral surface) for examination of the maxillary teeth on the side next to the cassette. This view is called a right dorsal–left ventral oblique (Rt20°D-LeVO) or left dorsal–right ventral oblique (Le20°D-RtVO) view. The mandibular teeth may be examined by directing the x-ray beam from below (approximately 20 degrees ventral to the lateral surface). This view is called a right ventral–left dorsal oblique (Rt20°V-LeDO) or left ventral–right dorsal (Le20°V-RtDO) view.

In most skull studies a grid should be used. Alternatively, the exposure may be made through the back of the cassette (see p. 69).

Figure 21–2 illustrates the radiographic anatomy of the caudal part of an equine head in Le-RtL standing/horizontal view.

Figure 21–3 illustrates the radiographic anatomy of the caudal part of an immature equine head to show the normal open sutures.

Figure 21–4 illustrates the radiographic anatomy of the paranasal sinuses in Le-RtL standing/horizontal view. Note the fluid line in the maxillary sinus due to traumatic hemorrhage. The fluid levels are easily identified in this view where a horizontally directed x-ray beam was used.

Figure 21–5 illustrates the radiographic anatomy of the maxillary teeth of a mature equine in Le-RtL standing/horizontal view.

Figure 21–6 illustrates the radiographic anatomy of the mandibular teeth of a 2-year-old equine in Le-RtL standing/horizontal view.

Figure 21–7 illustrates the radiographic anatomy of the rostral aspect of the head of a one-year-old equine in Le-RtL standing/horizontal view.

Figure 21–8 illustrates the radiographic anatomy of the guttural pouches, nasopharynx and epiglottis region of an equine in Le-RtL standing/horizontal view.

Right Caudal–Left Rostral (Rt30°Cd-LeRO) or Left Caudal–Right Rostral (Le30°Cd-RtRO) Oblique View. This view is specifically designed to examine the frontal sinus region. The side of the head to be examined is placed away from the cassette. The patient stands partially facing the cassette cabinet or cassette holder so that the longitudinal axis of the body is 60 degrees from the cassette surface (Fig. 21–9). Alternatively, the x-ray beam may be directed at an angle of 30 degrees caudal to the lateral surface of the head while remaining perpendicular to the cassette surface, thereby avoiding grid cut.

Text continued on page 492.

481

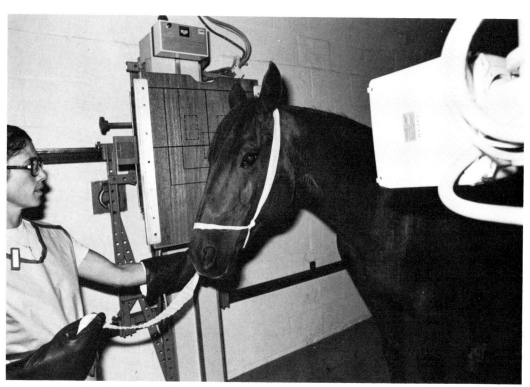

Figure 21–1. Position for left-right lateral (Le-RtL standing/horizontal) view of the equine head.

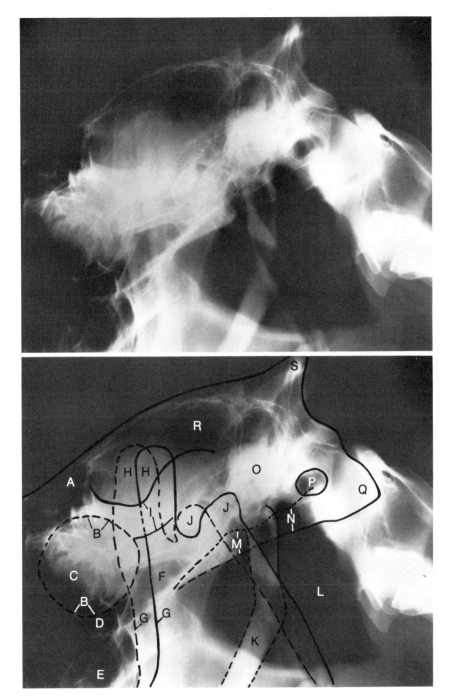

Figure 21–2. Left-right lateral (Le-RtL standing/horizontal) view of an equine head (caudal part).

A. Frontal sinus
B. Oribit
C. Ethmoid turbinates
D. Palatine sinus
E. Maxillary sinus
F. Sphenoid sinus
G. Rami of mandible
H. Coronoid processes
I. Zygomatic arch
J. Mandibular condyles

K. Stylohyoid bones
L. Guttural pouch (diverticulum of auditory tube)
M. Basisphenoid bone
N. Basilar part of occipital bone
O. Petrous temporal bones
P. Tympanic bullae
Q. Occipital condyle
R. Cranial vault
S. Nuchal crest

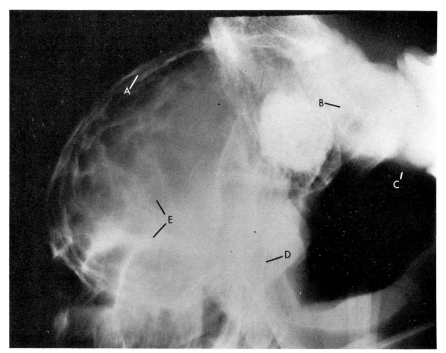

Figure 21–3. Left-right lateral (Le-RtL standing/horizontal) view of the skull of nine-week-old foal to illustrate normal open sutures.
A. Coronal suture between the parietal and frontal bones
B. Lambdoidal suture between the parietal and occipital bones
C. Suture between the squamous part and the lateral parts of the occipital bone
D. Spheno-occipital suture between the basisphenoid bone and the basilar part of the occipital bone
E. Sutures between the zygomatic processes of the frontal bones and the zygomatic processes of the temporal bone

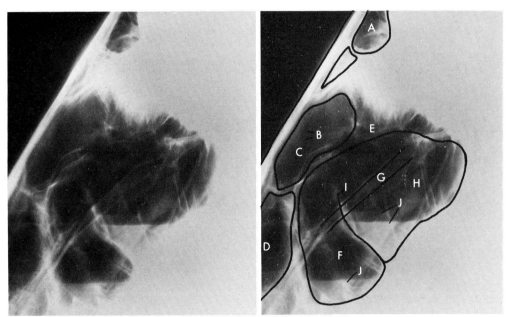

Figure 21–4. Left-right lateral (Le-RtL standing/horizontal) view of paranasal sinuses in an equine. Note the fluid line (*J*) in the maxillary sinus (hemorrhage due to trauma).

A. Frontal sinus
B. Nasal turbinates
C. Sinus of the nasal turbinates
D. Recess of the nasal turbinates
E. Ethmoid turbinates
F. Maxillary sinus (rostral compartment)
G. Infraorbital canal
H. Maxillary sinus (caudal compartment)
I. Septum between maxillary sinus compartments
J. Fluid levels within the maxillary sinus (hemorrhage)

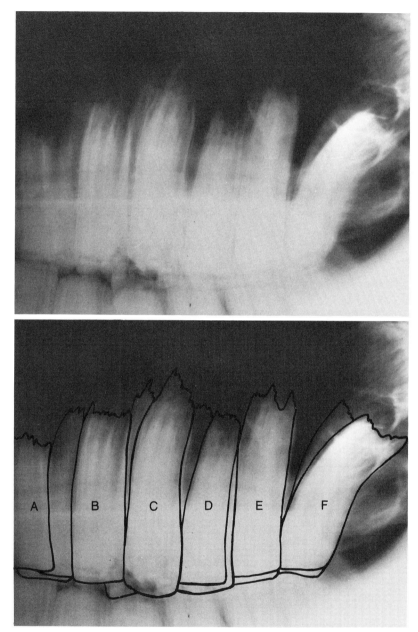

Figure 21–5. Left-right lateral (LeRtL standing/horizontal) view of maxillary teeth of a mature equine.
A. Second premolar
B. Third premolar
C. Fourth premolar
D. First molar
E. Second molar
F. Third molar

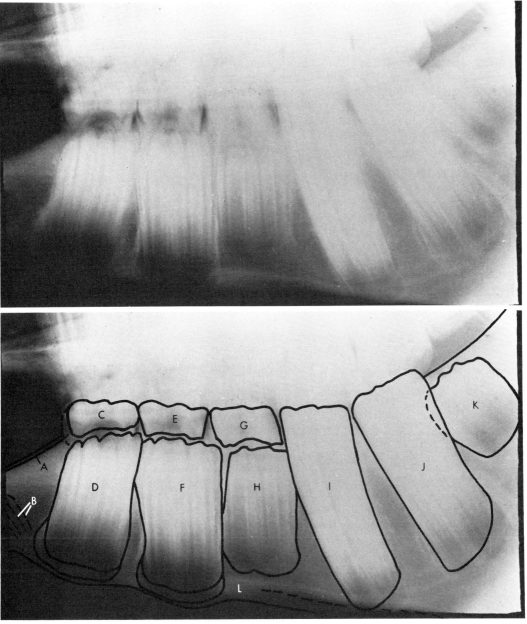

Figure 21–6. Left-right lateral (Le-RtL standing/horizontal) view of the mandibular teeth of a two-year-old equine.

A. Interalveolar margin of the mandible
B. Mandibular canals
C. Second deciduous premolar
D. Second premolar (unerupted)
E. Third deciduous premolar
F. Third premolar (unerupted)
G. Fourth deciduous premolar
H. Fourth premolar (unerupted)
I. First molar
J. Second molar
K. Third molar (unerupted)
L. Body of the mandible

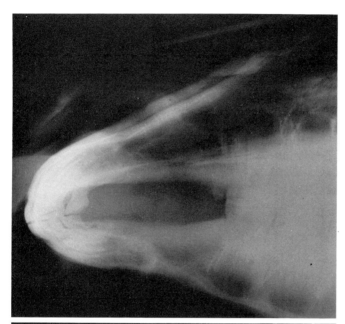

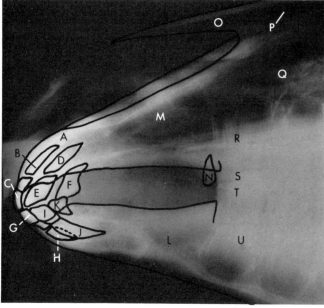

Figure 21–7. Left-right lateral (Le-RtL standing/horizontal) view of the rostral aspect of the head of a one-year-old equine.
A. Body of incisive bone
B. First maxillary incisor (unerupted)
C. First deciduous maxillary incisor
D. Second maxillary incisor (unerupted)
E. Second deciduous maxillary incisor
F. Third deciduous maxillary incisor
G. First deciduous mandibular incisor
H. First mandibular incisor (unerupted)
I. Second deciduous mandibular incisor
J. Second mandibular incisor (unerupted)
K. Third deciduous mandibular incisor
L. Body of the mandible
M. Nasal process of the incisive bone
N. First deciduous maxillary premolar
O. Nasal process of nasal bone
P. Dorsal nasal meatus
Q. Nasal turbinates
R. Second maxillary premolar (unerupted)
S. Second deciduous maxillary premolar
T. Second deciduous mandibular premolar
U. Second mandibular premolar (unerupted)

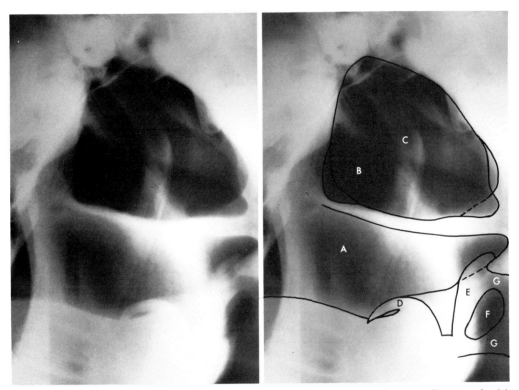

Figure 21–8. Left-right lateral (Le-RtL standing/horizontal) view of the guttural pouches, nasopharynx and epiglottis region of an equine.

A. Nasopharynx
B. Guttural pouches
C. Stylohyoid bones
D. Epiglottis
E. Arytenoid cartilage of the larynx
F. Lateral ventricles of the larynx
G. Laryngeal lumen

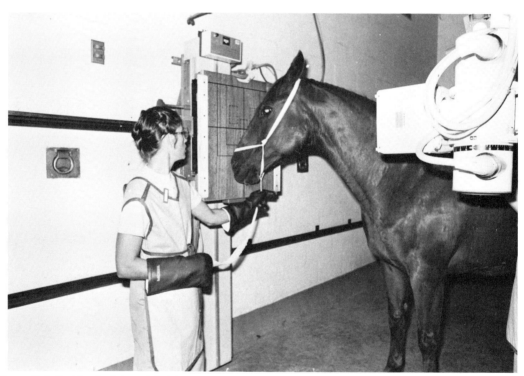

Figure 21–9. Position for left caudal–right rostral oblique (Le30°Cd-RtRO standing/horizontal) view of the left frontal sinus region of the equine.

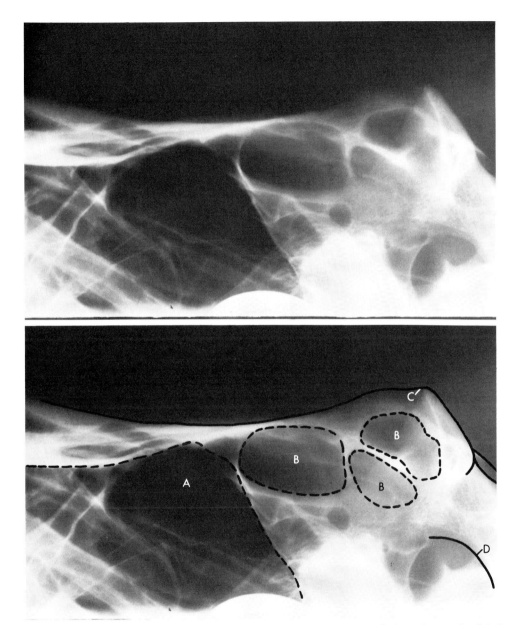

Figure 21–10. Left caudal–right rostral oblique (Le30°Cd-RtRO standing/horizontal) view of an equine left frontal sinus.

    A. Maxillary sinus
    B. Frontal sinus
    C. Supraorbital process
    D. Zygomatic process of the frontal bone

A grid should be used for most examinations. Alternatively, the exposure may be made through the back of the cassette (see p. 69).

Figure 21–10 illustrates the radiographic anatomy of the left frontal sinus of an equine in Le30°Cd-RtRO view.

REFERENCES

Getty, R.: Sisson and Grossman's The Anatomy of the Domestic Animals. 5th ed. Philadelphia, W. B. Saunders Co., 1975.
Schebitz, H. and Wilkens, H.: Atlas of Radiographic Anatomy of the Horse. Berlin, Paul Parey, 1975.

22

Thorax

Right-Left Lateral (Rt-LeL standing/horizontal) or Left-Right Lateral (Le-RtL standing/horizontal) View. Because of the size of the mature equine thorax, multiple radiographs are necessary to study the entire thorax in lateral view. This may require as many as four overlapping radiographs of the craniodorsal, caudodorsal, cranioventral and caudoventral areas with a 14 × 17 inch cassette. (Farrow, 1981; Morgan and Silverman, 1982). Usually, however, three radiographs are sufficient. In this case, the cranial and mid-thorax are examined with the cassette oriented vertically (17 inches high), and a third radiograph is made of the caudodorsal aspect with the cassette oriented horizontally (14 inches high). Exposure factors should be reduced for the examination of the caudodorsal area of the thorax.

The patient is allowed to stand normally with the side of interest against the cassette cabinet or cassette holder (Fig. 22–1). Usually the patient is examined with both right and left lateral views in order to improve radiographic detail on each side. Structures in the hemithorax that are close to the cassette will have better detail.

The x-ray beam is directed parallel to the floor and centered at the field of interest. Care must be taken to be sure that the x-ray beam and the cassette are properly aligned. This can best be accomplished before the patient is placed between the cassette and the tube head. The exposure is made during the inspiratory pause of the respiratory cycle. This is best accomplished by using rare earth phosphor screens and equipment with high ma capabilities.

Figure 22–2 illustrates the radiographic anatomy of the cranial aspect of an equine thorax in Le-RtL standing/horizontal view.

Figure 22–3 illustrates the radiographic anatomy of the middle portion of an equine thorax in Le-RtL standing/horizontal view.

Figure 22–4 illustrates the radiographic anatomy of the caudodorsal aspect of an equine thorax in Le-RtL standing/horizontal view.

Figure 22–5 illustrates the radiographic anatomy of a one-day-old equine thorax in Le-RtL view. This radiograph was produced in lateral recumbency with an overhead x-ray beam.

REFERENCES

Farrow, C. S.: Equine Thoracic Radiography. J.A.V.M.A, *179*(8):776, 1981.
Getty, R.: Sisson and Grossman's The Anatomy of the Domestic Animals. 5th ed. Philadelphia, W. B. Saunders Co., 1975.
Morgan, P., and Silverman, S.: Techniques of Veterinary Radiography. 3rd ed. Davis, Ca., Veterinary Radiology Associates, 1982.
Schebitz, H., and Wilkens, H.: Atlas of Radiographic Anatomy of the Horse. Berlin, Paul Parey, 1978.

Illustrations follow.

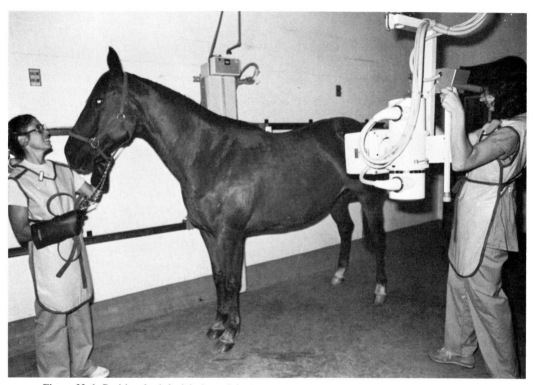

Figure 22–1. Position for left-right lateral (LeRtL standing/horizontal) views of the equine thorax

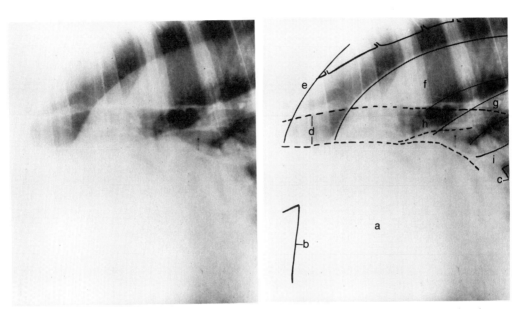

Figure 22–2. Left-right lateral (Le-RtL standing/horizontal) view of the cranial aspect of an equine thorax
a. Heart
b. Cranial border of the heart
c. Caudal border of the heart
d. Trachea
e. Blade of the scapula
f. Aorta
g. Caudal lobe pulmonary artery
h. Region of the carina
i. Caudal lobe pulmonary vein

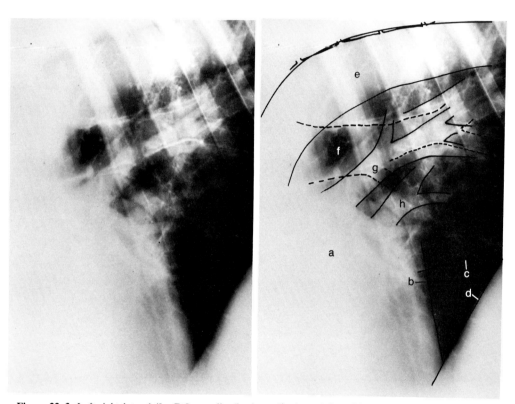

Figure 22–3. Left-right lateral (Le-RtL standing/horizontal) view of the midportion of an equine thorax.

    a. Heart
    b. Caudal border of the heart
    c. Ventral border of the caudal vena cava
    d. Diaphragm
    e. Aorta
    f. Region of the carina
    g. Caudal lobe pulmonary artery
    h. Caudal lobe pulmonary vein

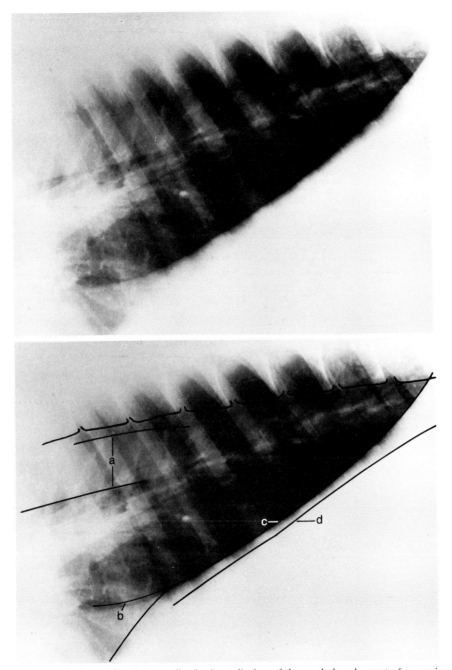

Figure 22–4. Left-right lateral (Le-RtL standing/horizontal) view of the caudodorsal aspect of an equine thorax.

a. Aorta
b. Dorsal aspect of the caudal vena cava
c. Right crus of the diaphragm
d. Left crus of the diaphragm

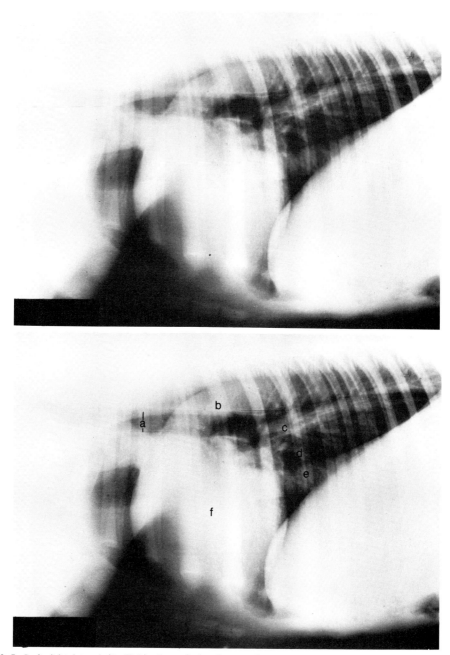

Figure 22–5. Left-right lateral (Le-RtL) view of the thorax of a one-day-old equine (produced in right lateral recumbency with an overhead x-ray beam).

    a. Trachea
    b. Aorta
    c. Pulmonary arteries
    d. Pulmonary veins
    e. Caudal vena cava
    f. Heart

Glossary

Angiocardiography—A contrast study of the cardiovascular system.

Angiography—A contrast study of the blood vessels.

Anode—The positive terminal of an x-ray tube that contains the target.

Arthrography—A contrast study of a joint.

Autotransformer—A transformer with insulated primary and secondary windings on one core.

Brachycephalic—Short-headed (such as in breeds like the Bulldog).

Bremsstrahlung x-ray Radiation—X-rays that are irradiated from a target atom as a result of electron-target atom attraction which changes the electron direction and decreases velocity, resulting in an energy loss that is irradiated as a continuous spectrum of x-rays, depending on the magnitude of direction change that occurs (see Fig. 1–5).

Bucky Mechanism—The Potter-Bucky mechanism (named after Dr. Hollis E. Potter, inventor of the movable grid, and Dr. Gustave Bucky, inventor of the grid)—usually shortened to "Bucky" in common usage. This device moves the grid at right angles to the grid strips during exposure so that the white line images of the lead strips are blurred and thereby made indistinguishable.

Cassettes—Light-tight metal cases that are designed to support a pair of intensifying screens and a sheet of x-ray film and to apply moderate pressure to insure good screen-film contact. The front of the cassette is made of plastic or low-atomic-number metal, such as magnesium, and the back of the cassette is a hinged metal lid (see Fig. 2–18).

Cathode—The negative terminal of an x-ray tube that contains a heated, electron-emitting surface.

Caudal—Denoting a position more toward the tail than some specific point of reference. This term applies to head, neck, trunk and limbs proximal to the antibrachiocarpal and tarsocrural (hock) joints.

Characteristic x-ray Radiation—X-rays that are irradiated from a target as a result of inner (K or L shell) orbital electron removal by an accelerated electron interaction. Outer orbital electrons then fill the vacated orbits in sequence, and the difference in their binding energies is irradiated. The term "characteristic" is derived from the fact that these radiations are characteristic for a given target atom, since the differences in orbital electron-binding energies are unique (see Fig. 1–5).

Cholecystography—A contrast study of the gallbladder.

Cineradiography—A motion picture filming of the output of image intensification fluoroscopy.

Collisional Interactions—Two types of collisional interactions may occur when a target is bombarded by electrons of the energy range used in medical radiography. Both types result in heat loss. (1) An incoming electron may excite an outer orbital electron of a target atom by passing in near proximity to its orbit, thus transferring energy. This allows the orbital

499

electron to increase its distance from the nucleus. When the excited orbital electron returns to its original orbit, energy is irradiated as heat. (2) If an incoming electron possesses sufficient energy to remove an outer electron from a target atom, the atom is ionized. The ejected electron and the incoming electron may undergo further interactions with target atoms. The total energy is eventually dissipated as heat.

Compton Absorption—That mode of electromagnetic energy absorption that is independent of the number of electrons per gram of absorbing material. This mode of x-ray absorption becomes increasingly important in the upper range of x-ray energies used in medical radiography (see Fig. 2–9).

Cone—A cylindrical device that is placed on the output window of the x-ray tube housing for purposes of restricting the size of the primary x-ray beam (see Fig. 2–13).

Contralateral—Situated on or pertaining to the opposite side.

Cranial—Denoting a position more toward the head than some specific point of reference. This term applies to the neck, trunk, and limbs proximal to the antibrachiocarpal and the tarsocrural (hock) joints.

Dacryocystorhinography—A contrast study of the nasolacrimal duct.

Developer Solution—A solution of reducing agents that continues the process initiated by the photon interaction that formed the latent image. Electrons made available from the reducing agents allow an increased number of reduced silver atoms (metallic silver) to form, which appear as black foci on the finished radiograph.

Diaphragm—A variable sized rectangular device that is placed on the output window of the x-ray tube housing for purposes of restricting the size of the primary x-ray beam (see Fig. 2–13).

Diaphysis—The shaft of a long bone.

Dolichocephalic—Long-headed (such as in breeds like Collies).

Dorsal—Pertaining to the back or denoting a position more toward the top surface of the head, neck, trunk and tail. This term replaces *cranial* when reference is made to the distal limbs.

Dorsoventral (DV) View—A radiograph produced by passing an x-ray beam from the dorsal to the ventral surface of the head, neck, trunk or tail.

Epiphysis—The ends of a long bone. Separated from the metaphysis by the physis during the growth of an animal.

Esophagram—A contrast study of the esophagus.

Filter—A thin sheet of aluminum that is placed over the output window of an x-ray tube for the purpose of removing the less energetic, less penetrating x-rays from the primary x-ray beam.

Fixer solution—Fixer solution removes the unexposed (unreduced) silver salts from the x-ray film emulsion after the development process. Sodium or ammonium thiosulfate is the principal chemical used in fixer solutions. These chemicals "clear" the film and leave only black metallic silver atoms in the emulsion. Fixer solutions also contain a hardener (usually salts of aluminum) to prevent excessive swelling and softening of the emulsion during washing and to reduce the drying time.

Fluoroscope—A device used to record an x-ray image on a fluorescent screen instead of film.

Focal-Film Distance (FFD)—The distance from the x-ray source (tube target) to the x-ray film surface.

Focal Spot—The area on the surface of the tungsten target that is bombarded by electrons during x-ray production (see Fig. 1–6).

Focused Grid—A grid composed of strips that are placed parallel to the primary x-ray beam and at increasing angles to the grid surface near the periphery of the grid (see Fig. 2–16). This design allows the primary beam to expose the periphery of the film with nearly the same intensity as the central ray.

Grid—A series of thin, linear strips of alternating radiodense and radiolucent materials, which are encased in a rectangular wafer (see Fig. 2–14) used to reduce scatter radiation.

Grid Cut—Absorption of excessive amounts of the primary x-ray beam caused by improper alignment of the grid and the x-ray beam. The beam must be placed perpendicular to the grid surface unless it is angled in the same direction as the lead strips in the grid.

Grid Efficiency—Grid efficiency is governed by the grid ratio. Grids with greater ratios remove scatter radiation more efficiently.

Grid Ratio—The ratio of the height of the strips to the distance between the radiodense strips.

"Heel Effect"—Unequal distribution of the x-ray beam intensity emitted from the x-ray tube. With a target angle of 20 degrees to the central x-ray beam, the distribution of beam intensity decreases rapidly toward the anode due to absorption of the x-ray beam by target and anode material (see Fig. 1–4).

Image Amplifiers—Electronic devices that are used to amplify a fluoroscopic image. The devices consist of a fluorescent screen that is bonded to a light-sensitive photocathode which produces low energy photoelectrons that are accelerated toward a small fluorescent anode (output viewing screen) (see Fig. 2–21). The net result of photoelectron acceleration and image concentration is image intensification.

Intensifying Screens—Sheets of luminescent chemicals applied to a supporting base, which fluoresce when irradiated and emit foci of light in areas in which x-rays have penetrated a patient, thereby exposing the x-ray film that is placed in close contact to the screens.

Ipsilateral—Situated on or pertaining to the same side.

Kilovolts (kv)—1000 volts. Kv as applied to radiographic technique indicates the voltage applied across an x-ray tube (from cathode to anode).

Latent Image—When the sensitive speck (silver sulfide incorporated within the silver halide crystals of x-ray film) acquires a negative charge from a liberated outer orbital electron of a silver halide atom during x-ray exposure, the positive silver ion is attracted to the sensitive speck, where it is reduced to a silver atom. This process is repeated several times, the number depending upon the number of x-rays interacting on a given area of film. Silver halide crystals, in which the sensitive specks have acquired silver atoms during x-ray exposure, are invisible and constitute the latent image.

Metaphysis—A zone of spongy bone located between the physis and diaphysis of long bones.

Milliampere (ma)—1/1000 ampere. Ma as applied to radiographic technique indicates the milliamperes of current flow from cathode to anode in an x-ray tube during the production of a radiograph.

Milliampere-seconds (mas)—The product of the value of milliamperes of current flow across the x-ray tube and the number of seconds the current is allowed to flow. It is thus a measure of the relative number of total x-rays generated during an exposure.

Myelography—A contrast study of the subarachnoid space of the spinal cord.

Oligocephalic—Normal-sized head (such as in breeds like the Beagle).

Parallel Grid—A grid composed of strips that are placed perpendicular to the grid surface (see Fig. 2–15).

Photoelectric Absorption—The mode of electromagnetic energy absorption that depends on the number of electrons per gram of absorbing material. This mode of absorption is very important in the energy range used in medical radiography and accounts for the differential absorption of x-rays by the various tissues of the body (see Fig. 2–9).

Physis—The cartilaginous growth plate that is located between the metaphysis and epiphysis of growing long bones.

Plantar Surface—This term replaces *caudal* when reference is made to the distal pelvic limb.

Radiative Interactions—If an incoming electron possesses sufficient energy to remove an inner (K or L shell) orbital electron from a target atom, radiative interaction occurs. The ejected electron is replaced by an outer orbital electron and the difference in binding energies is irradiated as characteristic x-ray radiation. If an incoming electron approaches the nucleus of a target atom and is attracted toward the positive nucleus, the incoming electron changes direction and loses velocity and the lost energy is irradiated as "bremsstrahlung" x-ray radiation.

Radiographic Contrast—Differences in the densities of the various subjects on a finished radiograph. These differences are a function of both film contrast and subject contrast.

Radiographic Density—The degree of blackness possessed by a finished radiograph. Density is a quantitative measure.

Radiographic Detail—The degree of sharpness of the individual shadows on a finished radiograph. Detail is essentially a visual quality.

Radiographic Fog—A general or local deposition of silver on a finished radiograph produced by extraneous radiation or chemical reaction. Fog decreases radiographic detail by imparting a gray appearance to the light areas of a finished radiograph.

Reciprocating Bucky—A movable grid that is driven by a solenoid that works against a spring tension on the opposite end of a slide mechanism. This mechanism oscillates continuously without manual loading.

Recipromatic Bucky—A movable grid that is driven by an electric motor.

Roentgen—A quantity of x- or gamma radiation such that the associated corpuscular emission per 0.001293 gm of air (1 cc of dry air at 0° C and 760 mm of Hg barometric pressure) produces, in the air, ions carrying one electrostatic unit of electrical charge of either positive or negative sign.

Roentgen Equivalent Man (rem)—A dose of any ionizing radiation absorbed per gram of living matter such that the relative biological effectiveness (rbe) is the same as 1 rad (radiation absorbed dose) of 200 to 250 kv x-rays. For diagnostic x-ray exposure the rem, rad and roentgen of exposure are equal.

Rostral—Denoting a position more near the tip of the nose than some specific point of reference on the head. This term replaces *cranial* when reference is made to the head.

Sagittal—Situated in the direction of the ventrodorsal plane or a section parallel to the long axis of the body.

Scale of Contrast—A description of the relative densities on a finished radiograph. A radiograph with an increased scale of contrast possesses more shades of gray and a radiograph with a short scale of contrast possesses a more nearly black and white image.

Scatter Radiation—That radiation that has interacted with the patient's tissues and is scattered multidirectionally. This radiation is reduced in energy compared with the primary x-ray beam.

Sialography—A contrast study of the salivary ducts and glandular ductules.

Spot Film—A radiograph produced during a fluoroscopic examination by a device that places an x-ray cassette in the fluoroscopic beam.

Target—An area on the surface of an x-ray tube anode that contains a focal spot.

Urethrogram—A contrast study of the urethra.

Urinary Cystography—A contrast study of the urinary bladder.

Urogram—A contrast study of the kidneys and ureters.

Ventral—Pertaining to the underside of the head, neck, trunk and tail.

Ventrodorsal (VD) View—A radiograph produced by passing an x-ray beam from the ventral to the dorsal surface of the head, neck, trunk or tail.

Videoradiography—The display of the output of image intensification fluoroscopy on a television screen. This image may also be recorded on magnetic video tape.

Volar Surface—This term replaces *caudal* when reference is made to the distal thoracic limb.

X-ray Film—A photographic film formed by layering a silver halide-containing emulsion on each side of a supporting polyester sheet (see Fig. 2–7).

X Rays—Electromagnetic radiations of wavelengths less than 100 Å produced by the interaction of an electron beam with a material such as tungsten.

Index

Page numbers in *italics* refer to illustrations; (t) indicates tables. Unless otherwise indicated, radiographic views are for small animals.

503